T0296909

Culture Media, Solutions, and Systems in Human ART

Culture Media, Solutions, and Systems in Human ART

Edited by
Patrick Quinn
Emeritus Vice-President, Research and Development,
SAGE IVF, A CooperSurgical Company,
Trumbull, CT, USA

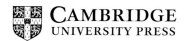

CAMBRIDGE
UNIVERSITY PRESS

University Printing House, Cambridge CB2 8BS, United Kingdom

One Liberty Plaza, 20th Floor, New York, NY 10006, USA

477 Williamstown Road, Port Melbourne, VIC 3207, Australia

314-321, 3rd Floor, Plot 3, Splendor Forum, Jasola District Centre, New Delhi - 110025, India

79 Anson Road, #06-04/06, Singapore 079906

Cambridge University Press is part of the University of Cambridge.

It furthers the University's mission by disseminating knowledge in the pursuit of education, learning and research at the highest international levels of excellence.

www.cambridge.org
Information on this title: www.cambridge.org/9781107619531

First published 2014

A catalogue record for this publication is available from the British Library

Library of Congress Cataloging in Publication data
Culture media, solutions, and systems in human ART / edited by Patrick Quinn.
    p.   cm.
Includes bibliographical references and index.
ISBN 978-1-107-61953-1 (Paperback)
I. Quinn, Patrick, 1946- editor of compilation.
[DNLM: 1. Reproductive Techniques, Assisted.   2. Culture Media.
3. Infertility–therapy.   4. Solutions.   WQ 208]
RC889
616.6´9206–dc23   2013044706

ISBN 978-1-107-61953-1 Paperback

To my wife Kay and my family for their
support and love throughout my career

Contents

Section 3 – Summary and conclusions

Contributors

Jay M. Baltz, PhD
Associate Scientific Director and Senior Scientist; Professor, Department of Obstetrics and Gynecology, University of Ottawa, and Ottawa Hospital Research Institute, Ottawa, Ontario, Canada

Diana Patricia Bernal, DVM
Cryopreservation Coordinator, Reproductive Biology Associates, Sandy Springs, GA, USA

William R. Boone, PhD, HCLD (ABB)
Director of Assisted Reproductive Technology Laboratories, Greenville Hospital System University Medical Center, Greenville, SC, USA

Ching-Chien Chang, PhD
Cryo-Egg Bank Director, Reproductive Biology Associates, Sandy Springs, GA, USA

Ri-Cheng Chian, MSc, PhD
Associate Professor, Department of Obstetrics and Gynecology, McGill University, Montreal, Quebec, Canada

Takeo Cho, BA
Global Sales Division Manager, Astec Co. Ltd., Fukuoka, Japan

Natalie A. Clark, MD
House Officer, Department of Obstetrics and Gynecology, University of Michigan, Ann Arbor, MI, USA

Joe Conaghan, PhD, HCLD
Laboratory Director, Pacific Fertility Center, San Francisco, CA, USA

Shan-Jun Dai, MD, PhD
Visiting Scholar, Department of Obstetrics and Gynecology, McGill University, Montreal, Quebec, Canada

Anna P. Ferraretti, MD, PhD
Scientific Director, S.I.S.Me.R. Reproductive Medicine Unit, Bologna, Italy

Luca Gianaroli, MD
CEO, S.I.S.Me.R. Reproductive Medicine Unit, Bologna, Italy

H. Lee Higdon III, PhD, HCLD (ABB)
Director of Research, Department of Obstetrics and Gynecology, Greenville Hospital System University Medical Center, Greenville, SC, USA

Theresa Jeary, BSc (Hons), MSc
Device Drug Combinations Expert and Technical Manager, Lloyds Register of Quality Assurance, UK

Eduardo Kelly, MD, MBA, ELD (ABB)
Director of Embryology Laboratories, Steptoe Medical Devices, Hingham, MA, USA

Michelle Lane, PhD
Repromed, Dulwich, and Research Centre for Reproductive Health, Discipline of Obstetrics and Gynaecology, University of Adelaide, South Australia, Australia

Henry J. Leese, BSc, PhD, FRCOG (ad eundem)
Professor of Biology Emeritus, Hull York Medical School, University of Hull, Hull, UK

M. Cristina Magli, MSc
R&D Director, S.I.S.Me.R Reproductive Medicine Unit, Bologna, Italy

Marius Meintjes, PhD
Scientific Director, Frisco Institute for Reproductive Medicine, Frisco, TX, USA

Kathleen A. Miller, BS, TS
Scientific Director, IVF Florida Reproductive Associates, Margate, FL, USA

Markus H. M. Montag, PhD
IVF Laboratory Director, Department of
Gynecological Endocrinology and Fertility
Disorder, University of Heidelberg,
Heidelberg, Germany; and Ilabcomm,
St. Augustin, Germany

André Monteiro da Rocha, PhD, DVM
Research Fellow, MStem Cell Laboratories,
Department of Obstetrics and Gynecology,
University of Michigan, Ann Arbor, MI, USA

David Mortimer, PhD
Oozoa Biomedical Inc., West Vancouver,
British Columbia, Canada

Sharon T. Mortimer, PhD
Oozoa Biomedical Inc., West Vancouver,
British Columbia, Canada

Zsolt Peter Nagy, MD, PhD
Scientific and Laboratory Director,
Reproductive Biology Associates,
Sandy Springs, GA, USA

Kamilla S. Pedersen, PhD
Customer Communication Manager,
Unisense FertiliTech A/S, Aarhus N,
Denmark

Thomas B. Pool, PhD, HCLD
Scientific and Laboratory Director, Fertility
Center of San Antonio, San Antonio, TX, USA

Patrick Quinn, PhD
Emeritus Vice-President, Research
and Development, SAGE IVF,
A CooperSurgical Company, Trumbull,
CT, USA

Niels B. Ramsing, PhD
Chief Scientific Officer, Unisense
FertiliTech A/S, Aarhus N, Denmark

Sarah A. Robertson, BSc, PhD
Professor of Reproductive Biomedicine
and Director, The Robinson Institute,
School of Paediatrics and Reproductive
Health, University of Adelaide, Adelaide,
Australia

Gary Daniel Smith, PhD, HCLD
Professor, Departments of Obstetrics and
Gynecology, Physiology, and Urology;
Director, MStem Cell Laboratories, University
of Michigan, Ann Arbor, MI, USA

Jason E. Swain, PhD, HCLD
Scientific Director, Department of
Obstetrics and Gynecology and
Reproductive Sciences Program,
University of Michigan, Ann Arbor,
MI, USA

Jeremy G. Thompson, PhD, FSRB
Associate Professor, The Robinson
Institute, School of Paediatrics and
Reproductive Health, University of
Adelaide, Adelaide, Australia

Yao Wang, MD, PhD
Visiting Scholar, Department of
Obstetrics and Gynecology,
McGill University, Montreal, Quebec,
Canada

Sarah-Louise Whitear, BSc, PhD
Graduate student, Department of Biology,
University of York, York, UK

Deirdre Zander-Fox, PhD
Repromed, Dulwich, and Research
Centre for Reproductive Health,
Discipline of Obstetrics and
Gynaecology, University of Adelaide,
South Australia, Australia

Foreword

Patrick Quinn came from humble beginnings as an Australian reproductive biologist with a strong interest in biochemistry. With the rapid expansion of in vitro fertilization (IVF) technologies worldwide, Patrick found his career motivating research shift into the area of preimplantation embryo culture in vitro. When he moved to the USA, he was able to convert his research interests into the full-scale demands of producing high quality media for use in assisted reproductive technologies. He has been extremely successful in the design and production of quality products that have met the high demands of maximizing embryo viability for research and clinical medicine. This book *Culture Media, Solutions, and Systems in Human ART* contains all the ingredients necessary to understand the requirements, pitfalls, and demands of commercial products. These media must meet the highest quality hurdles necessary for an extremely delicate process of maturing, fertilizing, and developing the embryo in the laboratory; the beginnings of human life.

Since the oocyte and early embryo are not merely passive traffickers in isotonic media, Quinn and his collaborating authors take the reader on a journey that all embryologists and students of cell biology should take. The needs of an oocyte to be fertilized properly, to activate the embryonic genome, and to convert the maternal oocyte cell machinery into a developmentally competent and fully functional organism is no mere spontaneous feat. There are many default pathways to abnormality and degeneration, and this book describes many of them. Knowing where this developmental process can go wrong creates the opportunity to ensure that an optimum environment can be created for the developing embryo.

There are excellent authors and coauthors who have contributed to the book; many of them are internationally recognizable from their excellent published research. Many are also involved in clinical IVF and provide a very practical perspective to the issues raised in various chapters. Perhaps this is not the last word written on the design and requirements of optimized IVF culture media but it does address the vast majority of matters that need consideration. A while ago I asked Patrick to design a simple IVF medium that could withstand the rigors of demand in primitive communities where electricity and refrigeration were luxuries that could not be counted on. He, as usual, responded with enthusiasm to meet my request and this is a work in progress. The book will help scholars and practitioners understand the environment they themselves need to work in, make requests of Patrick and his colleagues for situational improvements, and will continue to assist the field to evolve to that perfect "drop" that Patrick has in mind.

Alan Trounson PhD
President, California Institute for Regenerative Medicine, San Francisco
Emeritus Professor, Monash University, Melbourne, Australia

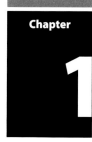

Chapter 1

Overview

Patrick Quinn

Introduction

In this book we have attempted to review current formulations of human assisted reproductive technology (ART) media and solutions, where they came from, and possible contentious areas such as deficiencies and the like that need further investigation, for example the epigenetic effects of media on offspring [1–3]. Most of these topics are contained in the first section of the book. In the second section, which we have entitled "Culture systems," not only the liquid products but also the devices used for in vitro culture of gametes and embryos and how they are used, for example incubators, time-lapse photography and other procedures proposed for determining the selection of the best quality embryos are the subjects of discussion for it does no good to have a good medium if it is not used effectively. Certain aspects of the ART laboratory environment have not been included but should still be considered to optimize the results from any ART program and here I am referring to the macroenvironment in the laboratory or general geographic locale. In particular, things such as toxins, volatile organic compounds, insecticides, building materials, and the like if not considered or recognized as potential detrimental factors could have a very negative impact on outcomes [4, 5].

As we are reminded by Biggers [6], the accomplishments of in vitro fertilization (IVF) and embryo transfer (ET) in humans and other mammals are not something that happened through the work of only a few but were achieved through the cumulative efforts of many workers in the field, past and present, and no doubt will continue in the future. One of the main aims of this work is to summarize these efforts, highlight some of the critical aspects that have been studied, and hopefully provide some inspiration to those who have just entered the field or are considering a career in the area. I can personally say that I am grateful that I have had the opportunity to work in the field of preimplantation mammalian embryology for over four decades, the culmination of which was the birth of our grandson who was conceived and developed for several days in media I had designed.

Progress in media development

When I first entered the field in the late 1960s, the ability to culture mouse embryos in a relatively well-defined medium was possible [7]. One of the primary breakthroughs was the use of Krebs–Ringer solution as the base medium for mouse embryo culture in vitro [8, 9]. This approach was justified in further studies that showed the benefit of using what was considered to be a close chemical imitation of the contents of the female reproductive tract fluids when formulating culture media for the embryos of various species [10–12]. Such a strategy has been called the "back to nature" approach. Another strategy is where every possible compound that the embryo may need over the whole preimplantation period is added to the medium and this is called the "let the embryo choose" approach [13]. A more detailed discussion of these two concepts is presented in Chapter 2. There are many reviews that detail how ART media have evolved and the results that have been obtained with them [14–16] and the reader is directed to these references for further information on this topic. Some of the more pertinent aspects of culture media formulation, how they are used, and their performance are the topics I wish to discuss in more detail and is the primary emphasis of the next chapter and the whole book overall.

Summary

The aim of this work is to describe the history, current status, and significance of culture media and solutions and the culture systems in which they are used for human ART. Various chapters describe culture media and solutions used in human ART, how they have been developed for in vitro human preimplantation embryo development, the function and importance of the various components in these media and solutions, and how systems and equipment in which the media and solutions are used can influence the outcomes obtained in human ART. Additionally, oocyte maturation in vitro, oocyte and embryo cryopreservation, and regulatory matters are discussed. We hope this book will be of interest to students, embryologists, physicians, patients, and other personnel involved in or with an interest in the fluid products used in human ART for the culture and handling of gametes, embryos, and reproductive tissues.

References

1. Dumoulin JC, Land JA, Van Montfoort AP, et al. Effect of in vitro culture of human embryos on birthweight of newborns. Hum Reprod 2010;25:605–12.

2. Eaton JL, Liebermann ES, Stearns C, et al. Embryo culture media and neonatal birthweight following IVF. Hum Reprod 2012;27:375–9.

3. Vergouw CG, Kostelijk EA, Doejaaren E, et al. The influence of the type of embryo culture medium on neonatal birthweight after single embryo transfer in IVF. Hum Reprod 2012;27:2619–26.

4. Cohen J, Gilligan A, Esposito W, et al. Ambient air and its potential effects on conception in vitro. Hum Reprod 1997;12:1742–9.

5. Thomas T. Culture systems: air quality. In: Smith GD, Swain JE, Pool TB, eds. Embryo Culture. Methods and Protocols. New York, Humana Press. 2012;313–24.

6. Biggers JD. IVF and embryo transfer: historical origin and development. Reprod Biomed Online 2012;25:118–27.

7. Arechaga J. Embryo culture, stem cells and experimental modification of the embryonic genome. An interview with Professor Ralph Brinster. Int J Dev Biol 1998;42:861–77.

8. Whitten WK. Culture of tubal mouse ova. Nature 1956;177:96.

9. Brinster RL. A method for in vitro cultivation of mouse ova from two-cell to blastocyst. Exp Cell Res 1963;32:205–8.

10. Tervit HR, Whittingham DG, Rowson LEA. Successful culture in vitro of sheep and cattle ova. J Reprod Fertil 1972;30:493–7.

11. Quinn P, Kerin JF, Warnes GM. Improved pregnancy rate in human in vitro fertilization with the use of a medium based on the composition of human tubal fluid. Fertil Steril 1985;44:493–8.

12. Gardner DK, Lane M, Calderon I, *et al.* Environment of the preimplantation human embryo in vivo: metabolite analysis of oviduct and uterine fluids and metabolism of cumulus cells. *Fertil Steril* 1996;**65**:349–53.

13. Summers MC, Biggers JD. Chemically defined media and the culture of mammalian preimplantation embryos: historical perspective and current issues. *Hum Reprod Update* 2003;**9**:557–82.

14. Biggers JD. Thoughts on embryo culture conditions. *Reprod Biomed Online* 2002;**4**:30–8.

15. Quinn P. Short culture: day 1/day 2/day 3 embryo culture. In: Nagy ZP, Varghese AC, Agarawal A, eds. *Practical Manual of In Vitro Fertilization. Advanced Methods and Novel Devices.* New York, Springer. 2012;133–40.

16. Gardner DK, Lane M. Extended culture in IVF. In: Nagy ZP, Varghese AC, Agarawal A, eds. *Practical Manual of In Vitro Fertilization. Advanced Methods and Novel Devices.* New York, Springer. 2012;141–50.

Media and embryo interactions

Patrick Quinn

Introduction

Over the past several decades the success rates of in vitro fertilization (IVF)/intracytoplasmic sperm injection (ICSI) assisted reproductive technology (ART) procedures using fresh non-donor oocytes with or without ICSI have increased. Quinn reported a linear increase in viable rates for IVF/ICSI procedures in Australia and New Zealand from 1992 to 2001 [1]; rates more than doubled from 10% to 24% per transfer (Figure 2.1). Pregnancy rates in gamete intrafallopian transfer (GIFT) remained constant at 21% over the same period, indicating that the primary reason for the increase in the IVF/ICSI patients during this time was due to improvements in the culture systems being used. Similar increases over the same time span were reported for US data [2]. These increases in success rates in the USA have continued with live births per embryo transfer for fresh embryos from non-donor eggs significantly increasing from 35.8% to 36.4% to 38.5% for the years 2002 to 2006 to 2010, respectively, with the average number of embryos transferred decreasing from 3.0 to 2.6 to 2.4 over this period [3]. These data taken as a whole can be interpreted to indicate that improvements in the laboratory system are responsible for the majority of the increased success rates. Various aspects of these improvements, both in the culture media and in the important interacting aspects of the culture systems are discussed below.

ART media formulations

This topic is one of the oldest, most studied and discussed in preimplantation mammalian embryology so the discussion below will be more of a summary of the situation as seen by this author. There are many reviews on the topic that provide further details [4–10] and, of course, several chapters in this book.

Mammalian ovulated oocytes, spermatozoa, and preimplantation embryos are very amenable to collection and culture in vitro. The gametes and embryos of most mammals carry very few endogenous nutrients and they have to gain their nutrients from the reproductive tract fluid. They will not survive for very long when placed into an isotonic solution devoid of nutrients. If we have some idea of the nutrients and other solutes required to sustain the embryo during the preimplantation period, we can attempt to imitate the in vivo environment in the reproductive tract in the in vitro situation. This has been the basis of the so-called imitative principle, more popularly called the "back to nature" strategy [11], for formulating tissue culture media in general and IVF media in particular.

Culture Media, Solutions, and Systems in Human ART, ed. Patrick Quinn. Published by Cambridge University Press. © Cambridge University Press 2014.

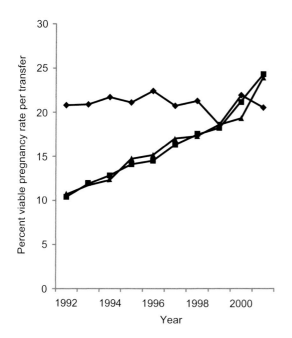

Figure 2.1 Reported viable pregnancy rates per completed procedure for IVF, ICSI, and GIFT in Australia and New Zealand from 1992 to 2001. Diamonds = GIFT; squares = IVF; triangles = ICSI. Reproduced from Quinn [1] with permission.

ART media need to provide hydration, ions, and nutrients and be able to dilute waste products.

Here is a list of potential ingredients:

1. Water
2. Inorganic ions: cations and anions – Na^+, K^+, Mg^{2+}, Ca^{2+}, Cl^-, SO_4^{2-}, PO_4^{3-}, HCO_3^-
3. Energy substrates – glucose, lactate, pyruvate, amino acids
4. Amino acids – non-essential amino acids, essential amino acids
5. Vitamins
6. Fatty acids or precursors
7. Nucleic acid precursors
8. Chelators – ethylenediaminetetraacetic acid (EDTA)
9. Antioxidants
10. Proteins or macromolecules
11. Polypeptide growth factors/hormones
12. Buffering system
13. Antibiotics.

A minimal mix of components would include a mix of electrolytes (cations and anions), energy substrates, amino acids, probably vitamins, oxygen (O_2) and carbon dioxide (CO_2), and a macromolecule such as albumin.

In addition the following aspects form an integral part of how culture media perform:

1. Oil overlay
2. Gas phase
3. Incubation chamber

4. Embryo density – embryo number per volume of medium
5. Contact supplies – culture dishes/microfluidic device, flasks, pipettes
6. Quality control (QC)
7. Quality assurance/management.

Water

The basic foundation of any culture medium is high quality water. When one looks over the past 50 years at the processing of water used to make culture media for embryos, a progression in the treatment to improve water quality is evident. In 1963, Brinster used deionized water [12]; in 1971, Whitten used water which was distilled from deionized tap water [13]. When I started my own mouse embryo lab in 1974 I followed the procedure I had learned in Wes Whitten's laboratory and used triple glass distilled water to make culture medium. Glassware was washed in 1% 7X detergent and glass tubes to be used for culture were then siliconized with 1% soluble silicone for at least 5 seconds before being rinsed 10 times in deionized water, five times in double glass distilled water, and then sterilized by dry heat [14]. When I started human IVF in the early 1980s, we initially used rainwater which was collected on a clean plastic sheet placed on the roof of the laboratory. The collected water was redistilled six times in glass [15]. Finally we used water that had been processed through a Millipore reverse osmosis unit and Milliq treatment system [16]. Most commercial ART companies now either purchase or have their own water purification system. The water must meet strict specifications, is USP/EP certified sterile, and is water for injection quality water. The specifications for such water can be found on line [17]. The water, together with all other components being used, needs to be QC tested prior to use in a clinical or research setting. Protocols for the mouse embryo assay (MEA) and human sperm motility assay are given in Quinn *et al.* [15].

Inorganic ions

This topic has been recently reviewed by Baltz [18] who has given a good historical perspective of the topic. The milestones for culture media for mammalian preimplantation embryo culture were the media formulated by Whitten [19] and Brinster [12] both of which were based on Krebs–Ringer Bicarbonate (KRB). KRB contains Na^+, K^+, Mg^{2+}, Ca^{2+}, Cl^-, SO_4^{2-}, PO_4^{3-}, and HCO_3^-. This was the basis for the inorganic salts in embryo culture media up until the mid 1980s. When I formulated my Human Tubal Fluid (HTF) medium [16] I did find that an excessive ratio of Na^+ to K^+, as in Tyrode's T6 medium that was being used for IVF at that time, inhibited mouse embryo development which was overcome when the K^+ concentration was increased in HTF to levels closer to Whitten's medium. A similar strategy was used during the development of KSOM medium [20]

By the late 1980s the phenomenon of the 2-cell block in hamster and mouse embryos and at other stages in other mammalian species was being studied [21] and it was found that phosphate and/or glucose was involved in the hamster, and that removal of phosphate in particular overcame this block. Removal of phosphate in human ART media resulted in good IVF outcomes [22]. This was probably due to the excessive stimulation of glycolysis by the high levels of glucose and phosphate in the media, as proposed by Schini and Bavister [21]. The addition of amino acids to media have negated this effect and most commercial ART media now contain between 0.25 and 0.35 mEq/L of phosphate ions.

Another modulation of inorganic ion content in media is with Ca^{2+} and Mg^{2+}. Both of these ions are required by embryos as shown by the reversal of compaction when embryos are placed in Ca/Mg-free medium prior to biopsy. However, it has been shown that in 1- and 2-cell hamster embryos an excessive uptake of Ca^{2+} occurred due to inappropriate handling, metabolic perturbations, and just by the act of collecting the embryos and placing them in culture, which reduced further development in vitro [23]. The increase in intracellular Ca^{2+} came from intracellular storage sites and also by influx from the medium through L-gated calcium channels but it could be lessened by increasing Mg^{2+} concentration in the medium. This strategy has been adopted by several commercial ART media companies. It must be remembered however that there is a Ca^{2+} spike in spermatozoa during the fertilization process so a lower Mg^{2+} concentration is required in fertilization medium [24]

The final inorganic ion component in media is HCO_3^-, which will be discussed further in the section on buffering systems.

Energy substrates

This is a huge and diverse topic that has been studied over the past 50+ years so the comments made will be brief and of a summary type. For readers who want more details I highly recommend recent reviews by Gardner [5], Gardner and Wale [25], and Leese [7]. For reference, see Figures 2.2 and 2.3, which are from Gardner and Wale [25] and show the major metabolic pathways and the compounds involved at the zygote and blastocyst stage, respectively.

Oocyte and early cleavage stage embryos do not utilize glucose but have low levels of oxidation of pyruvate. Hence the ATP:ADP ratio is high as there is low biosynthesis and limited cell division. ATP:ADP ratios fall as embryo development proceeds and there is an increase in energy demand. This change in ATP:ADP ratio with development was first reported by Quinn and Wales [26, 27] and subsequently confirmed by Leese et al. [28]. Quinn and Wales [27] also proposed that the lowering of ATP:ADP ratio at later stages of development would increase the utilization of glucose by glycolysis via an increase in the activity of the glycolytic enzyme phosphofructokinase, which is inhibited by high ATP levels, and also an increase in the tricarboxylic acid (TCA) cycle activity, which is also limited by high levels of ATP. Increased TCA cycle activity would then increase the rate of oxidative phosphorylation to provide greater amounts of ATP for biosynthesis and blastocoel cavity formation during the later stages of preimplantation development.

A more erudite summary of what happens in metabolism during preimplanataion development is given by Leese [7] and is worthy of quoting:

The Krebs cycle [also called the TCA cycle] and oxidative phosphorylation provide the main source of energy throughout the preimplantation period. Pyruvate is the central energy substrate during the first cleavage in those species in which energy source requirements of the embryo have been examined, although it is not obligatory for all species (e.g., porcine). Other substrates, notably, amino acids, lactate and endogenous fatty acids derived from triglyceride, combine with pyruvate to provide embryos with a range of potential energy sources through to, and including the blastocyst stage. These nutrients have numerous, overlapping, metabolic roles. Prior to the morula stage, glucose consumption and metabolism is low, although some glucose is necessary for intracellular signaling purposes. With blastocyst formation, large increases in O_2 consumption and the uptake and incorporation of carbon occur and there is a sharp increase in glycolysis, at least in

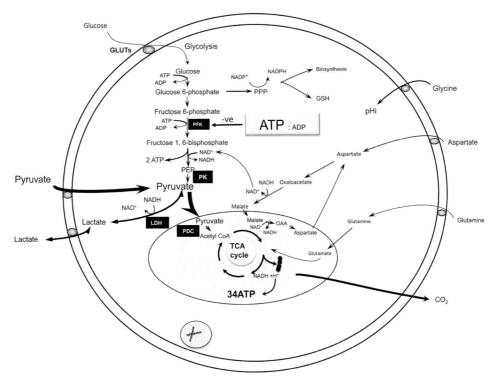

Figure 2.2 Metabolism of the pronucleate oocyte and cleavage stage embryo. The thickness of the lines in the figure represents the relative flux of metabolites through that pathway. GLUTs = glucose transporters; GSH = reduced glutathione; OAA = oxaloacetate; PDC = pyruvate dehydrogenase complex; PK = pyruvate kinase; PPP = pentose phosphate pathway. Reproduced from Gardner and Wale [25] with permission.

vitro. The embryo goes from a relatively inactive metabolic tissue at ovulation to a rapid metabolism at implantation. Mitochondria play a pivotal role during early development, as well as providing a cellular focus for metabolic events. We are almost totally ignorant of the metabolism of preimplantation embryos *in situ* (in the oviduct and uterus) and understanding of signal transduction within embryos is in its infancy as is the molecular dialog between embryos in culture and with the maternal tract in vivo.

A possible practical application of metabolic analysis of human embryos for selection of those more likely to implant and progress to live birth has been reported [29]. It was reported that by measuring glucose consumption of mouse blastocysts it was possible to determine prospectively which embryos were more likely to implant and develop. The embryos chosen for transfer were those with a glycolytic activity similar to that of in vivo-derived embryos [29]. Similar results were observed of the glucose uptake by human embryos on day 4 of development and it was also found that female embryos on day 4 had a significantly greater glucose uptake [30]. A prospective trial using this technology for the selection of viable human embryos for transfer is awaited.

On a practical note, care is needed with the storage of sodium pyruvate raw material. Pyruvate is a free radical scavenger but has limited aqueous stability [31], converting to parapyruvate, which is a metabolic inhibitor. Wales and Whittingham [32] found that the

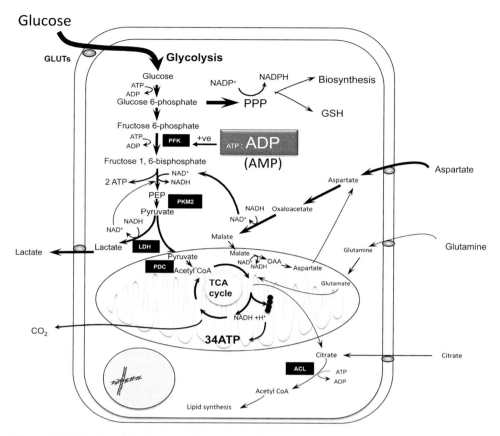

Figure 2.3 Metabolism of the blastocyst. The thickness of the lines in the figure represents the relative flux of metabolites through that pathway. ACL = acetyl-citrate lyase; GLUTs = glucose transporters; LDH = lactate dehydrogenase; OAA = oxaloacetate; PDC = pyruvate dehydrogenase complex. Reproduced from Gardner and Wale [25] with permission.

stability of pyruvate was improved and its embryotoxicity was reduced when it was stored below −40 °C. Swain and Pool [33] reported that ethyl pyruvate and, to a lesser extent, methyl pyruvate, more stable esterified forms of pyruvate, improved mouse embryo development in vitro. These esterified forms of pyruvate are also more membrane permeable and could therefore more easily enter mitochondria and stimulate NADH/NADPH production, thereby maintaining metabolism at physiological levels and reducing stress on the embryo.

Amino acids

This topic has been concisely reviewed by Gardner and Lane [5, 34]. Amino acids have varied and important roles during early mammalian embryo development which range from biosynthetic precursors and energy sources to osmolytes, intracellular pH buffers, antioxidants, chelators, and regulators of differentiation [5]. The addition of amino acids to culture media makes the development of embryos closer to that of in vivo rates [34]. As amino acids are present in reproductive tract fluids [35] it makes sense to include them in embryo culture media even though mouse embryos can develop to expanded blastocysts in vitro in the absence of amino acids. Steptoe *et al.* [36] used Ham's F10 medium, which contains amino acids, in some of their early work but as human IVF became more utilized in the 1980s, media without amino acids such as Tyrode's T6 and HTF became widely used. The works of Gardner and Lane (reviewed in [5]) brought the focus back on amino acids and all commercial ART media for human IVF contain amino acids. Not only do amino acids alleviate stress on embryos and oocytes during culture, their presence prevents efflux of endogenous amino acids from the embryo during handling procedures such as oocyte collection, micromanipulation, cryopreservation, and embryo transfer [37].

The concentration and necessity for all amino acids during all of the preimplantation period have been debated. The initial recommendation by Gardner and Lane based on mouse studies [38] was to use amino acids at the same concentration as that recommended in Eagle's medium and adding the non-essential group for the first 48 hours of culture and then including the essential along with the non-essential amino acids for the second 48 hours, that is, from day 3 until day 5/6 for human embryos. The authors also reported that exposure of mouse zygotes to essential amino acids impaired their development. We have also substantiated this negative effect of essential amino acids on mouse zygotes but not on 2-cell embryos (P. Quinn, unpublished observations, 2005). In 2000, Biggers *et al.* [39] reported that non-essential and essential amino acids at half the concentration in Eagle's medium gave improved development rates of mouse embryos and his laboratory have retained that concentration in their KSOM^{AA} medium [40]. On the other hand, Lane *et al.* reduced the concentration of only essential amino acids by one half [41]. This reduction in essential amino acids to one half of the previous concentration did significantly increase blastocyst cell number in mouse blastocysts, as well as the number of cells in the inner cell mass (ICM) and the proportion of total cells that were in the ICM. It should be noted that Gardner and Lane incorrectly reported a 10-fold higher concentration of tryptophan in their medium in several of their papers [41]. The correct concentration is 0.05 mM in Eagle's medium, as stated in the article by Lane et al. [41]. There have been few reports on the effects of individual amino acids on human IVF. One exception is the abstract from Mortimer *et al.* in 1998 [42] in which they found that after removal of isoleucine and phenylalanine from medium used for culture from the zygote to 4/8 cells, entry into the first cleavage division was faster and positive pregnancy and implantation rates were significantly higher.

The major negative effect of amino acids is their deamination, which releases ammonium most of which comes from spontaneous deamination and a smaller proportion from the metabolism of amino acids by embryos. See the paper of Lane *et al.* [41] to see an example of the differences in ammonium released by chemical deamination alone and by the addition of embryos to the same medium. The buildup of ammonium in vitro causes embryo retardation and fetal defects after implantation [43]. The problems with ammonium accumulation in medium can be lessened by renewing the medium at least every 48 hours and also substituting glutamine with the stable dipeptide alanyl-L-glutamine or glycyl-L-glutamine, which are stable at 37 °C. Eagle [44] showed that human and mouse cells in culture are able to substitute and use dipeptides for a missing essential amino acid. Despite the suggestion that glycyl-L-glutamine may be a better source of stable glutamine for mouse embryos [45], there is a report in which human IVF was performed using KSOM^{AA} containing either alanyl-L-glutamine or glycyl-L-glutamine and the alanyl-L-glutamine gave superior ART outcomes than glycyl-L-glutamine [46] This illustrates the risk of extrapolating from one species to another.

As well as studying the effects of amino acids added to culture media for embryo culture, the consumption and excretion of amino acids by preimplantation embryos has been studied. Most of this work has come from the laboratory of Leese and has included both human and non-human species [reviewed in 47]. In the human embryo, leucine was consumed at all stages from day 2/3 through to the blastocyst stage, indicating that this amino acid should be present in medium for all stages of development, whereas alanine and glutamate were consistently produced at all stages of development studied [48]. Because of the accumulation of alanine, I have omitted alanine from all of my culture media so that there is continued transamination of pyruvate into alanine by the enzyme transaminase, thereby removing toxic ammonium from the embryo. Such a process has been proposed by others [49] and it has been shown that mouse embryos can convert pyruvate carbon to alanine over the preimplantation period [50]

If the accumulation of ammonium in medium still occurs to a sufficient level to affect negatively embryo development, it would seem prudent to renew culture medium every 48 hours with either the same medium if one were using a 1-step protocol or with a medium specifically designed for culture to the blastocyst stage. This would make the logistic and cost of working with a sequential 2-step system or a single 1-step medium similar. There have been very few comparisons of the 1-step versus 2-step culture system with or without change over after the first 48 hours of culture. Gardner and Lane [34] and Biggers *et al.* [40] have made attempts to make the comparison of the two systems using mouse embryos. The results obtained of cleavage time, development rates to the blastocyst stage, blastocyst cell numbers, and fetal development after transfer were the opposite or no different between the two study groups. The studies were not exactly the same, with differences in the genetic makeup of the embryos; with Biggers *et al.* using superovulated CF1 females mated to F1 hybrid males [51] and Gardner and Lane using embryos from CF1 × CF1 or F1 × F1 crosses [34], depending on location. Biggers *et al.* [40] based some of their observations on development for 5 days of culture (144 hours post human chorionic gonadotropin [hCG]), which is 24 hours beyond the normal time that a blastocyst is considered to be developed and ready for embryo transfer. Differences in the media between the Gardner and Biggers groups, apart from carbohydrate levels and some electrolytes, were the concentrations of non-essential and essential amino acids and the absence of essential amino acids in Gardner's G1 medium. Biggers *et al.* also used 0.01 mM EDTA throughout culture [40], whereas Gardner and Lane used 0.01 mM EDTA only during the first 48 hours [34]. A criticism of the design used by Gardner and Lane [34] was that embryos were transferred to fresh medium after the initial 48 hours of culture to minimize any buildup of ammonium in the comparative KSOM^{AA}, which at that time contained glutamine rather than a stabilized dipeptide containing glutamine, for example alanyl-L-glutamine or glycyl-L-glutamine. The exchange of medium at 48 hours of culture was also necessary in the Gardner sequential series of G1 and G2 medium. Surprisingly, the inclusion of 1.0 mM glutamine in the KSOM$_g^{AA}$ medium used by Biggers *et al.* [40] was reported to have no adverse effects on outcomes. So, the question at least with a mouse model of whether a 1-step medium without renewal after the first 48 hours of culture is as good as a 2-step sequential series with exchange at 48 hours remains unanswered. If indeed a switch to fresh medium because of a buildup of ammonium is required and it is unclear to this author whether Gardner and Lane [51] mean even in the presence of alanyl-L-glutamine even though they claim that ammonium is produced in significant amounts by human blastocysts [34], then it would appear that the purported logistical benefits of a decrease in technical time and cost of using a 1-step monoculture system are obviated. There has been one study with human IVF where embryos were cultured in a 1-step continuous medium and compared with those cultured in a 2-step sequential medium using a sibling embryo protocol [52]. Outcomes were similar for transfers on day 3 but on day 5, there were a greater number of blastocysts available for transfer from the continuous single 1-step medium compared with the 2-step sequential media. These results warrant further similar studies.

Vitamins

One of the first human ART media in the recent past that contained vitamins was G2 and was based on positive results obtained with mouse blastocysts [53] when the vitamins in Eagle's medium were added to medium. In studies of hamster embryos, only the water-soluble vitamin pantothenate was found to stimulate the development of zygotes to the blastocyst stage [54], whereas in rabbits, several other water-soluble vitamins were found to stimulate the expansion and hatching of blastocysts [55]. Based on these data, in addition to the G2 medium, several other ART media companies have added vitamins to all or some of their media. For example, Cook IVF has added calcium pantothenate to both their Cleavage and Blastocyst media [18]. It is also believed that Vitrolife have removed several of the vitamins from their G2 medium perhaps based on the report that nicotinamide (also known as niacinamide) inhibits mouse embryo development in vitro and reduces subsequent development after transfer [56]. Obviously the topic of vitamins needs further study to determine which, if any, vitamins would help in ART media.

Fatty acids

Fatty acids can act as energy sources for the culture of 1-cell rabbit zygotes [57]. It has also been reported that fatty acids inhibited mouse IVF but restored mouse zygote development to blastocysts in vitro when added back to fatty acid-free bovine serum albumin (BSA) [58]. Mouse embryos can also synthesize phospholipids from choline [59]. The ova and embryos of some species can survive and undergo some mitotic divisions in the absence of any exogenous nutrients; the degree of this accomplishment is dependent on the endogenous fat content of the oocyte, so mouse oocytes with very few endogenous nutrients cannot survive for more than a few hours in the absence of exogenous nutrients (reviewed by Leese [7]). It is likely that human oocytes and embryos would be more like mouse oocytes and embryos than those of more robust species such as the rabbit, pig, sheep and cattle.

It is likely that embryos can utilize fatty acids that are bound to the protein supplement added to media so this should be taken into account when using recombinant albumin and other macromolecules devoid of fatty acids. Also, the reverse applies to fertilization in vitro because the fatty acid content of albumin may influence the results, the results being better with a lower fatty acid content.

Nucleic acid precursors

Very little work, if any, has been done on this topic. The ribose subunits of nucleic acids would come from the pentose phosphate pathway, hence the need for some glucose in culture medium at all preimplantation stages (see Figures 2.2 and 2.3). Whether exogenous precursors are needed is unknown but good ART results occur without any exogenous purines and pyrimidines.

Chelators and antioxidants

This topic has been recently reviewed by Combelles and Hennet [60] and Guerin *et al.* [61]. Reactive oxygen species (ROS) are generated by oxidative phosphorylation and other factors in the culture system including metallic ions, light, excess glucose, and spermatozoa. ROS have deleterious effects on lipids, protein, DNA, and mitochondria and can cause ATP depletion, apoptosis, and fragmentation in embryos which are all associated with impaired embryo development. [61]. Some components included in media, primarily amino acids, are chelators as are compounds such as glutathione and citrate. The problem with many chelators that act as antioxidants and have a reducing side chain is they have a very short half-life and would not be suitable in a commercial product; for example, cysteine is rapidly oxidized after a 10 minute incubation in culture medium [61]. Whether L-carnitine, which has been shown to have protective beneficial effects on mouse embryos [62, 63], can remain stable in commercially prepared ART media is not known. When comparing several ROS scavenging enzymes, EDTA, and O_2 concentrations used for culture of mouse embryos it was reported that 5% O_2 had the best overall results with regard to blastocyst formation, hatching rates, and cell numbers while EDTA increased blastocyst formation but they had fewer cells than control blastocysts. Catalase and superoxide dismutase (SOD) had no effect [64]. There is also evidence that pyruvate is an important antioxidant that can chemically remove damaging hydrogen peroxide in culture medium and preserve the viability of 2-cell mouse embryos that had been exposed to hydrogen peroxide in HEPES-buffered medium for 45 minutes [65]. Pyruvate similarly prevents peroxide-induced damage of in vitro cultured bovine embryos [66]. Pyruvate when added with lactate also prevents the effects of ROS when added to human spermatozoa [67]. Interestingly, it has been found that washed erythrocytes are a useful antioxidant resource as they contain scavenging enzymes such as SOD and catalase as well as glutathione and hemoglobin, which scavenges nitric oxide and suppresses ROS generation [68]. It was found that the addition of erythrocytes to mouse zygotes being cultured under high ROS or zygotes from aged mothers restored blastocyst development rates to those in positive controls.

Proteins or macromolecules

This topic is covered in Chapter 6.

Growth factors

There is a good recent review of this topic by Hedge and Behr [69]. Receptors for a number of growth factors (GFs) have been found on preimplantation embryos and the ligands for these receptors are present in the fluids of the reproductive tracts [69]. Growth factors added to human ART media have stimulated the formation of blastocysts [69]. So far, only one GF, granulocyte–macrophage colony-stimulating factor (GM-CSF) has been clinically tested and although there was some moderate increase in pregnancy rates and live births, using a mixture of GFs added to culture medium has been proposed rather than a single GF but more studies are required to determine dose and combination of GFs to use [69].

Buffering system

This topic is covered in Chapter 4.

Antibiotics

Antibiotics are added to all media used in tissue culture but nutritionally they are not necessary. They are added to avoid contamination from microorganisms. In ART an overlay of oil can isolate the medium from the external environment and this helps to avoid microbial contamination. Magli *et al.* reported that antibiotic supplementation of media used for in vitro production of human embryos with standard amounts of penicillin (100 IU/mL) and streptomycin (50 µg/mL) had an adverse effect on the embryonic growth [70]. Similarly, Zhou *et al.* found that penicillin and streptomycin adversely affected the development of pronucleate hamster embryos [71]. However, gentamicin (10 µg/mL) had no such detrimental effects on hamster embryo development. It was concluded that if antibiotics were to be used in culture medium, gentamicin would be the safest. Microbial contamination of semen is common even after the patient has had antimicrobial therapy [72] and therefore most ART programs include antibiotics in media for oocyte collection, sperm preparation, and insemination in vitro. Most commercial ART companies provide their media with antibiotics, which is 10 µg/mL gentamicin, but they will make antibiotic-free medium upon request.

Oil overlay

Both Brinster [12] and Whitten [13] used oil washed with medium not containing protein and bubbled with a gas mixture containing 5% CO_2 in air (Brinster) or 5% CO_2: 5% O_2: 90% nitrogen (N_2) (Whitten). This protocol is similar to many of those used today by people who want to wash ART oil if it has not already been done so by the commercial supplier. Some of the benefits of using an oil overlay include the culture of gametes and embryos in small volumes that allow their ready assessment with minimization of pH, temperature, and osmotic fluctuations. Some culture technologies such as microfluidic culture (see Chapter 15) and glass capillary tubes [73] do not require oil but the vast majority of human ART cycles use drops of medium under oil. Most commercial ART oil suppliers wash the oil and filter sterilize it. Various aspects of oil have been reviewed by Morbeck and Leonard [74]. One of the most promising protocols coming out of Morbeck's laboratory is a modified mouse embryo assay using morphokinetics (MKs) to assess embryo sensitivity to toxins. It was found that although toxic oil samples passed the standard MEA test, the MK assay was able to differentiate the toxic oil between the 4- to 8-cell stage, at least 48 hours before the end of the traditional MEA [75].

Gas phase

In 1971 Whitten reported that in his culture system no mouse zygotes formed blastocysts under 20% O_2 whereas 100% did so under 5% O_2 [13]. These results were subsequently confirmed except that some embryos (~25%) did reach the blastocyst stage under 20% O_2 [14]. Follow-on studies showed that fetal retardation occurred in those embryos under 20% O_2 but not in 5% O_2. [76]. Subsequently there have been numerous reports of the beneficial effect of 5% O_2 on embryo development and the damage that 20% O_2 can cause in a number of species, including humans (reviewed by Wale and Gardner [77, 78] and

Gardner and Wale [25]). Despite these overwhelming data, many IVF clinics still use 20% O_2 to the detriment of their patients.

The other important component in the gas phase is the concentration of CO_2 and this is dealt with in Chapter 4 in regard to its influence on the pH of the medium.

Incubation chamber

There has been a steady progress in refinement in the incubators used in ART from large single door models to more refined benchtop models that can maintain temperature and the atmosphere in a reliable and consistent manner. The most important factor involved with incubators is to maintain the correct CO_2 concentration so that there are minimal excursions of pH in the media. Benchtop incubators usually have a system that purges the chamber after it has been closed so that there is a more rapid regain of the CO_2 concentration. One of the main problems with conventional incubators is that the frequency of door openings can cause wide variations in CO_2 and temperature levels. This is usually related to patient load in the program and can cause variation in success rates [79]. A practical approach to alleviate this problem is to monitor who and when they opened the door. It is also beneficial to use a working incubator in which media and dishes are stored as well as embryos that are to be further handled and to have other incubators that are used for longer-term culture and are only opened when necessary. What appears to be the final refinement of incubators are those that are closed during the whole culture period and time-lapse videography is used inside the incubator to monitor MK changes of the embryos (see Chapter 16).

Embryo density

This topic has been recently extensively reviewed [80]. As an example it has been found that in mice, embryos at higher density, that is, embryos per volume of medium, develop better than single embryos or when the embryos are cultured in larger volumes of medium; the presence of a sufficient concentration of autocrine trophic factors has been proposed as the positive agents involved [81, 82].

Contact supplies

It is accepted that all plasticware and other consumables such as gloves, media, chemicals, and oil that come into contact with gametes and/or embryos need to be part of the QC program to maintain the optimal environment for embryo culture. A record needs to be kept of all lots of material being used so that they can be checked if adverse results are obtained. Consumable supplies should be tested with a MEA and/or sperm motility assay that is sensitive enough to detect levels of toxicity that would impact the development of human embryos. As noted in the next section, a useful system to standardize and improve the MEA is a MK system that appears to be more sensitive and relies on quantitative parameters rather than the current qualitative assessment of embryo development.

Quality control/quality assurance

Lane *et al.* have given an extensive review of QC options for laboratory aspects of an ART program [83]. They point out the variability between government regulations of this process worldwide. The ultimate aim of QC in ART is to ensure repeatable embryo quality.

The format used for the management system should be a quality management system that can be audited much in the same way as an ISO/IEC accreditation. The MEA [15] and sperm motility assays were some of the first QC tests used in IVF labs and they have been the mainstay for QC in most ART labs worldwide. Although development rates of embryos were the first parameters used in the MEA, Lane *et al.* stress the importance of more refined parameters such as the use of cell number at the blastocyst stage, their allocation to ICM and trophectoderm, and birth rates after transfer as more robust parameters to use [83]. Most ART laboratories do not have the resources to undertake these types of assessment beyond just the culture of mouse embryos so a more sensitive MEA should be considered, for example using frozen/thawed embryos and culture in protein-free medium to avoid masking toxins. It is generally agreed that the 1-cell stage MEA is more sensitive than the 2-cell assay. Wolff *et al.* found that the MK parameters for mouse embryos using time-lapse videography was more sensitive than the traditional proportion of embryos reaching the expanded blastocyst stage by 96 hours [75]. The MK data detected toxic effects on embryos from added toxins or suspected toxic lots of oil within early cleavage stages and at a lower concentration than the blastocyst development rates. This study puts the QC application of the MEA using MK on a much sounder footing, using a much better quantitative than subjective qualitative assessment of embryo development in vitro. At the bare minimum an ART laboratory should use a human sperm motility assay in which sperm are cultured for an extended period of time, up to 5 days in some laboratories, under conditions that will retain adequate motility in control media in a consistent fashion.

Summary

A valuable resource for many of the topics that have been discussed are available in the article by Boone *et al.* [84].

The overall concept put forward is that mammalian preimplantation embryos can be cultured in vitro but that there is a multitude of factors required to maintain embryos in a homeostatic environment with as little stress as possible. All the components of this symphony have to interact harmoniously with one another. Culture media, their components therein, how they are incubated, under what conditions of temperature, atmosphere, density, etc. are all crucial parts of what is needed. It is also evident that even a "good" embryo may not result in a healthy child so we have to determine is this due to patients or some other factors outside of the laboratory, not involving culture media or how they are used. If attention is paid to all of the factors described so far, we will know that we have done all we can to achieve the ultimate goal of a healthy baby.

References

1. Quinn P. The development and impact of culture media for assisted reproductive technologies. *Fertil Steril* 2004;**81**:27–9.

2. Toner JP. Progress we can be proud of: U.S. trends in assisted reproduction over the first 20 years. *Fertil Steril* 2002;**78**:943–50.

3. Centers for Disease Control and Prevention. Assisted Reproductive Technology (ART) Report. ART Success Rates. 2010. http://apps.nccd.cdc.gov/art/Apps?nationalSummaryReport.aspx (accessed June 24, 2013).

4. Gardner DK. Analysis of embryo metabolism and the metabolome to identify the most viable embryo within a cohort. In: Gardner DK, Rizk BRMB, Falcone T, eds. *Human Assisted Reproductive Technology: Future Trends in Laboratory and Clinical Practice.* Cambridge, Cambridge University Press. 2011;301–12.

5. Gardner DK. Dissection of culture media for embryos: the most important and less important components and characteristics. *Reprod Fertil Dev* 2008;**20**:9–18.

6. Biggers JD, Summers MC. Choosing a culture medium: making informed choices. *Fertil Steril* 2008;**90**:473–83.

7. Leese HJ. Metabolism of the preimplantation embryo: 40 years on. *Reproduction* 2012;**143**:417–27.

8. Pool TB. Recent advances in the production of viable human embryos in vitro. *Reprod Biomed Online* 2004;**4**:294–302.

9. Quinn P. Short culture: day 1/day 2/day 3 embryo culture. In: Nagy ZP, Varghese AC, Agarawal A, eds. *Practical Manual of In Vitro Fertilization. Advanced Methods and Novel Devices*. New York, Springer. 2012;133–40.

10. Quinn P. Culture systems: sequential. In: Smith GD, Swain JE, Pool TB, eds. *Embryo Culture. Methods and Protocols*. New York, Humana Press. 2012;211–30.

11. Leese HJ. Human embryo culture: back to nature. *J Assist Reprod Genet* 1998;**15**:466–8.

12. Brinster RL. A method for in vitro cultivation of mouse ova from two-cell to blastocyst. *Exp Cell Res* 1963;**32**:205–8.

13. Whitten WK. Nutrient requirements for the culture of preimplantation embryos in vitro. *Adv Biosci* 1971;**6**:129–41.

14. Quinn P, Harlow GM. The effect of oxygen on the development of preimplantation mouse embryos in vitro. *J Exp Zool* 1978;**206**:73–80.

15. Quinn P, Warnes GM, Kerin JK, *et al.* Culture factors in relation to the success of human in vitro fertilization and embryo transfer. *Fertil Steril* 1984;**41**:202–9.

16. Quinn P, Kerin JF, Warnes GM. Improved pregnancy rate in human in vitro fertilization with the use of a medium based on the composition of human tubal fluid. *Fertil Steril* 1985;**44**:493–8.

17. Certificate of Analysis. Description: USP/EP Certified Sterile. WFI-Quality Water.

http://cellgro.com/media/docs/files/items//25065053.pdf (accessed June 29, 2013).

18. Baltz JM. Media composition: salts and osmolality. In: Smith GD, Swain JE, Pool TB, eds. *Embryo Culture. Methods and Protocols*. New York, Humana Press. 2012;61–80.

19. Whitten WK. Culture of tubal mouse ova. *Nature* 1956;**177**:96.

20. Biggers JD, Lawitts JA, Lechene CP. The protective action of betaine on the deleterious effect of NaCl on preimplantation mouse embryos in vitro. *Mol Reprod Dev* 1993;**34**:380–90.

21. Schini SA, Bavister BD. Two-cell block to development of cultured hamster embryos is caused by phosphate and glucose. *Biol Reprod* 1988;**39**:1183–92.

22. Quinn P. Enhanced results in mouse and human embryo culture using a modified human tubal fluid medium lacking glucose and phosphate. *J Assist Reprod Genet* 1995;**12**:97–105.

23. Lane M, Boatman DE, Albrecht RM, *et al.* Intracellular divalent cation homeostasis and developmental competence in the hamster preimplantation embryo. *Mol Reprod Dev* 1998;**50**:443–50.

24. Rogers BJ, Yanagimachi R. Competitive effect of magnesium on the calcium-dependent acrosome reaction in guinea pig spermatozoa. *Biol Reprod* 1976;**15**:614–19.

25. Gardner DK, Wale PL. Analysis of metabolism to select viable human embryos for transfer. *Fertil Steril* 2013;**99**:1062–72.

26. Quinn P, Wales RG. Adenosine triphosphate content of preimplantation mouse embryos. *J Reprod Fertil* 1971;**25**:133–5.

27. Quinn P, Wales RG. The effect of culture in vitro on the levels of adenosine triphosphate in preimplantation mouse embryos. *J Reprod Fertil* 1973;**32**:231–41.

28. Leese HJ, Biggers JD, Mroz EA, *et al.* Nucleotides in a single mammalian ovum or preimplantation embryo. *Anal Biochem* 1984;**140**:443–8.

29. Lane M, Gardner DK. Selection of viable mouse blastocyst prior to transfer using a metabolic criterion. *Hum Reprod* 1996;**11**:1975–8.

30. Gardner DK, Wale PL, Collins R, *et al.* Glucose consumption of single post-compaction human embryos is predictive of embryo sex and live birth outcome. *Hum Reprod* 2011;**26**:1981–6.

31. Woo YJ, Taylor MD, Cohen JE, *et al.* Ethyl pyruvate preserves cardiac function and attenuates oxidative injury after prolonged myocardial ischemia. *J Thorac Cardiovasc Surg* 2004;**127**:1262–9.

32. Wales RG, Whittingham DG. Decomposition of sodium pyruvate in culture medium stored at 5 °C and its effects on the development of the preimplantation mouse embryo. *J Reprod Fertil* 1971;**24**:126.

33. Swain JE, Pool TB. Supplementation of culture media with esterified forms of pyruvate improves mouse embryo development. *Fertil Steril* 2008;**90**(Suppl):S47.

34. Gardner DK, Lane M. Extended culture in IVF. In: Nagy ZP, Varghese AC, Agarawal A, eds. *Practical Manual of In Vitro Fertilization: Advanced Methods and Novel Devices.* New York, Springer. 2012;141–50.

35. Tay JI, Rutherford AJ, Killick SR, *et al.* Human tubal fluid: production, nutrient composition and response to adrenergic agents. *Hum Reprod* 1997;**12**:2451–6.

36. Steptoe PC, Edwards RG, Purdy JM. Human blastocysts grown in culture. *Nature* 1971;**229**:132–3.

37. Kolajora M, Baltz JM. Volume-regulated anion and organic osmolyte channels in mouse zygotes. *Biol Reprod* 1999;**60**:964–72.

38. Gardner DK, Lane M. Culture and selection of viable blastocysts: a feasible proposition for human IVF? *Hum Reprod Update* 1997;**3**:367–82.

39. Biggers JD, McGinnis LK, Raffin M. Amino acids and preimplantation development of the mouse in protein-free potassium simplex optimized medium. *Biol Reprod* 2000;**63**:281–93.

40. Biggers JD, McGinnis LK, Lawitts JA. One-step versus two-step culture of mouse preimplantation embryos: is there a difference? *Hum Reprod* 2005;**20**:3376–84.

41. Lane M, Hooper K, Gardner DK. Effect of essential amino acids on mouse embryo viability and ammonium production. *J Assist Reprod Genet* 2001;**18**:519–25.

42. Mortimer D, Henman M, Peters K, *et al.* Inhibitory effects of isoleucine and phenylalanine upon early human embryos. *Abstracts of the 14th Annual Meeting of the ESHRE, Goteborg* 1998, pp. 218 Abstract P-178.

43. Lane M, Gardner DK. Increase in postimplantation development of cultured mouse embryos by amino acids and induction of fetal retardation and encephaly by ammonium ions. *J Reprod Fertil* 1994;**102**:305–12.

44. Eagle H. Utilization of dipeptides by mammalian cells in tissue culture. *Proc Soc Exp Biol Med* 1955;**89**:96–9.

45. Biggers JD. Enhanced effect of glycyl-L-glutamine on mouse preimplantation embryos in vitro. *Reprod Biomed Online* 2004;**9**:59–69.

46. Quintans CJ, Donaldson MJ, Massaldi AM, *et al.* Human IVF outcome in media containing either alanyl-L-glutamine or glycyl-L-glutamine. *Fertil Steril* 2005;**84**(Suppl 1)S456.

47. Sturmey RG, Brison DR, Leese HJ. Innovative techniques in human embryo viability assessment: embryo viability by measurement of amino acid turnover. *Reprod Biomed Online* 2008;**17**:486–96.

48. Houghton FD, Hawkhead JA, Humpherson PG, *et al.* Non-invasive amino acid turnover predicts human embryo developmental capacity. *Hum Reprod* 2002;**17**:999–1005.

49. Booth PJ, Humpherson PG, Watson TJ, *et al.* Amino acid depletion and appearance during porcine preimplantation embryo development in vitro. *Reproduction* 2005;**130**:655–68.

50. Quinn P, Wales RG. Uptake and metabolism of pyruvate and lactate during

preimplantation development of the mouse embryo in vitro. *J Reprod Fertil* 1973;**35**:273–87.

51. Gardner DK, Lane M. Towards single embryo transfer. *Reprod Biomed Online* 2003;**6**:470–81.

52. Reed ML, Hamic A, Thompson DJ, *et al.* Continuous uninterrupted single medium culture without medium renewal versus sequential media culture: a sibling embryo study. *Fertil Steril* 2009;**92**:1783–6.

53. Lane M, Gardner DK. Amino acids and vitamins prevent culture-induced metabolic perturbations and associated loss of viability of mouse blastocysts. *Hum Reprod* 1998;**13**:991–7.

54. McKiernan SH, Bavister BD. Culture of one-cell hamster embryos with water soluble vitamins: pantothenate stimulates blastocyst production. *Hum Reprod* 2000;**15**:157–64.

55. Kane MT. The effects of water-soluble vitamins on the expansion of rabbit blastocysts in vitro. *J Exp Zool* 1988;**245**:220–3.

56. Tsai FCH, Gardner DK. Nicotinamide, a component of complex culture media, inhibits mouse embryo development in vitro and reduces subsequent developmental potential after transfer. *Fertil Steril* 1994;**61**:376–82.

57. Kane MT. Fatty acids as energy sources for culture of one-cell rabbit ova to viable morulae. *Biol Reprod* 1979;**20**:323–32.

58. Quinn P, Whittingham DG. Effect of fatty acids on fertilization and development of mouse embryos in vitro. *J Androl* 1982;**3**:440–4.

59. Pratt HPM. Phospholipid synthesis in the preimplantation mouse embryo. *J Reprod Fertil* 1980;**58**:237–48.

60. Combelles CMH, Hennet ML. Medium composition: antioxidants/chelators and cellular function. In: Smith GD, Swain JE, Pool TB, eds. *Embryo Culture. Methods and Protocols.* New York, Humana Press. 2012;129–59.

61. Guerin P, El Mouatassin S, Menezo Y. Oxidative stress and protection against reactive oxygen species in preimplantation embryos and its surroundings. *Hum Reprod Update* 2001;**7**:175–89.

62. Abdelrazik H, Sharma R, Mahfouz R, *et al.* L-carnitine decreases DNA damage and improves the in vitro blastocyst development rate in mouse embryos. *Fertil Steril* 2009;**91**:89–96.

63. Mansour G, Abdelrazik A, Sharma RK, *et al.* L-carnitine supplementation reduces oocyte cytoskeleton damage and embryo apoptosis induced by incubation in peritoneal fluid from patients with endometriosis. *Fertil Steril* 2009;**91**:2079–86.

64. Orsi, NM, Leese HJ. Protection against reactive oxygen species during mouse preimplantation development: role of EDTA, oxygen tension, catalase, superoxide dismutase and pyruvate. *Mol Reprod Dev* 2001;**59**:44–53.

65. O'Fallon JV, Wright RW. Pyruvate revisted: a non-metabolic role for pyruvate in preimplantation embryo development. *Theriogenology* 1995;**43**:288.

66. Morales H, Tilquin P, Rees JF, *et al.* Pyruvate prevents peroxide-induced injury of in vitro preimplantation bovine embryos. *Mol Reprod Dev* 1999;**52**:149–57.

67. de Lamirande E, Gagnon C. Reactive oxygen species and human spermatozoa. II. Depletion of adenosine triphosphate plays an important role in the inhibition of sperm motility. *J Androl* 1992;**13**:379–86.

68. Fukuhara R, Fujii S, Nakamura R, *et al.* Erythrocytes counteract the negative effects of female ageing on mouse preimplantation embryo development and blastocyst formation. *Hum Reprod* 2008;**23**:2080–5.

69. Hegde A, Behr B. Media composition: growth factors. In: Smith GD, Swain JE, Pool TB, eds. *Embryo Culture. Methods and Protocols.* New York, Humana Press. 2012;177–98.

70. Magli MC, Gianaroli L, Fiorentino A, *et al.* Improved cleavage rate of human embryos cultured in antibiotic-free medium. *Hum Reprod* 1996;**11**:1520–4.

71. Zhou H, McKiernan SH, Ji W, *et al.* Effects of antibiotics on development in vitro of hamster pronucleate ova. *Theriogenology* 2000;**54**:999–1006.

72. Huyser C, Fourie F, Oosthuizen M, *et al.* Microbial flora in semen during in vitro fertilization. *J In Vitro Fert Embryo Transf* 1991;**8**:260–4.

73. Thouas GA, Jones GM, Trounson AO. The 'GO' system – a novel method of microculture for in vitro development of mouse zygotes to the blastocyst stage. *Reproduction* 2003;**126**:161–9.

74. Morbeck DE, Leonard PH. Culture systems: mineral oil overlay. In: Smith GD, Swain JE, Pool TB, eds. *Embryo Culture. Methods and Protocols.* New York, Humana Press. 2012;325–31.

75. Wolff HS, Fredrickson JR, Walker DL, *et al.* Advances in quality control: mouse embryo morphokinetics are sensitive markers of in vitro stress. *Hum Reprod* 2013;**28**:1776–82.

76. Harlow GM, Quinn P. Foetal and placental growth in the mouse after pre-implantation development in vitro under oxygen concentrations of 5 and 20%. *Aust J Biol Sci* 1979;**32**:363–9.

77. Wale PL, Gardner DK. Oxygen regulates amino acid turnover and carbohydrate uptake during the preimplantation period of mouse embryo development. *Biol Reprod* 2012;**87**:24, 1–8.

78. Wale PL, Gardner DK. Time-lapse analysis of mouse embryo development in oxygen gradients. *Reprod Biomed Online* 2010;**21**:402–10.

79. Abramczuk JW, Lopata A. Incubator performance in the clinical in vitro fertilization program: importance of temperature conditions for the fertilization and cleavage of human oocytes. *Fertil Steril* 1986;**46**:132–4.

80. Reed ML. Culture systems:embryo density. In: Smith GD, Swain JE, Pool TB, eds. *Embryo Culture. Methods and Protocols.* New York, Humana Press. 2012;273–312.

81. Lane M, Gardner DK. Effect of incubation volume and embryo density on the development and viability of mouse embryos in vitro. *Hum Reprod* 1992;**7**:558–62.

82. Canseco RS, Sparks AET, Pearson RE, *et al.* Embryo density and medium volume effects on early murine embryo development. *J Assist Reprod Genet* 1992;**9**:454–7.

83. Lane M, Mitchell M, Cashman KS, *et al.* To QC or not to QC: the key to a consistent laboratory? *Reprod Fertil Dev* 2008;**20**:23–32.

84. Boone WR, Higdon HL, Johnson JE. Quality management issues in the assisted reproduction laboratory. *J Reprod Stem Cell Biotechnol* 2010;**1**:30–107.

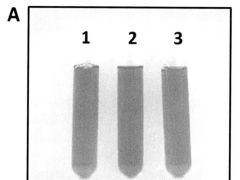

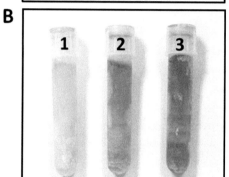

Figure 4.2 Apparent pH change of media contained the indicator phenol red buffered with (1) phosphate, (2) phosphate and HEPES, or (3) HEPES. (A). pH at room temperature. (B) pH following direct plunge into liquid nitrogen. Phosphate buffered media appear to become acidic, while HEPES-buffered media appears to become alkaline. Combining HEPES and PBS appears to stabilize pH and may be useful as a buffering system for cryopreservation procedures (adapted from Will *et al.* [81], with permission).

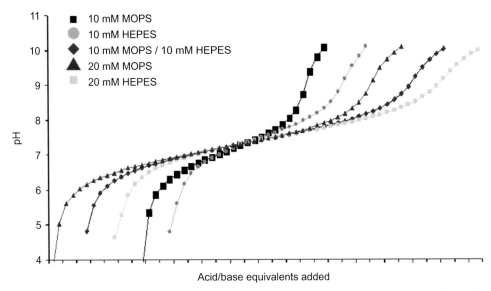

Figure 4.3 Combination of pH buffers allows for lowering of individual buffer concentrations, while simultaneously allowing for adjustment of pK$_a$, or optimal buffering, to the desired range. Multiple buffers and varying ratios can be utilized. This approach can help to formulate a buffering system for specific IVF procedures, yielding optimal pH buffering based on cell type or procedure/temperature utilized (adapted from Swain and Pool [67], with permission).

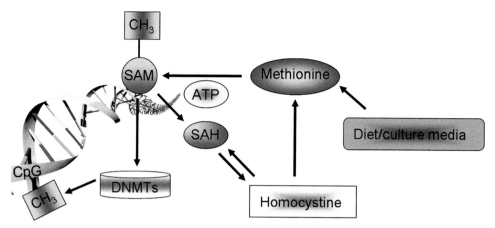

Figure 8.4 Schematic depicting the methionine pathway leading to DNA methylation. Figure adapted from Sergio and Lamprecht Nature Review 2003. SAM (S-adenosyl methionine), ATP (adenosine triphosphate) DNMT (DNA methyltransferase), SAH (S-adenosyl homocystine), CH₃ (methyl group), CpG (CpG island with the DNA strand).

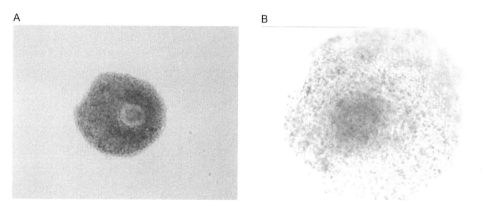

Figure 12.1 Human cumulus–oocyte complex (COC) before and after maturation in culture in a designed IVM medium. (A) The COC was collected immediately from a small follicle (3 mm in diameter) without gonadotropin priming; (B) the same COC was cultured in IVM medium for 24 hours. Note the size of COC expansion before and after maturation in culture (two photos with the same magnification ×200).

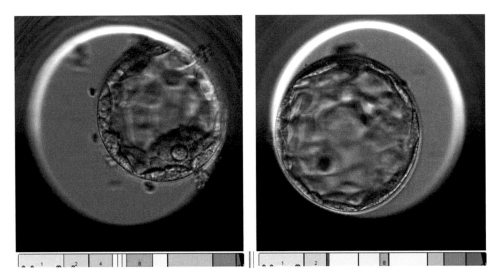

Figure 16.10 Uneven cell numbers and asynchronous division. The bars below the images depict a timeline for embryo development. The numbers (1, 2, 4, or 8) indicate the cell number in the respective periods. The stages with an extended duration due to DNA replication corresponding to 1, 2, 4, or 8 cells are shown in shades of green. Transient stages such as 3, 5, 6, or 7 cells due to lack of synchrony are shown in yellow. Stages of compaction and blastulation are indicated in blue. The blastocyst on the right is more expanded than the left one. However, time-lapse images of the embryo to the left revealed synchronous divisions from the 2-cell stage to the 4-cell stage and a relatively fast progression from the 4- to 8-cell stage. In contrast, the embryo to the right immediately divided from the 2- to the 6-cell stage and spent a long time in the 6- to 7-cell stage prior to reaching the 8-cell stage, which was of short duration. Although the time interval from the onset of the 2-cell stage until the end of the 8-cell stage is identical in both embryos, the one at the left has a better history of even cell numbers and synchronous cleavage cycles. The asynchronous cell division of the right-hand embryo could indicate a lower quality and the embryo to the left should probably be preferred for transfer.

Chapter

3

Female tract environment and its relationship to ART media composition

Henry J. Leese and Sarah-Louise Whitear

Introduction

A plethora of media are available for the culture of human preimplantation embryos conceived by assisted reproductive technologies (ART). However, after examining randomized controlled trials on the influence of culture media on laboratory and clinical outcomes, Youssef *et al.* concluded that "There is little evidence in the literature indicating which culture medium is best for human preimplantation embryos." [1].

This study is interesting for its breadth of coverage: databases from the last 25 years were searched but out of 376 shortlisted studies only 37 met the criteria for proper meta-analysis and of these, only four had data on live births. Moreover, it is unlikely that robust information comparing the laboratory performance of different media will become available since the chance of sufficient surplus human embryos being provided to facilitate studies of the necessary statistical power is remote [2].

In the absence of such evidence, it is timely to revisit the possibility of basing the composition of media for the culture of gametes and early embryos on the environment to which they would normally be exposed in the female reproductive tract [3]. A strong rationale for this approach is provided by data from a wide variety of species showing that embryos develop better in vivo than in vitro; a finding particularly well-illustrated by Merton and colleagues [4] in a review of factors influencing embryo development in cattle. As the data in Figure 3.1 illustrate, embryo development increases progressively as the key processes: egg maturation, fertilization, and early development, are carried out in vivo rather than in vitro. Data consistent with this conclusion were reviewed by Lonergan *et al.* [5]. For example, culture of in vitro-produced bovine zygotes in the ewe oviduct dramatically increases the quality of the resulting blastocysts and in a reciprocal experiment, culture in vitro of in vivo-produced bovine zygotes leads to the production of poor quality blastocysts. Moreover, increasing evidence points to the conclusion that the decline in embryo health is proportional to the time spent in culture [6], suggesting that it is desirable to transfer embryos on day 2 or 3 rather than at the blastocyst stage. The challenge therefore becomes one of mimicking the physical and chemical environment within the lumen of the oviduct (Fallopian tube or "tube" in women), where fertilization and the cleavage stages of development normally occur. It is also worth noting, as emphasized by Lonergan *et al.* [5], that the oviduct is able to support the complete development of zygotes into blastocysts; an ability that even allows the embryos of some species to be cross-fostered in the oviducts of another species, highlighting the considerable autonomy at the preimplantation embryo; something considered later in this review.

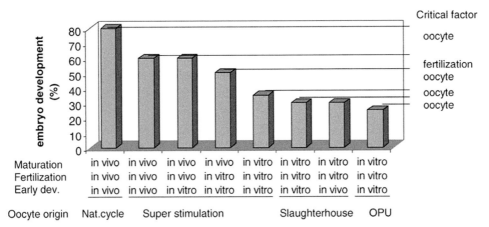

Figure 3.1 Effect on embryo production of the origin of the oocyte and the successive steps of maturation, fertilization and early development performed in vivo and/or in vitro. The source of the respective decreases is noted at the right of the figure. Reprinted from Merten *et al.* [4], with permission from Elsevier. OPU = ovum pick-up.

Development of a "back to nature" embryo culture medium
Collection and analysis of reproductive tract fluids

The first obstacle in achieving this objective is to obtain data on the composition of human Fallopian tubal fluid. This, in turn, requires the collection of tubal fluid, for which a number of methods have been used as summarized in reviews by Aguilar and Reyley [7] and Leese and colleagues [8]. The technique most likely to provide physiological data is that of direct sampling of the fluid in the tubal lumen during surgical operations. This method was used by Borland *et al.* to provide picoliter samples of fluid which were analyzed for electrolytes by electron probe microanalysis [9]. Direct sampling under surgery was also used by Gardner *et al.* to generate human Fallopian tubal samples for analysis of glucose, pyruvate, and lactate concentrations which were measured ultramicrofluorometrically [10].

It has been suggested that sampling the "bulk fluid" in the oviduct lumen does not reflect the true concentrations of ions and nutrients in the vicinity of the embryo due to the convoluted nature of the endosalpinx which may harbor "microenvironments" [2]. In response, it can be argued that no current technique is able to sample the microenvironment adjacent to any cell in the body – say, within 1–2 μm, which ideally is required – and that sampling the tubal lumen provides a better indication of the embryo's environment than no data at all. In addition, the tubal epithelial cells are lined by cilia, the beating of which, in addition to the contraction of the myosalpinx, can be expected to induce mixing within the microenvironments and minimize the buildup of unstirred layers. Moreover, human tubal fluid is not produced in copious amounts; arguably, the environment within the human tube is better described as "moist," such that samples withdrawn by micropipette may come close to approximating the true environment.

Historically, prolonged cannulation of the Fallopian tube of women over a period of 2–8 days was used to collect human tubal fluid (summarized by Tay *et al.* [11]) but the technique risked the development of inflammation at the site of cannulation, was unlikely to generate fluid physiologically over many days, and nowadays would not receive ethical approval. Dickens *et al.* developed an alternative method for collecting luminal fluid using human tubes removed at hysterectomy [12]. In this technique, an artery serving the tube was cannulated and the vasculature perfused with Medium 199. A cannula was then tied into the tubal lumen, and after a short delay a fluid which can be considered as "close to physiological" accumulated linearly for at least 2 hours. Fluids collected in this manner were analyzed for glucose, pyruvate, and lactate [12] and amino acid [11] content. A culture medium based on the composition of this fluid sustained rates of human early embryo development in vitro [13] and pregnancy rates in clinical in vitro fertilization (IVF) [14] comparable to commercial media formulations/standard clinical practice. While the vascular perfusion method contributed novel information on the physiology of human tubal fluid formation, including its modulation by adrenergic agents, the technique was technically very demanding, limited by the rather short duration of experiments and the availability of appropriate tissue (premenopausal, non-pathological human Fallopian tubes).

In order to overcome these problems and discover more about the influence of the estrous cycle, and the difference between oviduct and uterine fluids and the mechanisms underlying their formation, we turned to an animal model of the oviduct *in situ*. In this, heifers were anesthetized and a cannula tied into the proximal end of the oviduct or uterus. The cannulae were attached to a calibrated tube in which oviduct or uterine fluid began to appear within a few minutes of cannulation and continued to do so at a linear rate for the duration of the experiments (4 hours). This enabled oviduct fluid to be collected on days 0, 2, 3, 4, and 6 and uterine fluid on days 6, 8, and 14 of the estrous cycle. These fluids were analyzed for electrolytes and pH [15], and the nutrients pyruvate, glucose, and lactate [16] and amino acids [17].

Development of a novel medium for culturing bovine zygotes

On the basis of these data, we devised a new medium: Bovine Oviduct Medium for Embryo Culture (BOMEC), the composition of which is given in Leese *et al.* [8]. The development of in vitro-produced bovine zygotes in BOMEC was compared with control zygotes grown in SOF medium [18]. Blastocyst rates were slightly higher in SOF (28% vs. 24%, $P < 0.05$) while there was a trend for cell numbers to be higher in BOMEC (151 for BOMEC vs. 135 for SOF: not significant). By contrast, the time taken for zygotes to complete first cleavage (a marker of subsequent viability in a variety of species [19]) was considerably shorter for those grown in BOMEC vs. SOF (Figure 3.2).

Although these data suggest that a culture medium based on the composition of oviduct fluid is conducive to bovine preimplantation development they should be interpreted with caution and further work would be required to establish the capacity of BOMEC to give rise to healthy offspring following embryo transfer. In this context, Walker *et al.* cultured sheep zygotes in a medium containing oviduct fluid concentrations of amino acids and reported increased development to the blastocyst stage and a greater proportion of embryos developing to day 13 following transfer (day 0) [20], while Hill *et al.*, using a similar medium for bovine zygotes, found improved development to blastocysts, but no evidence of increased viability post-transfer [21].

Macromolecular components in embryo culture media

The review so far has been concerned with the electrolyte and nutrient composition of female reproductive tract fluids. There is the difficult question of other components,

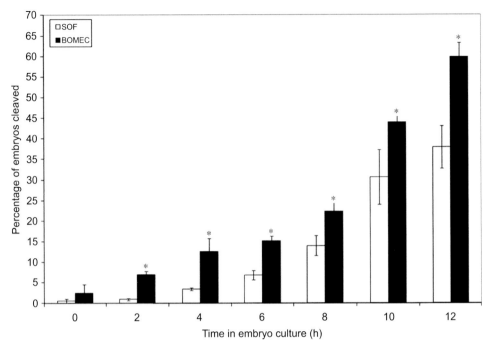

Figure 3.2 The time taken for bovine zygotes to complete the first cleavage division in BOMEC or SOF embryo culture medium.
*BOMEC and SOF significantly different ($P < 0.05$).
S.-L. Whitear and H. J. Leese (unpublished).

notably, macromolecules and cell signaling molecules, notably, cytokines [22], and which, if any, of these should be added and at what concentration. In the case of somatic cell culture, this issue would be addressed by the inclusion of serum or a serum substitute and the addition of further growth factors as appropriate. In the case of embryos, patient's serum, though widely added to culture media in the early years of IVF, is no longer considered a desirable supplement, due to its ill-defined nature and association with the "large offspring syndrome" in cattle and sheep [23]. While serum addition is not advocated, it is appropriate to add human serum albumin as a macromolecule to facilitate embryo handling since it is the most abundant protein in oviduct fluid and acts as a carrier of fat-soluble vitamins, hormones, bioactive lipids, and autocrine embryotropins [24, 25]. By contrast, the addition of single growth factors risks producing an unbalanced situation since the embryo will normally be exposed not to one, but numerous, such factors, which interact with one another at the receptor level and at the level of downstream signaling to produce pleiotropic effects. Moreover, these molecules are likely to be synthesized in a highly regulated but dynamic manner.

One solution to this dilemma is to exploit the fact that early embryos exhibit considerable autonomy and produce autocrine/paracrine factors which enhance their survival in vitro and are most likely involved in survival in the female tract [26, 27]. This challenging area, cognitively and technically, has been expertly summarized by O'Neill [25, 28]. The action of putative embryotrophic signals may be facilitated by culturing in microdrops

(1–5 µL), minimizing their loss by dilution and allowing embryos to autoregulate. This would seem to be a prudent approach bearing in mind our ignorance of the molecular cell biology of autocrine/paracrine signaling, rather than attempting to mimic the complex extracellular milieu by the addition of an arbitrary mixture of growth factors.

Environmental temperature

There is good evidence that the temperature in the ovarian follicle and lumen of the oviduct is below core body temperature by between 1 and 2 °C; a phenomenon particularly well-illustrated in the striking thermographic images of pig follicles produced by Hunter [29]. It has been proposed that culture at a reduced temperature will encourage "quiet metabolism" and promote embryo viability [30]. If this is the case, then arguably, human eggs and early embryos should be cultured at a temperature of ~36.0–36.5 °C rather than at 37–37.5 °C as currently practiced. However, before this is attempted there needs to be research using surplus human embryos to define the optimum temperature for their development to blastocysts in culture, followed by a randomized trial of the effect of reduced temperature(s) on the outcome of clinical IVF.

Physical environment within the oviduct

This is a difficult area to address since it is impossible to recreate the physical aspects of the oviductal environment: the presence of ciliated and non-ciliated (secretory) cells, fluid viscosity [31], etc. in culture. One approach is to grow embryos on cultured oviduct epithelial cells, but this faces two fundamental problems. The first is how to accommodate the differing nutrient requirements of two different cell types in the same culture dish; the preimplantation embryo, whose requirements appear relatively simple, and somatic cells, where complex media are essential. The second is to account for the changes in phenotype which occur when somatic cells are isolated, that is, epithelial cells from the reproductive tract "dedifferentiate" in culture [32], but it is rare to see this issue addressed. By the same token it is even rarer for embryo–somatic cell co-culture studies to include a control experiment to discover whether comparable embryo development can be achieved using cells from tissues other than those derived from the female reproductive tract. The utility and problems of co-culture work have been expertly summarized by Orsi and Reischl [33]. Developments in microfluidics offer a further possibility to get closer to the in vivo situation; especially those systems in which it is possible to confine an embryo(s) within a small volume of medium to allow for autocrine/paracrine effects but then allow for fluid to flow over the embryos, to encourage mixing, which will occur physiologically and minimize the accumulation of end-products [34].

Does the autonomy of the early embryo rule out the need for an oviduct?

It might seem strange to question the physiological need for the existence of the tissue which creates the environment one wishes to replicate. However, the semi-autonomous nature of the embryo has long been commented on [35] and one way of addressing this issue is to ask to what extent the "demand" for nutrients matches their "supply" by the oviduct.

Evidence that oviduct function *is* a function of gamete/early embryo requirements is as follows:

- Oviduct fluid formation in the rabbit is consistent with the need to sustain the embryo up to day 3, when there is a reduction in fluid volume and nutrients with passage of the embryo into the uterus [36].
- Human oviduct and uterine fluid nutrient concentrations are consistent with the use of pyruvate during early cleavage, with an increase in glucose consumption at the blastocyst stage [10].
- Nutrient concentrations in peri-ovulatory oviductal fluid of pigs are consistent with a strategy of protecting embryos from high glucose post-ovulation [37].
- Reduction in oviductal lumen temperature would promote "quiet" metabolism in the early embryo, which, it has been proposed, is related positively to viability [30].
- The oviduct epithelium is sensitive to candidate signaling molecules: (e.g., ATP, platelet activating factor [PAF], cyclic AMP) released by sperm and early embryos [38].
- Temporal patterns of oviductal gene and protein expression are consistent with gamete and preimplantation embryo development [39].
- The oviduct regulates sperm storage and movement [40].
- An abnormal oviductal environment compromises embryo development [41].

This issue has been considered by Hunter [42] in a provocatively titled review: "The Fallopian tubes in domestic mammals: how vital is their physiological activity?," which emphasizes the role of oviduct sperm reservoirs, temperature gradients, microenvironments, and local communication between the regions of the reproductive tract.

Taken overall, this evidence indicates that oviduct supply and gamete/embryo demand *are* compatible and that the female tract facilitates development but that the issue is confounded by the issue of embryo autonomy and adaptability. However, one could argue that IVF and related technologies have been successful because of the capacity of early embryos to adapt to an unnatural environment.

Efficacy and safety of embryo culture media

Leese *et al.* [8] building on the concept of Harding [43] proposed that the oviduct epithelium could be seen as the final component in a supply chain that linked maternal diet at one end with the consumption of nutrients by the early embryo at the other. When considered in this way, the oviduct (and uterine) epithelia assume the role of "gatekeepers" protecting the embryo from perturbation in maternal nutritional status. Such a function is lost in vitro and there is a very considerable literature showing convincingly that modification of the environment of the early embryo in culture can lead to deleterious consequences for the offspring [23, 44, 45]. A particularly striking example of this phenomenon is provided by the work of Dumoulin *et al.* [46], who reported that culture of human IVF embryos in different media resulted in a shift in birthweight of the offspring.

These and the other data considered in this review argue for minimizing the time for which an IVF embryo is maintained in vitro and using as benign a culture medium as possible. These objectives may be achieved by transferring embryos at the cleavage stage on day 2 or day 3 post-fertilization and mimicking as far as possible, their natural environment.

Acknowledgements
We thank Roger Sturmey for his most constructive comments on the manuscript.

References
1. Youssef M, Mantikou E, Gaber H, *et al.* Could culture media for human preimplantation embryos affect IVF/ICSI outcomes? A systematic review. *Hum Reprod* 2011;**24**(Suppl 1):i68.

2. Summers MC, Biggers JD. Chemically defined media and the culture of mammalian preimplantation embryos: historical perspectives and current issues *Hum Reprod Update* 2003;**9**:557–82.

3. Leese HJ. Human embryo culture: back to nature. *J Assist Reprod Genet* 1998;**15**:466–7.

4. Merton JS, de Roos APW, Mullaart E, *et al.* Effect on embryo production of the origin of the oocyte and the successive steps of maturation, fertilization and early development performed in vivo and/or in vitro in cattle. *Theriogenology* 2003;**59**:651–74.

5. Lonergan P, Fair T, Corcoran D, Evans ACO. Effect of culture environment on gene expression and developmental characteristics in IVF-derived embryos. *Theriogenology* 2006;**65**:137–52.

6. Market-Velker B, Fernandez AD, Mann MR. Side-by-side comparison of five commercial media systems in a mouse model: suboptimal in vitro culture interferes with imprint maintenance. *Biol Reprod* 2010;**83**:938–50.

7. Aguilar J, Reyley M. The uterine tubal fluid: secretion, composition and biological effects. *Anim Reprod* 2005;**2**:91–105.

8. Leese HJ, Hugentobler SA, Gray SM, *et al.* Female reproductive tract fluids: composition, mechanism of formation and potential role in the developmental origins of health and disease. *Reprod Fert Dev* 2008;**20**:1–8.

9. Borland RM, Hazra S, Biggers JD, *et al.* Elemental composition of fluid in the human Fallopian tube. *J Reprod Fertil* 1980;**58**:479–82.

10. Gardner DK, Lane M, Calderon I, *et al.* Environment of the preimplantation human embryo in vivo: metabolite analysis of oviduct and uterine fluids and metabolism of cumulus cells. *Fertil Steril* 1996;**65**:349–53.

11. Tay JI, Rutherford AJ, Killick SR, *et al.* Human tubal fluid: production, nutrient composition and response to adrenergic agents. *Hum Reprod* 1997;**12**:2451–6.

12. Dickens, CJ, Maguiness, SD, Comer MT, *et al.* Human tubal fluid: formation and composition during vascular perfusion of the Fallopian tube. *Hum Reprod* 1995;**10**:505–8.

13. Houghton FD, Hawkhead JA, Humpherson PG, *et al.* Non-invasive amino acid turnover predicts human embryo developmental capacity. *Hum Reprod* 2002;**17**:999–1005.

14. Brison DR, Houghton FD, Falconer D, *et al.* Identification of viable embryos in IVF by non-invasive measurement of amino acid turnover. *Hum Reprod* 2004;**19**:2319–24.

15. Hugentobler SA, Morris DG, Sreenan JM, *et al.* Ion concentrations in oviduct and uterine fluid and blood serum during the estrous cycle in the bovine. *Theriogenology* 2007;**68**:538–48.

16. Hugentobler SA, Humpherson PG, Leese HJ, *et al.* Energy substrates in bovine oviduct and uterine fluid and blood plasma during the oestrous cycle. *Mol Reprod Dev* 2007;**75**:496–503.

17. Hugentobler SA, Diskin MG, Leese HJ, *et al.* Amino acids in oviduct and uterine fluid and blood plasma during the estrous cycle in the bovine. *Mol Reprod Dev* 2007;**74**:445–54.

18. Gardner DK, Lane H, Spitzer A, *et al.* Enhanced rates of cleavage and development for sheep zygotes cultured to the blastocyst stage in vitro in the absence of serum and somatic cells: amino acids, vitamins and culturing embryos in groups

stimulate development. *Biol Reprod* 1994;**50**:390–400.

19. Booth, PJ, Watson, TJ, Leese HJ. Prediction of porcine blastocyst formation using morphological, kinetic, and amino acid depletion and appearance criteria determined during the early cleavage of in vitro-produced embryos. *Biol Reprod* 2007;**77**:765–79.

20. Walker SK, Hill JL, Kleemann DO, *et al.* Development of ovine embryos in synthetic oviductal fluid containing amino acids at oviductal fluid concentrations. *Biol Reprod* 1996;**55**:703–8.

21. Hill JL, Wade MG, Nancarrow CD, *et al.* Influence of ovine oviductal amino acid concentrations and an ovine oestrus-associated glycoprotein on development and viability of bovine embryos. *Mol Reprod Dev* 1997;**47**:164–9.

22. Robertson SA, Chin PY, Glynn DJ, *et al.* Peri-conceptual cytokines – setting the trajectory for embryo implantation, pregnancy and beyond. *Am J Reprod Immunol* 2011;**66**(Suppl 1):2–10.

23. Leese HJ, Donnay I, Thompson JG. Human assisted conception; a cautionary tale. Lessons from domestic animals. *Hum Reprod* 1998;**4**(Suppl 4):184–202.

24. Menezo Y, Guerin P. The mammalian oviduct: biochemistry and physiology. *Eur J Obstet Gynecol* 1997;**73**:99–104.

25. O'Neill C. The potential roles for embryotrophic ligands in preimplantation embryo development. *Hum Reprod Update* 2008;**14**:275–88.

26. Stokes PJ, Abeydeera LR, Leese HJ. Development of porcine embryos *in vivo* and *in vitro*; evidence for embryo 'cross talk' *in vitro*. *Dev Biol* 2005;**284**:62–71.

27. Gopichandran N, Leese HJ. The effect of paracrine/autocrine interactions on the in vitro culture of bovine preimplantation embryos. *Reproduction* 2006;**131**:269–77.

28. Jin XL, O'Neill C. Regulation of the expression of proto-oncogenes by autocrine embryotropins in the early mouse embryo. *Biol Reprod* 2011;**84**:1216–24.

29. Hunter RFH. Temperature gradients in female reproductive tissues and their potential significance. *Anim Reprod* 2009;**6**:7–15.

30. Leese HJ, Baumann CG, Brison DR, *et al.* Metabolism of the viable mammalian embryo: quietness revisited. *Mol Hum Reprod* 2008;**14**:667–72.

31. Hunter RH, Hunter P, Gadea J, *et al.* Considerations of viscosity in the preliminaries to mammalian fertilization. *J Assist Reprod Genet* 2011;**28**:191–7.

32. Comer MT, Leese HJ, Southgate J. Induction of a differentiated ciliated cell phenotype in primary cultures of Fallopian tube epithelium. *Hum Reprod* 1998;**13**:3114–20.

33. Orsi NM, Reischl JB. Mammalian embryo co-culture: trials and tribulations of a misunderstood method. *Theriogenology* 2007;**67**:441–58.

34. Swain JE, Smith GD Advances in embryo culture platforms: novel approaches to improve preimplantation embryo development through modifications of the microenvironment. *Hum Reprod Update* 2011;**17**:541–57.

35. Mclaren A. *Mammalian Chimaeras.* Cambridge, Cambridge University Press, 1976.

36. Leese HJ. Metabolic control during preimplantation mammalian development. *Hum Reprod Update* 1995;**1**:63–72.

37. Nichol R, Hunter RHF, Gardner DK, *et al.* Concentrations of energy substrates in oviductal fluid and blood plasma of pigs during the peri-ovulatory period. *J Reprod Fertil* 1992;**96**:699–707.

38. Downing SJ, Chambers EL, Maguiness SD, *et al.* Effect of inflammatory mediators on the electrophysiology of the human oviduct. *Biol Reprod* 1999;**61**:657–64.

39. Holt WV, Fazeli A. The oviduct as a complex mediator of mammalian sperm function and selection. *Mol Reprod Dev* 2010;**77**:934–43.

40. Suarez SS. Regulation of sperm storage and movement in the mammalian oviduct. *Int J Dev Biol* 2008;**52**:455–62.

41. Jefferson WN, Padilla-Banks E, Goulding EH, *et al*. Neonatal exposure to genistein disrupts ability of mouse female reproductive tract to support preimplantation embryo development and implantation. *Biol Reprod* 2009;**80**:425–31.

42. Hunter RH. The Fallopian tubes in domestic mammals: how vital is their physiological activity? *Reprod Nutr Dev* 2005;**45**:281–90.

43. Harding JE. The nutritional basis of the fetal origins of adult disease. *Int J Epidemiol* 2001;**30**:15–23.

44. Thompson JG, Mitchell M, Kind KL. Embryo culture and long-term consequences. *Reprod Fertil Dev* 2007;**19**:43–52.

45. Watkins AJ, Papenbrock T, Fleming TP. The preimplantation embryo: handle with care. *Semin Reprod Med* 2008;**26**:175–85.

46. Dumoulin JC, Land JA, Van Montfoort AP, *et al*. Effect of in vitro culture of human embryos on birthweight of newborns. *Hum. Reprod* 2010;**25**:605–12.

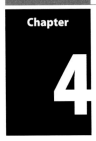

Chapter

4

Buffering systems in IVF

Natalie A. Clark and Jason E. Swain

Introduction

A pH buffer is a substance that acts as a weak acid and/or a weak base so that the pH of the solution to which it is added will be resistant to a change in pH in response to various insults. This occurs through accepting or donating hydrogen ions, which are ultimately responsible for establishing pH.

In cell culture, including in vitro fertilization (IVF), the most common buffer used in media is sodium bicarbonate. In conjunction with carbonic acid formed from the dissolving of carbon dioxide (CO_2) into the media when placed into the incubator, the external pH of media (pH_e) can be maintained as long as the levels of CO_2 remain constant. However, maintenance of CO_2 levels is problematic with repeated incubator openings/closings for cell observation as well as for manipulations performed at room atmosphere. Though some laboratories use isolettes or portable working incubators to maintain elevated CO_2 and pH_e for various procedures, these devices can be expensive and cumbersome. For procedures performed in room atmosphere, such as gamete collection, intracytoplasmic sperm injection (ICSI), cryopreservation, and embryo transfer, many labs choose to utilize handling media with reduced bicarbonate levels and inclusion of other pH buffers to maintain stable pH_e outside the incubator.

In an attempt to improve the selection of available pH buffers Good and colleagues developed a series of new biological pH buffers. These new compounds were largely zwitterionic aliphatic amines, or altered amino acids, the majority consisting of N-substituted taurine and glycine (Table 4.1). Zwitterions have the ability to act as either an acid or a base, and therefore are excellent buffers of pH. In the development of these new compounds, various criteria were set to ensure their usefulness for biological research. These included:

1. **pK_a**. Because most biological reactions take place at near-neutral pH between 6 and 8, ideal buffers would have pK_a values in this region to provide maximum buffering capacity there.

2. **Solubility**. For ease in handling, and because biological systems are in aqueous systems, good solubility in water is required. Low solubility in non-polar solvents (fats, oils, and organic solvents) is also considered beneficial, as this will tend to prevent the buffer compound from accumulating in non-polar compartments in biological systems, such as cell membranes.

Culture Media, Solutions, and Systems in Human ART, ed. Patrick Quinn. Published by Cambridge University Press. © Cambridge University Press 2014.

Table 4.1. List of pH buffers and their corresponding pK$_a$ values that may be suitable for use with gametes and embryos. pK$_a$, or optimal buffering capacity, changes with temperature and should be considered when choosing a buffer.

Common name	pK$_a$ @ 20 °C	pK$_a$ @ 37 °C	Temp effect ΔpH/ΔTemp	Full compound name
Tris [soe +]	8.3	7.82	−0.028	Tris(hydroxymethyl)methylamine
Tricine [s]	8.15	7.79	−0.021	N-Tris(hydroxymethyl)methylglycine
HEPPSO	7.9	7.73	−0.010	N-Hydroxyethylpiperazine-N′-2-hydroxypropanesulfonic acid
POPSO	7.85	7.63	−0.013	Piperazine-N,N′-bis (2-hydroxypropanesulfonic acid) dihydrate
TAPSO [s]	7.7	7.39	−0.018	3-[N-Tris(hydroxymethyl) methylamino]-2-hydroxypropanesulfonic acid
DIPSO [oe]	7.6	7.35	−0.015	2,3[N-Bis(hydroxyethyl)amino]-2-hydroxypropanesulfonic acid
HEPES [soe +]	7.55	7.31	−0.014	4-2-Hydroxyethyl-1-piperazineethanesulfonic acid
TES [so +]	7.5	7.16	−0.020	2{[Tris(hydroxymethyl)methyl]amino} ethanesulfonic acid
Phosphate [soe * +]	7.21	7.19	−0.001	
MOPS [soe +]	7.15	6.93	−0.013	3-(N-Morpholino)propanesulfonic acid
BES [s]	7.15	6.88	−0.016	N,N-Bis(2-hydroxyethyl)-2-aminoethanesulfonic acid
MOPSO	6.95	6.70	−0.015	3-(N-Morpholino)-2-hydroxypropanesulfonic acid
PIPES [so]	6.8	6.66	−0.008	Piperazine-N,N′-bis(2-ethanesulfonic acid)
Bicarbonate [soe * +]	6.38	6.30	−0.005	
MES [s]	6.15	5.96	−0.011	2-(N-Morpholino)ethanesulfonic acid

Lettered superscripts on the common buffer name indicates which cell type it has been tested with (s = sperm, o = oocyte, e = embryo). + indicates a commercial product for use in IVF is available with the buffer included, though this may be in conjunction with another buffer in a combination buffering system. * indicates a polyprotic acid with multiple pK$_a$ values. Values obtained from Ferguson et al. [1], Good et al. [2], Good and Izawa [3].

3. **Membrane impermeability**. Ideally, a buffer will not readily pass through cell membranes.
4. **Minimal salt effects**. Highly ionic buffers may cause problems or complications in some biological systems.
5. **Dissociation**. Buffer dissociation should be minimally affected by buffer concentration, temperature, and ionic composition of the medium.

6. **Well-behaved cation interactions**. If the buffers form complexes with cationic ligands, the complexes formed should remain soluble. Ideally, at least some of the buffering compounds will not form complexes.
7. **Stability**. The buffers should be chemically stable, resisting enzymatic and non-enzymatic degradation.
8. **Optical absorbance**. Though of less concern in use with gametes and embryos for IVF, buffers should not absorb visible or ultraviolet light at wavelengths longer than 230 nm so as not to interfere with commonly used spectrophotometric assays.
9. **Ease of preparation**. Buffers should be readily prepared from inexpensive materials and easily purified.

Buffers are generally selected based on their optimal pH buffering capacity or pK_a value. This is the log of the acid dissociation constant (K_a), or the point where equilibrium is reached and equal portions of acid and conjugate base exist in solution, thus providing the highest buffering, or ability to resist pH change. Because many biological processes or laboratory assays are only functional over a small range of pH_e, to maintain efficiently the pH_e within this working window, ideally the buffer utilized will have a pK_a value close to the working pH_e of the solution. When this occurs, a lower buffer concentration can be utilized, which is often safer than using higher concentrations. Additionally, in general, the protonized form of amine or zwitterionic buffers is less likely to be inhibitory or reactive than the non-protonated form [3]. Thus, in these cases it is usually safer to select a buffer with a pK_a value slightly above the desired pH_e.

As mentioned, buffers can have effects other than buffering pH [1–4]. Numerous studies, conducted primarily in somatic cell culture, demonstrate undesired actions of various pH buffers. For example, one of the buffers used in commercial IVF handling media, MOPS, has been noted to interfere with taurine uptake in tumor cell lines [5], interact with DNA in cellular preparations [6], and interfere with chloride conductance in neurons [7]. Similar such findings also exist with other buffers, including the common buffer HEPES. However, limited data on these buffers in regard to their impact on gametes or embryos exist. This is likely important because, though procedures in assisted reproductive technology (ART) using buffered handling media generally entail only brief exposures, even brief exposure to inappropriate handling media can be detrimental to embryo development [8–10]. Therefore, attempting to isolate the potential impact of the specific buffer from other aspects of the media is warranted and may help improve the culture system. Further warranting this examination of buffer impact, undesired effects and interactions may be cell-type specific. Thus, in an attempt to summarize what is known, and to improve upon current approaches, various pH buffers and their use with gametes and embryos are discussed.

Oocytes

Due to a lack of robust pH regulatory mechanisms, oocytes are generally considered to be a remarkably sensitive cell type in respect to pH, and this is particularly evident in the denuded mature oocyte [11–14]. The pH_e of culture media greatly influences oocyte maturation, even with brief exposures, with acidification and alkalization both being problematic. When pH_e rose above 7.45 during oocyte isolation for 30–45 minutes, mouse oocyte meiotic progression decreased and degeneration increased [15]. In culture for 3 hours at pH 6.8, oocyte nucleotide synthesis in the presence of follicle-stimulating hormone (FSH) was ~50% lower than at pH 7.4 [16]. Thus, periodic fluctuations of the pH_e are likely harmful, as these can then be translated into deleterious intracellular perturbations. As such, it is readily apparent that buffers used to stabilize pH_e are critical to the optimization of oocyte culture systems and further examination and refinement is essential to improve IVF outcomes. Currently, oocytes are exposed to media and buffers most frequently in retrieval procedures as well as fertilization utilizing ICSI. Unfortunately, few comparative studies have been performed to assess the impact various biological buffers have on oocytes.

In the past, handling media in IVF have frequently utilized phosphate buffered solutions (PBS), and some laboratories continue to use this media for oocyte retrieval. Consideration behind the use of PBS includes its pK_a (7.2) and buffering capacity, perhaps cost, as well as concern with other available buffers. However, use of phosphate buffer tends to precipitate polyvalent cations, while simultaneously acting as a metabolite or inhibitor in cells. Indeed, elevated levels of phosphate may compromise gamete and embryo metabolic activity, disrupt organelle distribution, and interfere with intracellular ionic homeostasis, including internal pH (pH_i) [17–19]. Data also demonstrate that phosphate yields very low rates of fertilization in hamster oocytes when compared with other buffers [20]. Whether this is due to impact on the sperm or the oocyte is unclear. As such, some speculation remains that, although PBS may be sufficient in terms of pH and temperature stability, detrimental influences on the oocyte mitigate its utility as an ideal buffer in IVF.

More commonly used buffers for oocyte manipulations are the Good's buffers, including HEPES and MOPS. By far, HEPES is the most well-studied buffer for use in IVF. Its pK_a value of 7.31 at 37 °C gives it excellent buffering capacity over the range commonly used for handling gametes and embryo (7.2–7.4). In regard to oocyte maturation, one early study reported that 10% HEPES used during mouse oocyte maturation caused oocyte degeneration [15]. Another study found that increasing HEPES from 20 to 25 mM did not affect spontaneous mouse oocyte maturation, but did suppress the ability to induce FSH-stimulated meiosis in pharmacologically inhibited oocytes with dcAMP but not hypoxanthine [16]. These two studies highlight the importance of examining confounding variables in the system when trying to determine the impact of only the pH buffer on cells, and also suggest buffer concentration may be an important factor as well. Importantly, both these studies were conducted in MEM medium, which contains riboflavin. Early somatic cell studies citing HEPES toxicity demonstrated that detrimental effects stemmed from light exposure and interactions with riboflavin [21]. This offers an easy explanation for oocyte degeneration. Additionally, the fact that HEPES did not impact spontaneous maturation of mouse oocytes, and only showed suppressive effects with one of two pharmacological inhibitors [16], further demonstrates the need to rule out confounding factors present in the culture media when trying to truly examine impact of a single pH buffer.

Lower rates of oocyte fertilization have been demonstrated when IVF in rodent species is performed in HEPES, or other synthetic organic buffered media [20, 22]. Again, it is unclear if potential impact is on the oocyte directly. However, those studies indicating lower fertilization rates in the presence of HEPES are likely due to the simultaneous reduction in bicarbonate concentrations, as bicarbonate is required for normal fertilization, likely through effects on sperm capacitation [22, 23].

Importantly, many studies indicate that HEPES is able to support efficiently oocyte maturation and fertilization from various species at room atmosphere [16, 22, 24–26]. In other studies, HEPES at various concentrations from 2.5 to 25 mM used in elevated CO_2 environments has been used to mature oocytes and fertilize eggs successfully, yielding rates similar to media with no HEPES present [23, 27]. Given the wealth of positively supporting data, at the present time, it can be concluded that HEPES is a reasonable buffer for oocyte culture.

The Good's buffer, MOPS, is much less well studied than HEPES in regard to its impact on the oocyte. One study has noted the ability of MOPS buffered media to mature successfully mouse oocytes at a concentration of 20 mM [16]. MOPS buffer was also used in media to fertilize guinea pig oocytes [22]. Another study indicated that MOPS buffer used for oocyte microinjection had no negative impact on pronuclear or blastocyst formation [28]. A later study using MOPS for oocyte microinjection showed no impact on oocyte pH_i [29]. These studies seem to indicate no detriment or benefit of MOPS compared to other buffers. Despite its low pK_a value at 37 °C, the buffer is now included in commercial handling media and used successfully for human ART procedures including oocyte handling and vitrification.

TES may have the single best buffering capacity for use in ART with a pK_a of 7.16 at 37 °C, as this is the closest to the pH_i of oocytes. However, although TES has been used extensively for molecular assays, it has received little use in IVF. In an attempt to avoid use of CO_2, TES was used as the buffer in a medium used to fertilize hamster oocytes. At 42 mM, TES permitted 55.8% fertilization, similar to that obtained with HEPES, though both were inferior to media buffered with bicarbonate and it was noted that anomalies were observed in pronuclei formed in TES buffered medium [20]. Similar results were obtained following IVF using TES for guinea pig oocytes [22]. However, again, this may be due to insufficient bicarbonate in the medium. TES has been examined for use with mouse oocyte microinjection and had no significant impact on pH_i, similar to MOPS and HEPES [29]. Additionally, TEST, a combination buffer consisting of TES and Tris buffers, is commonly used with sperm. At least one study has examined the impact of TEST on the storage of oocytes. Zona-intact hamster ova were stored in TEST-yolk buffer at 4 °C and were subsequently used for the sperm penetration assay, yielding 100% penetration similar to fresh ova [30]. As such, little data are available for the use of Good's buffers besides HEPES in oocyte culture; however, TES may be a reasonable alternative to HEPES in situations where bicarbonate buffer systems are not desirable options.

In the first report of a combination buffering system for use with oocyte ICSI, a HEPES: MOPS buffer at a 1:1 ratio totaling 10 mM final concentration was used successfully to hold and microinject human oocytes, and yielded similar rates of fertilization, embryo multinucleation, and resulting blastocyst formation compared to a HEPES-only medium [31]. Thus, these two buffers, or their combination, may be suitable for use in human IVF. A commercially available handling medium is now available that utilized a ratio of HEPES and MOPS to optimize pK_a and buffering capacity for use with human gamete and embryos.

Other buffers considered for use in oocyte handling and culture include PIPES and DIPSO. PIPES was noted to support mouse oocyte maturation in vitro to metaphase II at 20 mM, though there appeared to be interaction with hypoxanthine, as inhibition of germinal vesicle breakdown was reduced in the presence of the buffer compared to MOPS, HEPES, or DIPSO [16]. DIPSO was used in the same study of mouse oocyte maturation and showed no adverse effects on spontaneous maturation to metaphase II at 20 mM [16]. Tris and TAPSO have been used to fertilize guinea pig eggs and did not appear to offer any significant difference in outcomes compared to other buffers such as TES, MOPS, or HEPES [22]. Additional studies are required to determine the true impact of all of these alternative buffers on oocyte development and function.

Sperm

The greatest amount of information regarding impact of various pH buffers for use in ART procedures exists with sperm, primarily from a variety of domestic species. These buffers are used in media formulated for extending, washing, and preserving semen at low temperature, with impact on motility, fertilization capacity, and other molecular measurements often used as measures of buffer efficacy.

Many of the same buffers examined for use with oocytes have received attention for use with sperm, including phosphate. Decreased motility of boar sperm was observed when stored in phosphate buffered diluents, compared to various zwitterion buffered media [32]. Authors proposed this may be due to metabolic disruption, possibly via mediation of the Crabtree effect [33]. Additionally, as previously mentioned, use of media buffered with phosphate yielded very low rates of fertilization in hamster oocytes compared to other buffers tested [20].

Another common buffer used mostly for molecular assays is Tris. When used alone, Tris-HCl buffer in boar sperm diluents yielded significantly lower sperm motility following storage at 37 °C or 5 °C compared to seven Good's buffers studied (MES, PIPES, BES, MOPS, TES, HEPES, Tricine). Furthermore, Tris-HCl also resulted in the greatest amount of sperm membrane damage, as indicated by the increased release of glutamine oxaloacetate transaminase (GOT) from sperm, in comparison to other buffers studied [32]. However, the combination of Tris with other buffers has been used extensively in diluents and in cryopreservation solutions for mammalian sperm, including human. Perhaps the most well-known example of this is Tris and TES (TEST) [34, 35]. Other examples of Tris titrated combination buffers used with sperm include BES:Tris (BEST), HEPES:Tris (HEPEST), MOPS:Tris (MOPST) and PIPES:Tris (PIPEST) [36]. When used to titrate pH_e of media with various zwitterionic buffers, Tris resulted in higher bovine sperm motility after freezing than titration with other bases such as NaOH [32]. Titrating various buffer solutions with Tris has also been shown to have no adverse effect on post-thaw motility of bull sperm [37], but significantly impaired motility of turkey sperm [38], suggesting perhaps some species-specific sensitivity to Tris.

In a similar fashion, when combined with citrate, Tris:Citrate buffer combination has been used to freeze semen from a variety of domestic species including ram [39, 40], boar [32], bull [37], and turkey [38], though post-thaw motility and acrosome integrity was often lower than that obtained from other zwitterionic buffers studied, such as HEPES, TES, and PIPES [39, 40]. Tris:citrate buffer was also used to successfully freeze human spermatozoa [41, 42]. In early attempts to achieve fertilization in vitro in hamster, Bavister examined the use of Tris:citrate buffer (25 mM). Though an excellent pH buffer, and despite the fact that it stimulated sperm motility, no fertilization was obtained from 207 oocytes inseminated [20]. Because fertilization is obtained with Tris in combination with other buffers as mentioned above, a likely explanation for the lack of fertilization observed in Tris: citrate is the chelation of calcium ions by citrate.

More commonly examined buffers for use with mammalian sperm include the zwitterionic Good's buffers. HEPES, MOPS, TRIS, and TAPSO all permitted guinea pig sperm capacitation and acrosome reaction [22]. Lower rates of fertilization observed are likely due to the inadequate amounts of bicarbonate used in the study. HEPES has routinely been shown to be a safe and effective buffer when compared with other buffers for storage of sperm from a variety of species at various temperatures [32, 39, 43]. HEPES maintained boar sperm membrane integrity following storage at 5 °C and resulted in the lowest amount of GOT release. This effect was not significantly different from BES, TES, and PIPES, but was significantly better than MOPS, MES, and Tricine [32]. Additionally, HEPES has been shown to be efficacious for use with human sperm. HEPES-buffered media in room atmosphere gave similar rates of human intrauterine insemination (IUI) pregnancy compared to bicarbonate-buffered media [44]. Use of HEPES up to 50 mM, when used with elevated bicarbonate in the laboratory incubator, supported human sperm motility and permitted normal decondensation following microinjection into hamster ova, compared to bicarbonate-only buffered media [45].

Another Good's buffer, MOPS, was one of several buffers tested in diluents for cryopreservation of boar, ram, turkey, and bull sperm [32, 37, 38, 46, 47]. MOPS yielded similar motility after storage at 37 °C compared to other buffers, but MOPS was one of the top three buffers in regard to maintaining motility after storage at lower temperatures [32, 37, 38]. However, MOPS was one of the worst three buffers in maintaining membrane integrity, as measured by GOT release [32].

By itself, the Good's buffer TES was successfully used for cryopreservation of ram spermatozoa and yielded post-thaw motility similar to five other zwitterions buffered media (HEPES, HEPES:Tris, MES:Tris, PIPES, PIPES:Tris) [39]. TES was judged as one of the two best buffers used in diluents for storage or freezing boar sperm. Sperm exposed to TES yielded some of the highest rates of sperm motility following storage at 5 °C and lowest levels of GOT release compared to other buffers studied [32]. Perhaps the most apparent use of TES has been for sperm storage, as a component of a combination buffer in conjunction with Tris (TEST) [35, 37], which, when combined with egg yolk (TYB) has been used extensively for sperm storage at low temperature or freezing, including that of human [48–51]. Use of TYB medium maintained the capability of sperm to bind for the sperm penetration assay. Interestingly, it was found that in some samples, the percent penetration was improved by exposure to the TYB buffer [52]. This improved penetration has been verified and 42 hours was better than 18 hours [53]. Preincubation in TYB at ~5 °C improved results of the acrosome reaction test [54, 55], sperm penetration assay [52–58], and binding in the hemizona assay [59]. Finally, and perhaps more importantly, incubation of human sperm in TYB for 2 or 24 hours at 4 °C prior to insemination has been reported to increase fertilization rates in couples with poor or prior failed fertilization in IVF cases [60, 61]. Though these impacts cannot be attributed to TES or TRIS buffer alone [62], the results do indicate TEST is an apparently safe buffering system and does not compromise sperm function.

PIPES, another zwitterionic Good's buffer, used at ~39.6 mM after dilution yielded higher post-thaw motility and acrosome integrity than the controls in Tris:citrate buffer (120 mM:38 mM after dilution), with comparable rates of pregnancy following insemination of ewes [43]. PIPES was also used as a buffer in diluents for cryopreservation of boar sperm, where it yielded sperm motility after storage at 37 °C similar to six other zwitterionic buffers, but yielded significantly lower sperm motility when used at 5 °C in comparison to BES, MOPS, TES, HEPES, and Tricine [32].

MES was used as a buffer in diluents for cryopreservation of boar sperm, where it yielded similar sperm motility after storage at 37 °C compared to six other zwitterionic buffers, but yielded significantly lower sperm motility when used at 5 °C in comparison to BES, MOPS, TES, HEPES, and Tricine [32]. However, in another study, MES at 50 mM was the superior buffer of those tested and maintained bull sperm motility at 5 or 37 °C [63].

BES is a modified taurine molecule and one of the original Good's buffers. With a pK$_a$ of 6.90 at 37 °C, the buffer was used as a buffer in diluents for cryopreservation of boar sperm, where it yielded similar sperm motility after storage at 37 °C and was one of the top five buffers in regard to maintaining motility after storage at 5 °C, similar to MOPS, TES, HEPES, and Tricine [32] Additionally, BES was one of the top three buffers used successfully for storage and freezing of turkey and bull sperm [37, 38].

Tricine is a modified glycine molecule. With a pK$_a$ of 7.80 at 37 °C, Tricine has been used as a buffer in diluents for cryopreservation of boar sperm. When compared with the other zwitterionic buffers, Tricine performed similarly to TES and HEPES in respect to preserving boar sperm motility, but did result in significantly higher release of GOT after plunging into liquid nitrogen for cold storage [32].

Embryos

Embryos are potentially exposed to buffers at various stages of their development. Depending on a particular laboratory's protocol, embryos may be exposed to handling media with a pH buffer during embryo transfer. Alternatively, all laboratories expose embryos to a biological pH buffer when performing various cryopreservation procedures, though this aspect carries with it other particular concerns in regard to temperature and will be discussed in more detail later. Exposure to buffers during these procedures can occur during cleavage or blastocyst stages, and thus requires consideration when assessing buffer efficacy in IVF.

Perhaps one of the best methods to assess impact of a particular pH buffer on the embryos is performing extended culture in the presence of the buffer. As even brief exposure to inappropriate handling media has been shown to compromise hamster and rabbit embryo development [8, 9], a longer exposure period likely offers a means to observe more readily any detrimental impact. These sort of extended embryo culture studies performed in handling media have only been conducted with a few buffers such as HEPES and MOPS in animal models. More in-depth analysis, use of alternate model systems, and exploration of additional buffers may be helpful in further defining any potential detrimental impacts.

In the case of phosphate buffered media and impact of embryos, exposure for ~41 minutes during oocyte and embryo manipulation resulted in lower blastocyst formation and aberrant gene expression in bovine embryos when compared with zwitterionic buffers studied, such as MOPS and HEPES [10]. However, in these studies, results could not be attributed to phosphate alone, as the basal media and energy substrate composition also apparently differed between treatments. When examined in the context of the same basal medium, culture of embryos in phosphate buffered media resulted in significantly lower blastocyst formation and live birth rates in mice following transfer in comparison to a HEPES-buffered medium [64]

Culturing embryos at room atmosphere for extended periods in zwitterions buffered media, such as HEPES, has been reported for various species [26, 64–67], though some report compromised blastocyst development [68, 69]. In these cases demonstrating detrimental effects of HEPES, differences in development are likely due, at least in part, to the simultaneous reductions in CO_2 levels and bicarbonate concentrations of the handling medium compared to traditional media used in the laboratory incubator. Embryo development is supported in the presence of HEPES when bicarbonate is present, but not when bicarbonate is absent [64]. Bicarbonate levels influence blastocyst development, possibility through activity of various HCO_3^--dependent transporters [70]. Additionally, elevated CO_2 of the incubator is utilized by embryos as a carbon source for various biochemical processes [71–73], and is likely beneficial over culture at room atmosphere. Therefore, when embryos are cultured at room atmosphere and compared with controls cultured in 5% CO_2, differences in development cannot be attributed to HEPES alone. Indeed, when CO_2 and bicarbonate levels are accounted for as variables, media with up to 50 mM HEPES yielded similar rates of mouse blastocyst development and cell number compared to media without HEPES [67].

Few reports on the efficacy of MOPS and embryo culture exist. Mouse blastocysts have been successfully cultured in the presence of up to 50 mM MOPS with no apparent detriment over 96 hours [67]. Additionally, MOPS supported high rates of bovine blastocyst formation following relatively brief exposure during routine handling procedures and yielded a similar gene expression profile to that of embryos exposed to HEPES, most similar to in vivo-derived embryos [10]. Additionally, combining HEPES and MOPS for embryo culture demonstrated that the use of both buffers at 10 mM provided buffering at a point between HEPES or MOPS alone and also yielded similar blastocyst formation and cell number compared to use of the individual buffers [67].

Evidence for the impact of zwitterionic buffers other than MOPS or HEPES on mammalian embryo development is scarce. The zwitterionic buffer DIPSO was successfully used to culture mouse embryo blastocysts over 96 hours at concentrations of 25 or 50 mM of DIPSO in the presence of 25 mM $NaHCO_3$ in ~5% CO_2, yielding similar rates of development and resulting cell number compared to control media with no buffer, as well as other buffers, HEPES and MOPS [67]. Additionally, in the first examples of a tri-buffered media utilized for mammalian preimplantation embryos, the combination of HEPES, MOPS, and DIPSO at 6.7 mM each supported mouse blastocyst development, while allowing for the adjustment of pK_a and lowering of individual buffer concentrations compared to mono-buffered media [67]. The buffer TES was used to handle bovine zygotes and embryos for ~41 minutes during in vitro processing, and resulted in lower blastocyst development and an altered gene expression profile compared to HEPES or MOPS [10]. However, studies using mouse embryos indicate that 21 mM TES was able to support mouse blastocyst formation from the 1-cell stage at rates similar to bicarbonate-only buffered media, HEPES or MOPS (Figure 4.1). Because of its beneficial pK_a value, future examination of TES's efficacy is likely warranted.

Cryopreservation

Cryopreservation of gametes and embryos presents a particular dilemma and potential concern when using zwitterionic buffers. Although widely used in ART, it is often not appreciated that temperature affects pK_a of these synthetic organic buffers, as well as the actual pH of the media. In general, as temperature increases, pH and pK_a values decrease (Table 4.1) [1, 2]. This has been measured for buffers and handling media commonly used

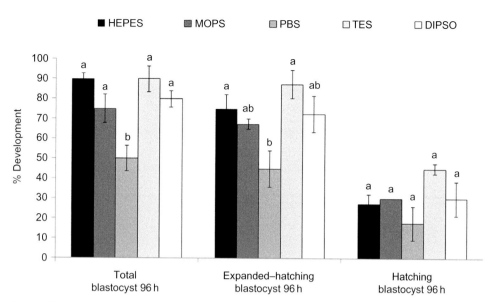

Figure 4.1 As previously demonstrated by somatic cell lines, different buffers can differentially impact cell development. Buffers such as MOPS, HEPES, and DIPSO and TES at 21 mM have been shown to support mouse embryo development at comparable rates following 96 hours of continuous culture from 1 cell. Phosphate appears to negatively impact embryo development.

in IVF [67]. As an example, MOPS was presumably selected as buffer for inclusion in commercial IVF handling media as an alternative to HEPES and associated toxicity concerns, but also because its pK_a of pH 7.2 is the closest of the 20 zwitterionic buffers to the pH_i of embryos of 7.12 [70]. Thus, MOPS would seemingly offer the best pH buffering of available options. However, the pK_a of 7.2 for MOPS is at 25 °C. Many laboratories warm their handling media to 37 °C, a temperature at which the pK_a for MOPS is actually 7.02. This is low, considering many labs set their media pH around 7.3. Similarly, the opposite holds true. As the temperature lowers, pK_a and pH rises. Thus, the same buffer used for procedures performed at 37 °C may not be the best buffer for procedures performed at cooler temperatures, such as those experienced during cryopreservation. Another important consideration in regard to buffers and temperature includes how much pK_a and pH change in response to temperature. Both MOPS and HEPES display approximately equal changes in pK_a in response to temperature changes between 25 °C and 37 °C (0.18 and 0.17, respectively). However, other buffers change more significantly.

One buffer that may raise concern in the context of pH change secondary to temperature is phosphate. Concerns exist in regard to the potential acidification of phosphate buffered media when frozen [74, 75]. Using spectrophotometric methods, it has been observed that the apparent pH of PBS decreases significantly upon slow rate freezing [75]. In examination of the color of PBS with phenol red used during slow rate freezing, at −80 °C the authors noted the "color is yellow, indicating severe acidification" (Figure 4.2) [74]. Whether this is a true pH change, or simply an effect of the concentration of solutes in the remaining liquid phase as ice crystals remains unclear. Regardless, PBS has been utilized extensively for successful cryopreservation, particularly vitrification, in various species and apparently provides excellent results when utilized with human blastocysts [76]. However,

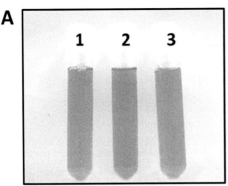

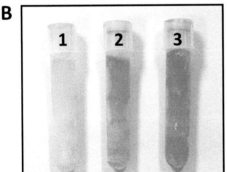

Figure 4.2 Apparent pH change of media contained the indicator phenol red buffered with (1) phosphate, (2) phosphate and HEPES, or (3) HEPES. (A). pH at room temperature. (B) pH following direct plunge into liquid nitrogen. Phosphate buffered media appear to become acidic, while HEPES-buffered media appears to become alkaline. Combining HEPES and PBS appears to stabilize pH and may be useful as a buffering system for cryopreservation procedures (adapted from Will *et al.* [81], with permission). See plate section for color version.

comparative studies examining the efficacy of PBS in cryosolutions to other buffers is scarce. One study examining slow rate freezing with dimethyl sulfoxide (DMSO) appeared to demonstrate that PBS was successfully able to cryopreserve human embryos better than HEPES, although embryo numbers were low and precluded statistical analysis [74]. In contrast, using vitrification with DMSO, PBS impaired embryo development and inner cell mass numbers in comparison to HEPES- or bicarbonate-buffered media [77]. Considering the impact of phosphate on gamete and embryo metabolism as well as apparent acidification with cooling, there may be more appropriate buffers for use with cryopreservation.

Several reports exist that examine the impact of zwitterionic buffers and their effects on sperm cryopreservation in various domestic animal species. These studies demonstrate that some buffers are superior in maintaining post-thaw sperm motility and membrane integrity [32, 37, 38, 46, 47]. Various rationales for these observed differences can be put forth, with change in pH as one plausible explanation. Unfortunately, comparative studies examining the influence of various buffers during oocyte and embryo cryopreservation is lacking. One preliminary abstract reported MOPS to be superior to HEPES for embryo vitrification, though the exact reason for this remains unclear and the comparison was not made during the same time period to rule out confounding variables [78]. This potential for differential effects of buffers during cryopreservation remains a valid area of continued research, as pH buffers may significantly impact the cryopreservation process in ways other than pH buffering. As an example, the structure of the TES molecule is similar to known cryoprotective agents, containing a central amide group, with three side hydroxyl groups and a double oxygen bond. Thus, it is conjectured that in addition to its pH buffering capability, TES perhaps also offers additional protection as a cryoprotectant [79]. If this is the case, the use of zwitterionic buffers in slow rate cooling or vitrification media needs to be evaluated in a comparative fashion, as not all buffers may perform similarly.

Cryopreservation presents unique considerations into the need for temperature-stable buffers. As noted previously, periodic fluctuations of pH_e can be traduced into deleterious intracellular perturbations [70], and these are most readily apparent in cells that lack robust pH_i regulatory mechanisms, such as denuded mature oocytes and cryopreserved/thawed embryos [80]. In these cases, maintenance of an appropriate and stable pH_e may be particularly crucial, especially considering the impact of temperature on pH_e of buffered media. Additionally, more concern may exist with slow rate protocols due to extended periods of media exposure in comparison to rapid vitrification. In these cases use of a single buffer may not provide optimal pH stability, rather, a combination of multiple buffers, such as phosphate and HEPES, may permit formation of a temperature-independent cryosolution with stable pH (Figure 4.2). Regardless of the buffer chosen, it is crucial to maintain an appropriate and constant temperature to avoid changes in pH. Due to this relationship, many studies detailing the effects of temperature on cellular structure and function, such as oocyte meiotic spindle organization, cannot rule out a role for pH in the regulation of these processes. These relationships between temperature and pH, influence of buffers, and impact on gametes has begun to receive attention [82] and continued research is prudent.

Conclusion and future directions

Buffers of pH are critical factors of an IVF culture system. Utilization of these compounds helps stabilize pH_e for procedures outside the laboratory incubator and minimize stress imposed upon gametes and embryos. Zwitterionic buffers, such as HEPES and MOPS, appear to be superior to buffers such as phosphate. Additionally, closer examination of additional buffers such as DIPSO or TES may be useful, as their pK_a values lend themselves to buffering in the range used for embryo culture.

Importantly, concern does exist with use of some buffers. This may be cell type and concentration dependent. Therefore, examination of methods to improve upon current approaches is warranted. To this end, further exploration of combination buffer systems with new buffers may lead to further improvements in the IVF culture system. Combination buffers have proven useful for sperm preparation in the past, and emerging data demonstrate their efficacy during embryo culture [31, 67, 81, 83]. These combinatorial systems can utilize different buffers to adjust and optimize pK_a, or provide optimal buffering, while allowing use of reduced buffer concentrations to alleviate toxicity concerns (Figure 4.3). In addition to the use of separate buffers, combination buffer systems can also use different forms of the same buffer, including different salt conjugated forms or free acid preparations. These allow for the refinement of the final working pH_e without the need for titrating with HCl or NaOH during preparation, which may improve consistency in media formulation [81]. Additionally, combination buffer systems may provide a means to improve cryopreservation media, allowing for compensation of pH changes due to temperature [75, 82]. Important to the endeavor of optimizing the buffering system for gametes and embryos is determining the optimal pH_e for culturing gametes and embryos. Once this value is established, a combination buffer system could be formulated with a pK_a value slightly above this pH_e for optimal buffering.

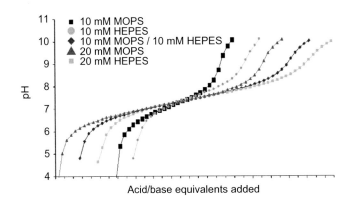

Figure 4.3 Combination of pH buffers allows for lowering of individual buffer concentrations, while simultaneously allowing for adjustment of pK_a, or optimal buffering, to the desired range. Multiple buffers and varying ratios can be utilized. This approach can help to formulate a buffering system for specific IVF procedures, yielding optimal pH buffering based on cell type or procedure/ temperature utilized (adapted from Swain and Pool [67], with permission). See plate section for color version.

Another area of research regarding improvement of buffers in IVF entails examination of the total concentration used. Generally 21 mM HEPES or MOPS are used in medium with ~4 mM sodium bicarbonate. However, the rationale for the concentration is not entirely clear. A plausible explanation would seem to be that most culture media in the past had a bicarbonate concentration of 25 mM. When bicarbonate levels are reduced to 4 mM, keeping the Na-conjugated buffer at 21 mM helps maintain media osmolality. Data suggest that lower concentrations of buffer may be adequate to maintain stability of pH_e, especially if pK_a values can be optimized via combining buffers [84]. This reduction in concentration may help alleviate possible toxicity concerns.

Additional benefit of pH buffers may arise from their use within media used in the incubator. Though bicarbonate concentration and external CO_2 levels will primarily regulate pH_e stability, addition of zwitterionic buffers can help further stabilize pH_e. This may be useful for culture approaches using extremely small volumes, including emerging microfluidic technology.

It is clear that there exists potential to improve upon current IVF handling media. Further experiments examining biochemical, molecular, and genetic endpoints will aid in this endeavor. Employing these approaches may lend itself to formulation of various specialized handling media used for specific procedures, constructed with specific buffer combinations and specific pH_e/pK_a for specific cell types.

Acknowledgements

The authors would like to thank Rusty Pool for his insight and assistance with preparation of this manuscript.

References

1. Ferguson WJ, Braunschweiger KI, Braunschweiger WR, *et al*. Hydrogen ion buffers for biological research. *Anal Biochem* 1980;**104**(2):300–10.

2. Good NE, Winget GD, Winter W, *et al*. Hydrogen ion buffers for biological research. *Biochemistry* 1966;**5**(2):467–77.

3. Good NE, Izawa S. Hydrogen ion buffers. *Methods Enzymol* 1972;**24**:53–68.

4. Eagle H. Buffer combinations for mammalian cell culture. *Science* 1971;**174**(8):500–3.

5. Wersinger C, Rebel G, Lelong-Rebel IH. Characterisation of taurine uptake in human KB MDR and non-MDR tumour

cell lines in culture. *Anticancer Res* 2001;**21**(5):3397–406.

6. Stellwagen NC, Bossi A, Gelfi C, *et al*. DNA and buffers: are there any noninteracting, neutral pH buffers? *Anal Biochem* 2000;**287**(1):167–75.

7. Schmidt J, Mangold C, Deitmer J. Membrane responses evoked by organic buffers in identified leech neurones. *J Exp Biol* 1996;**199**(Pt 2):327–35.

8. Farrell PS, Bavister BD. Short-term exposure of two-cell hamster embryos to collection media is detrimental to viability. *Biol Reprod* 1984;**31**(1):109–14.

9. Escriba MJ, Silvestre MA, Saeed AM, *et al*. Comparison of the effect of two different handling media on rabbit zygote developmental ability. *Reprod Nutr Dev* 2001;**41**(2):181–6.

10. Palasz AT, Brena PB, De la Fuente J, *et al*. The effect of different zwitterionic buffers and PBS used for out-of-incubator procedures during standard in vitro embryo production on development, morphology and gene expression of bovine embryos. *Theriogenology* 2008;**70**(9):1461–70.

11. Fitzharris G, Baltz JM. Granulosa cells regulate intracellular pH of the murine growing oocyte via gap junctions: development of independent homeostasis during oocyte growth. *Development* 2006;**133**(4):591–9.

12. FitzHarris G, Siyanov V, Baltz JM. Granulosa cells regulate oocyte intracellular pH against acidosis in preantral follicles by multiple mechanisms. *Development* 2007;**134**(23):4283–95.

13. Erdogan S, FitzHarris G, Tartia AP, *et al*. Mechanisms regulating intracellular pH are activated during growth of the mouse oocyte coincident with acquisition of meiotic competence. *Dev Biol* 2005;**286**(1):352–60.

14. Phillips KP, Petrunewich MA, Collins JL, *et al*. The intracellular pH-regulatory HCO_3^-/Cl^- exchanger in the mouse oocyte is inactivated during first meiotic metaphase and reactivated after egg activation via the MAP kinase pathway. *Mol Biol Cell* 2002;**13**(11):3800–10.

15. Bagger PV, Byskov AG, Christiansen MD. Maturation of mouse oocytes in vitro is influenced by alkalization during their isolation. *J Reprod Fertil* 1987;**80**(1):251–5.

16. Downs SM, Mastropolo AM. Culture conditions affect meiotic regulation in cumulus cell-enclosed mouse oocytes. *Mol Reprod Dev* 1997;**46**(4):551–66.

17. Barnett DK, Clayton MK., Kimura J, *et al*. Glucose and phosphate toxicity in hamster preimplantation embryos involves disruption of cellular organization, including distribution of active mitochondria. *Mol Reprod Dev* 1997;**48**(2):227–37.

18. Barnett DK, Bavister BD. Inhibitory effect of glucose and phosphate on the second cleavage division of hamster embryos: is it linked to metabolism? *Hum Reprod* 1996;**11**(1):177–83.

19. Lane M, Ludwig TE, Bavister BD. Phosphate induced developmental arrest of hamster two-cell embryos is associated with disrupted ionic homeostasis. *Mol Reprod Dev* 1999;**54**(4):410–17.

20. Bavister B, Analysis of culture media for in vitro fertilization and criteria for success. In: Mastroianni L, Biggers J, eds. *Fertilization and Embryonic Development In Vitro*. New York: Plenum Press, 1981.

21. Zigler JS Jr., Lepe-Zuniga JL, Vistica B, *et al*. Analysis of the cytotoxic effects of light-exposed HEPES-containing culture medium. *In Vitro Cell Dev Biol* 1985;**21**(5):282–7.

22. Bhattacharyya A, Yanagimachi R. Synthetic organic pH buffers can support fertilization of guinea pig eggs, but not as efficiently as bicarbonate buffer. *Gamete Res* 1988;**19**(2):123–9.

23. Lee MA, Storey BT. Bicarbonate is essential for fertilization of mouse eggs: mouse sperm require it to undergo the acrosome reaction. *Biol Reprod* 1986;**34**(2):349–56.

24. Byrd SR, Flores-Foxworth G, Applewhite AA, *et al*. In vitro maturation of ovine oocytes in a portable incubator. *Theriogenology* 1997;**47**(4):857–64.

25. Behr BR, Stratton CJ, Foote WD, *et al*. In vitro fertilization (IVF) of mouse ova in

HEPES-buffered culture media. *J In Vitro Fert Embryo Transf* 1990;**7**(1):9–15.

26. Hagen DR, Prather RS, Sims MM, *et al.* Development of one-cell porcine embryos to the blastocyst stage in simple media. *J Anim Sci* 1991;**69**(3):1147–50.

27. Geshi M, Yonai M, Sakaguchi M, *et al.* Improvement of in vitro co-culture systems for bovine embryos using a low concentration of carbon dioxide and medium supplemented with beta-mercaptoethanol. *Theriogenology* 1999;**51**(3):551–8.

28. Hagemann LJ. Pronuclear injection of mops-buffered medium does not affect bovine embryo development. *Theriogenology* 1995;**43**(1):229.

29. Edwards LJ, Williams DA, Gardner DK. Intracellular pH of the preimplantation mouse embryo: effects of extracellular pH and weak acids. *Mol Reprod Dev* 1998;**50**(4):434–42.

30. Syms AJ, Johnson AR., Lipshultz LI, *et al.* Effect of aging and cold temperature storage of hamster ova as assessed in the sperm penetration assay. *Fertil Steril* 1985;**43**(5):766–72.

31. Swain J, Ord V, Taylor D, *et al.* Use of two zwitterionic buffers in IVF handling media supports mouse blastocyst development and normal human oocyte fertilization following ICSI. In: *Proceedings from the 15th Annual World Congress on In Vitro Fetilization.* Geneva, Switzerland, 2009.

32. Crabo BG, Brown KI, Graham EF. Effect of some buffers on storage and freezing of boar spermatozoa. *J Anim Sci* 1972;**35**(2):377–82.

33. Koobs DH. Phosphate mediation of the Crabtree and Pasteur effects. *Science* 1972;**178**(57):127–33.

34. Veeck LL. TES and Tris (TEST)-yolk buffer systems, sperm function testing, and in vitro fertilization. *Fertil Steril* 1992;**58**(3):484–6.

35. Jeyendran RS, Gunawardana VK, Barisic D, *et al.* TEST-yolk media and sperm quality. *Hum Reprod Update* 1995;**1**(1):73–9.

36. Garcia MA, Graham EF. Development of a buffer system for dialysis of bovine

spermatozoa before freezing. III. Effect of different inorganic and organic salts on fresh and frozen-thawed semen. *Theriogenology* 1989;**31**(5):1039–48.

37. Graham EF, Crabo BG, Brown KI. Effect of some zwitter ion buffers on the freezing and storage of spermatozoa. I. Bull. *J Dairy Sci* 1972;**55**(3):372–8.

38. Brown KI, Graham EF, Crabo BG. Effect of some hydrogen ion buffers on storage and freezing of turkey spermatozoa. *Poult Sci* 1972;**51**(3):840–9.

39. Molinia FC, Evans G, Maxwell WM. In vitro evaluation of zwitterion buffers in diluents for freezing ram spermatozoa. *Reprod Nutr Dev* 1994;**34**(5):491–500.

40. Molinia FC, Evans G, Maxwell WM. Incorporation of penetrating cryoprotectants in diluents for pellet-freezing ram spermatozoa. *Theriogenology* 1994;**42**(5):849–58.

41. Weidel L, Prins GS. Cryosurvival of human spermatozoa frozen in eight different buffer systems. *J Androl* 1987;**8**(1):41–7.

42. Prins GS, Weidel L. A comparative study of buffer systems as cryoprotectants for human spermatozoa. *Fertil Steril* 1986;**46**(1):147–9.

43. Molinia FC, Evans G, Maxwell WM. Fertility of ram spermatozoa pellet-frozen in zwitterion-buffered diluents. *Reprod Nutr Dev* 1996;**36**(1):21–9.

44. Byrd W, Ackerman GE, Bradshaw KD, *et al.* Comparison of bicarbonate and HEPES-buffered media on pregnancy rates after intrauterine insemination with cryopreserved donor sperm. *Fertil Steril* 1991;**56**(3):540–6.

45. Swain JE, Pool TB. Supplementation of culture media with zwitterionic buffers supports sperm function and embryo development within the elevated CO_2 levels of the laboratory incubator *J Clin Embryol* 2008;**11**(2):14.

46. El-Alamy MA, Foote RH. Freezability of spermatozoa from Finn and Dorset rams in multiple semen extenders. *Anim Reprod Sci* 2001;**65**(3–4):245–54.

47. Garcia MA, Graham EF. Development of a buffer system for dialysis of bovine

spermatozoa before freezing. I. Effect of zwitterion buffers. *Theriogenology* 1989;**31**(5):1021–8.

48. Zavos PM, Goodpasture JC, Zaneveld LJ, *et al.* Motility and enzyme activity of human spermatozoa stored for 24 hours at +5 degrees C and −196 degrees C. *Fertil Steril* 1980;**34**(6):607–9.

49. Jaskey DG, Cohen MR. Twenty-four to ninety-six-hour storage of human spermatozoa in test-yolk buffer. *Fertil Steril* 1981;**35**(2):205–8.

50. Jeyendran RS, Van der Ven HH, Kennedy W, *et al.* Comparison of glycerol and a zwitter ion buffer system as cryoprotective media for human spermatozoa. Effect on motility, penetration of zona-free hamster oocytes, and acrosin/proacrosin. *J Androl* 1984;**5**(1):1–7.

51. McCoshen JA, Wodzicki A, Tyson JE. Effectiveness of human semen frozen in TEST-yolk-buffered medium on AID outcome. *Fertil Steril* 1984;**42**:162–3.

52. Bolanos JR, Overstreet JW, Katz DF. Human sperm penetration of zona-free hamster eggs after storage of the semen for 48 hours at 2 degrees C to 5 degrees C. *Fertil Steril* 1983;**39**(4):536–41.

53. Johnson AR, Syms AJ, Lipshultz LI, *et al.* Conditions influencing human sperm capacitation and penetration of zona-free hamster ova. *Fertil Steril* 1984;**41**(4):603–8.

54. Yang YS, Rojas FJ, Stone SC. Acrosome reaction of human spermatozoa in zona-free hamster egg penetration test. *Fertil Steril* 1988;**50**(6):954–9.

55. Bielfeld P, Jeyendran RS, Holmgren WJ, *et al.* Effect of egg yolk medium on the acrosome reaction of human spermatozoa. *J Androl* 1990;**11**(3):260–9.

56. Carrell DT, Bradshaw WS, Jones KP, *et al.* An evaluation of various treatments to increase sperm penetration capacity for potential use in an in vitro fertilization program. *Fertil Steril* 1992;**57**(1):134–8.

57. Chan SY, Tucker MJ. Comparative study on the use of human follicular fluid or egg yolk medium to enhance the performance of human sperm in the zona-free hamster

oocyte penetration assay. *Int J Androl* 1992;**15**(1):32–42.

58. Falk RM, Silverberg KM, Fetterolf PM, *et al.* Establishment of TEST-yolk buffer enhanced sperm penetration assay limits for fertile males. *Fertil Steril* 1990;**54**(1):121–6.

59. Lanzendorf SE, Holmgren WJ, Jeyendran RS. The effect of egg yolk medium on human sperm binding in the hemizona assay. *Fertil Steril* 1992;**58**(3):547–50.

60. Paulson RJ, Sauer MV, Francis MM, *et al.* A prospective controlled evaluation of TEST-yolk buffer in the preparation of sperm for human in vitro fertilization in suspected cases of male infertility. *Fertil Steril* 1992;**58**(3):551–5.

61. Katayama KP, Stehlik E, Roesler M, *et al.* Treatment of human spermatozoa with an egg yolk medium can enhance the outcome of in vitro fertilization. *Fertil Steril* 1989;**52**(6):1077–9.

62. Jacobs BR, Caulfield J, Boldt J. Analysis of TEST (TES and Tris) yolk buffer effects on human sperm. *Fertil Steril* 1995;**63**(5):1064–70.

63. Jones RC, Foote RH. Effect of osmolality and phosphate, 'tris', 'tes', 'mes', and 'hepes' hydrogen ion buffers on the motility of bull spermatozoa stored at 37 or 5 degreesC. *Aust J Biol Sci* 1972;**25**(5):1047–55.

64. Mahadevan MM, Fleetham J, Church RB, *et al.* Growth of mouse embryos in bicarbonate media buffered by carbon dioxide, hepes, or phosphate. *J In Vitro Fert Embryo Transf* 1986;**3**(5):304–8.

65. Ozawa M, Nagai T, Kaneko H, *et al.* Successful pig embryonic development in vitro outside a CO_2 gas-regulated incubator: effects of pH and osmolality. *Theriogenology* 2006;**65**(4):860–9.

66. Ali J, Whitten WK, Shelton JN. Effect of culture systems on mouse early embryo development. *Hum Reprod* 1993;**8**(7):1110–14.

67. Swain JE, Pool TB. New pH-buffering system for media utilized during gamete and embryo manipulations for assisted reproduction. *Reprod Biomed Online* 2009;**18**(6):799–810.

68. Walker SK, Lampe RJ, Seamark RF. Culture of sheep zygotes in synthetic oviduct fluid medium with different concentrations of sodium bicarbonate and HEPES. *Theriogenology* 1989;**32** (5):797–804.

69. Iwasaki T, Kimura E, Totsukawa K. Studies on a chemically defined medium for in vitro culture of in vitro matured and fertilized porcine oocytes. *Theriogenology* 1999;**51**(4):709–20.

70. Phillips KP, Leveille MC, Claman P, *et al.* Intracellular pH regulation in human preimplantation embryos. *Hum Reprod* 2000;**15**(4):896–904.

71. Graves CN, Biggers JD. Carbon dioxide fixation by mouse embryos prior to implantation. *Science* 1970;**167** (924):1506–8.

72. Quinn P, Wales RG. Fixation of carbon dioxide by pre-implantation mouse embryos in vitro and the activities of enzymes involved in the process. *Aust J Biol Sci* 1971;**24**(6):1277–90.

73. Quinn P, Wales RG. Fixation of carbon dioxide by preimplantation rabbit embryos in vitro. *J Reprod Fertil* 1974;**36** (1):29–39.

74. Quinn P, Kerin JF. Experience with the cryopreservation of human embryos using the mouse as a model to establish successful techniques. *J In Vitro Fert Embryo Transf* 1986;**3**(1):40–5.

75. Sieracki NA, Hwang HJ, Lee MK, *et al.* A temperature independent pH (TIP) buffer for biomedical biophysical applications at low temperatures. *Chem Commun (Camb)* 2008;(7):823–5.

76. Stachecki JJ, Garrisi J., Sabino S, *et al.* A new safe, simple and successful vitrification method for bovine and human blastocysts. *Reprod Biomed Online* 2008;**17**(3):360–7.

77. Vasuthevan S, Ng SC, Edirisinghe R, *et al.* The evaluation of various culture media in combination with dimethylsulfoxide for ultrarapid freezing of murine embryos. *Fertil Steril* 1992;**58**(6):1250–3.

78. El-Danasouri I, Selman H, Strehler E, *et al.* Comparison of MOPS and HEPES buffers during vitrification of human embryos. *Hum Reprod* 2004;**14**:i136.

79. Jeyendran RS, Graham E. An evaluation of cryoprotective compounds on bovine spermatozoa. *Cryobiology* 1980;**17**(5): 458–64.

80. Lane M, Lyons EA, Bavister BD. Cryopreservation reduces the ability of hamster 2-cell embryos to regulate intracellular pH. *Hum Reprod* 2000;**15** (2):389–94.

81. Will MA, Clark NA, Swain JE. Biological pH buffers in IVF: help or hindrance to success. *J Assist Reprod Genet* 2011;**28**:711–24.

82. Clark NA, Swain J, Ding J, Smith GD. Cryo solution buffering capacity during temperature reduction and experimental separation of temperature and pH influences on mouse oocyte. *Fertil Steril* 2011;**96**(3 Suppl):S74.

83. Swain JE. Optimizing the culture environment in the IVF laboratory: impact of pH and buffer capacity on gamete and embryo quality. *Reprod Biomed Online* 2010;**21**(1):6–16.

84. Will M, Swain JE. Reducing concentration and combining zwitterionic buffers in IVF handling media allows for optimization of pH buffering capacity and supports mouse blastocyst development. *Fertil Steril* 2012;**97**(35):P29.

Chapter

5

Essential features in media development for spermatozoa, oocytes, and embryos

David Mortimer and Sharon T. Mortimer

Introduction

Over the past 30 years many historical reviews of the development of culture media for mammalian (more specifically, eutherian) in vitro fertilization (IVF) and embryo culture have been published describing the general principles and practices employed as well as the experimental evidence upon which formulations have evolved [1–11]. In compliance with the publisher's limitation on the number of references, only key references have been cited in this chapter. Interested readers will need to refer to these earlier reviews for further background.

During the 1960s and 1970s almost all research on eutherian fertilization and embryo culture was on experimental and domesticated species, work that contributed greatly to the successful achievement of human IVF [4]. This opened a new era in clinical reproductive biomedicine, with workers striving to replace the use of culture media designed to support somatic cells (e.g., Earle's, Tyrode's, and Ham's F10 media) with formulations more suited to human gametes and embryos. Co-culture of embryos using various cell types such as bovine uterine fibroblasts, granulosa cells, and Vero (African green monkey kidney epithelium-derived) cells was popular in some laboratories from the late 1980s until the end of the 1990s, but the publication of draft documents by the US Food and Drug Administration in the late 1990s stating that embryos exposed to such conditions must be considered as xenografts, followed by the formal publication of the US Public Health Service *Guideline on Infectious Disease Issues in Xenotransplantation*, January 29, 2001, all but eliminated any clinical application of such technology [12, 13].

Almost every medium developed for human assisted reproductive technology (ART) purposes has been based on research using in vivo-generated mouse zygotes. This process involves the superovulation and then mating of female mice, with the zygotes being flushed from the oviducts post-mortem on day 1. Using mouse zygotes derived from IVF has not been employed – in spite of it being a physiologically better model – due to its increased technical complexity and reduced efficiency. Beyond in vivo-generated zygotes being generally hardier than IVF-derived zygotes, there are also issues with the need for proper formulation of the flushing medium to recover them from the oviduct. Gardner and Lane showed that even a brief 5-minute exposure to a flushing medium devoid of amino acids induced compromised developmental potential [14], a study whose full relevance is often not appreciated: that the findings from many earlier (and later?) studies where a properly formulated flushing medium was not used could have been significantly affected by artifact.

Culture Media, Solutions, and Systems in Human ART, ed. Patrick Quinn. Published by Cambridge University Press. © Cambridge University Press 2014.

This chapter will summarize the authors' work over a 15-year period (1982–97) that resulted in the only culture medium system for human ART use that was not based on experiments using mouse embryos [15], and discuss general principles that govern the formulation of media for the handling and culture of human gametes and embryos.

General approach

Rather than trying to formulate or optimize culture media by extensive empirical improvement, including the sophisticated simplex optimization approach [16], we chose to try and re-create the in vivo environment, that is, that of the Fallopian tube [17, 18]. Several embryo culture media have employed this approach, including Ménézo's "B2" medium based on bovine oviduct fluid [19], Tervit's "Synthetic Oviduct Fluid" medium or "SOF" [20], and Quinn's "Human Tubal Fluid" medium or "HTF" [21]. The background data for those media were derived from studies on the composition of female tract fluid, primarily oviductal fluid but also often uterine fluid and even follicular fluid, and that of blood plasma or serum. Differences in the composition of ampullary and isthmic fluid, as well as uterine fluid – along with the known changes in metabolic requirements of the various developmental stages between the unfertilized oocyte and the blastocyst – are the real basis for the concept of "sequential" media, pre-dating its application in commercial ART media [22–24] by many years. If the oocyte/zygote/cleavage stage embryo/blastocyst experiences different microenvironments in vivo, then a "best practice" approach to optimizing culture conditions in vitro should duplicate such changes to reduce metabolic and other sources of stress. Further discussion on the issue of sequential versus "one-step" media will be presented later.

Early formulation work

Formulation work on a culture medium for studies on human sperm physiology began in 1982, employing all the then-available data on human oviduct fluid composition, supplemented with information firstly from other primates, secondly from other eutherian species, and thirdly from human blood plasma (or serum where plasma-derived information was unavailable). This research culminated in 1986 with a more-or-less defined medium, that is, it included human serum albumin (HSA) and was not supplemented with blood serum (see Table 5.1). This "synthetic tubal fluid" medium or "STF" was used in the author's laboratory at the University of Calgary for extensive studies on human sperm capacitation and the acrosome reaction, including demonstrating a role for taurine as a promoter of capacitation [17]. Unfortunately, STF's perceived complexity compared to the then-standard human IVF media such as Tyrode's T6 medium, Earle's Balanced Salt Solution, "EBSS," and the new Quinn's HTF medium, all of which were used with serum supplementation, precluded its use in routine human IVF.

Following the first author's move to Sydney IVF, a research program was initiated to develop a culture medium for human ART (i.e., fertilization as well as embryo culture in vitro) that would produce embryos with better developmental potential, and hence lead to an increase in IVF clinical pregnancy rate – which stood at 11.0% in Australia in 1991 (range: 3.6–27.3% [26]) – concomitant with minimizing the risk of high-order multiple pregnancies. Because the project began in 1991, the media were given the sobriquet "M91." The early M91 system included Fertilization, Cleavage, and Blastocyst Media variants, based on the same salts "backbone" as STF, although NaCl was modified to maintain the desired

Table 5.1. Formulation of synthetic tubal fluid (STF) medium

Component	Concentration	Amount	Notes
NaCl	106.00 mM	6.194 g/l	
KCl	4.69 mM	0.350 g/l	
KH_2PO_4	0.37 mM	0.050 g/l	
Na_2HPO_4	1.48 mM	0.210 g/l	
$NaHCO_3$	10.00 mM	0.840 g/l	
$MgSO_4 \cdot 7H_2O$	0.20 mM	0.050 g/l	
$MgCl_2 \cdot 6H_2O$	1.00 mM	0.203 g/l	
Glucose	5.55 mM	1.000 g/l	
Glycine	1.33 mM	0.100 g/l	
HEPES (free acid)	10.00 mM	2.383 g/l	
NaOH (5N solution)	9.00 mM	1.80 ml/l	
$Ca(lactate)_2 \cdot 2H_2O$	3.00 mM	0.763 g/l	
Taurine	0.07 mM	0.0083 g/l	(1 ml of 83 mg/10 ml)
Glutamine	0.68 mM	0.100 g/l	
Na pyruvate	1.00 mM	0.110 g/l	
Estradiol	300 pg/ml	10 µl of 30 µg/ml	Dissolved in analytical absolute ethanol
Progesterone	1.5 ng/ml	10 µl of 150 µg/ml	
Albumin, human serum	30 mg/ml	(as needed)	Cohn fraction V
Essential amino acids		20 ml/l	50X MEM concentrate [25]
Non-essential amino acids		10 ml/l	100X MEM concentrate [25]
Vitamins		10 ml/l	100X MEM concentrate [25]
Phenol red	5 µg/ml	1 ml/l of 0.5% (w/v)	

Reproduced from Mortimer [17] with permission.

osmolarity as additional substances were added or their concentrations changed. All variants employed low phosphate (0.35 mEq/L) and calcium and lactate were added as 2.0 mM calcium lactate so as to avoid sodium lactate syrup (see "Lactate," below). Sodium pyruvate was present at 0.2 mM, and glucose at 3.0 mM in all variants except Cleavage Medium, which was glucose-free. Taurine and glycine were included as osmolytes, and gentamicin (0.01 g/mL) was used instead of penicillin and streptomycin. A "handling buffer" was formulated by adding 20 mM HEPES, reducing the bicarbonate to 10 mEq/L, and adjusting the NaCl content to maintain osmolarity.

Based on published research [1] glutamine, isoleucine, phenylalanine, and methionine were included in the original M91 formulations (2.0, 0.2, 0.1, and 0.05 mM, respectively) although the latter three, being essential amino acids, were later removed. All M91 media had osmolarities in the range 285–295 mOsm, and the pH was adjusted to 7.2–7.4 after gassing. Although the early studies used 5% carbon dioxide (CO_2)-in-air, later series employed 6% CO_2/5% oxygen (O_2), balance nitrogen to achieve better pH stability and reduced O_2 tension [27].

The entire project employed only human embryos: polyspermic or unipronucleate zygotes, supernumerary day 2 embryos, and cryopreserved embryos that were donated for research. No experiments on mouse embryos were performed. After initial work (1991–3) had confirmed that M91 was able to support human embryo development in vitro at least as well as the HTF medium in routine clinical use, evolving formulations of M91 were evaluated clinically against HTF using a periodic crossover basis, with the M91 media typically being used in 3-week blocks (the time required to use a batch of medium). Early findings included a significantly higher IVF fertilization rate in M91 of 63.9% compared to HTF at 49.8% ($P < 0.001$).

Evolutions in the media formulations during this time included:

- Subsequent to the findings of Gardner and Lane [14], non-essential amino acids (NEAA) were included in Fertilization and Cleavage Media at the start of clinical evaluation studies, and essential amino acids (EAA) were added to Blastocyst Medium. These amino acids were obtained as Eagle's Minimum Essential Medium (MEM) concentrates, NEAA at 100× and EAA at 50× as in STF medium; a similar approach was also taken in Gardner's original G1 and G2 media [22].
- Glutamine was reduced to 0.01 mM, a change that reduced the granularity of zygotes.
- Based on findings from an "early cleavage" quality assurance exercise, isoleucine, phenylalanine, and methionine were removed from the basal formulation (but remained in the EAA supplement), which resulted in a significant increase in pregnancy rate (β human chorionic gonadotropin [β-hCG] positive per embryo transfer) from 32.9% (27/82) to 52.1% (73/140), $\chi^2 = 6.957$, $P = 0.0083$. Embryo fragmentation also decreased significantly, with 52% of M91 embryos having <10% fragmentation compared to 33% of HTF embryos ($P < 0.001$).
- NEAA were added to Blastocyst Medium.

Also, with the introduction of the prototype K-MINC benchtop incubators (Cook Australia, Eight Mile Plains, Qld, Australia) in 1996, the later stages of the project also included a comparison of the efficacy of the more stable temperature and gas control, as well as low-O_2 tension, afforded by these incubators compared to traditional CO_2-in-air "big-box" Forma 3336 incubators. Figure 5.1 summarizes the overall improvements achieved comparing the traditional HTF/Forma system with the M91/MINC system. Embryo implantation rate, which is the best overall indicator of culture system performance, increased from 7.1% to 38.5% ($P < 0.0001$).

Finally, prior to Sydney IVF's commercialization of M91 with Cook Australia, phenol red was removed, and vitamins were added to all variants using a 100× Eagle's MEM concentrate. Clearly, the Cook "Sydney IVF" media were not based on Quinn's HTF as has been misunderstood by some workers [28]. The "second-generation" media released by Cook in April 2007 reflected further developmental work performed at Sydney IVF after the

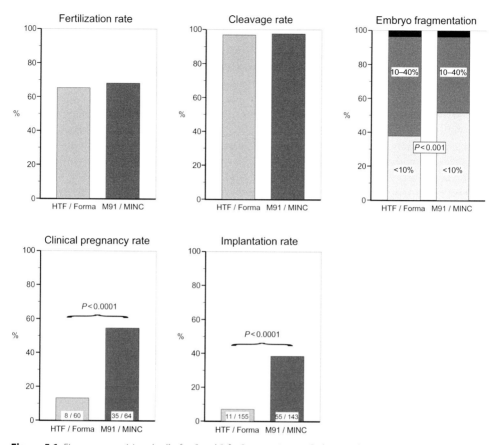

Figure 5.1 Figure summarizing the "before" and "after" comparison at Sydney IVF between the traditional culture system using HTF medium and Forma "big-box" incubators (60 treatment cycles performed during January–March 1996) and the M91v6 medium and Cook MINC benchtop incubator culture system (64 treatment cycles performed during August–October 1997). Data taken from Mortimer *et al.* [15].

authors' return to Canada, although in our hands this has not generated significant improvements in either embryo quality or pregnancy rates over the original media suite.

ART media: some chemical aspects

The following subsections consider various components and aspects of modern ART media, listed in alphabetical order for ease of reference.

Amino acids

When discussing "essential" and "non-essential" amino acids it must be remembered that these definitions were conferred in regard to the needs of somatic cells in culture [25]. For embryos, in vitro development of zygotes to the blastocyst stage is significantly improved by the presence of **NEAA** (plus glutamine) via promoting cleavage rate in precompaction embryos and then blastocoel development and blastocyst hatching from compaction onwards, while culture in the presence of *EAA* without glutamine significantly impairs blastocyst development during early cleavage, but stimulates inner cell mass development post-compaction [24, 29].

Changes in amino acid transport mechanisms during embryo development from the zygote to the blastocyst may account for stage-specific changes in the effects of amino acids on embryo development, making it inadvisable to simply add them all throughout the in vitro culture period [1], especially at the elevated concentrations found in Eagle's somatic cell media supplements. Indeed, the use of amino acids at reduced concentrations, or at concentrations reflecting those in oviduct fluid is becoming increasingly common in embryo culture media [30–32], and seems to avoid the observed toxicity of EAA during early cleavage.

Glutamine is able to counteract the inhibitory effects of the Crabtree effect on rodent embryos (glucose in the presence of inorganic phosphate) [1, 33], as well as serve as an organic osmolyte to counteract the negative effects that high sodium ion concentrations can have on embryos [34]. It can also serve as an alternative energy source in glucose-free media [35]. Because of concerns regarding glutamine's stability in solution (its breakdown generates ammonium ions), it is often added to modern media as a more stable dimeric form such as alanyl-glutamine (ALA-GLN) or glycyl-glutamine (GLY-GLN), as in Gibco's GlutaMAX™ cell culture media.

Glycine plays an important role as an osmolyte in protecting embryos from osmotic stress (see "Osmolytes," below), and is present in oviduct fluid at mM concentrations perhaps as high as 10 mM [31, 36, 37].

Taurine is another component that helps overcome early cleavage stage developmental blocks, and hypotaurine (a precursor of taurine) is essential for hamster embryos in vitro. Both inhibit Na^+/K^+-ATPases, whose activity during the early cleavage stages becomes deregulated in vitro, leading to intracellular electrolyte imbalances – and consequently their inhibition can help prevent this. But after compaction water uptake is essential for development of the blastocoel, and so inhibition of the ATPase would be detrimental – hence some authorities recommend only including taurine (at about 0.1 mM) in embryo media for the first 48 hours of culture [23]. However, taurine is often included in embryo media at 0.1–1.0 mM through to the blastocyst stage, while others have shown beneficial effects of substantially higher mM concentrations [38, 39]. These beneficial effects might be due to other effects of taurine, including its roles as an antioxidant and an osmolyte. Taurine also supports sperm physiology even at serum levels [17].

Although most human embryo culture media used until the mid 1990s did not systematically include amino acids, the findings that culturing mouse embryos in the absence of amino acids induced behavioral alterations in the resulting adult mice [40], as well as changes in gene expression patterns [41], make it clear that modern embryo media formulations should include them.

Ammonium ions

The instability of amino acids in solution (especially glutamine), especially during incubation at 37 °C, is considered a major source of ammonium ions that are detrimental to embryonic development due to intracellular acidification [42, 43]. Lower purity albumin can also contribute substantial amounts of ammonium ions to media during storage, and some authorities recommend that HSA should be dialyzed before use in manufacturing human ART media.

A general recommendation to avoid the possible accumulation of ammonium ions in culture medium at 37 °C is to change culture medium every 48 hours. As a matter of routine practice, this fits perfectly well with the way the vast majority of human IVF laboratories function, changing the medium at fertilization check on day 1, and again on day 3 when/if embryos go into "extended culture" for blastocyst development. This also fits with the typical use of sequential culture systems, employing fertilization, cleavage, and blastocyst media. Many of those laboratories that need to culture embryos on to day 6 to achieve good blastocyst development also change the embryos into fresh blastocyst medium on day 5.

Antioxidants and oxidative stress

There is a prolific literature on the deleterious effects of free radicals or reactive oxygen species (ROS) on gametes (especially spermatozoa) and embryos, although far less on specific techniques for counteracting them using antioxidants.

ROS often damage spermatozoa irreversibly, causing membrane damage that can affect their fertilizing ability to the extent that fertilization in vitro fails, and DNA fragmentation that can be so extreme that the limited repair mechanisms of the oocyte are inadequate to restore a functional genome [46–49]. While most andrology and IVF media have little antioxidant capacity to protect spermatozoa from ROS-induced damage during handling and processing under a high pO_2 (i.e., room air), the impact of ROS on sperm physiology and function in vitro can be largely avoided by using an appropriate sperm preparation method such as density gradient centrifugation [50, 51].

Oocytes and embryos in vivo are exposed to a low-O_2 environment within the female reproductive tract, generally estimated at 5–8% [44, 52], and their intrinsic ability to handle self-generated ROS is tailored to their mitochondrial oxidative phosphorylation activity running under such low pO_2 conditions. Exposure to atmospheric pO_2 levels (~158 mm Hg at sea level, that is, 20.8% O_2) causes the generation of supraphysiological ROS levels that damage cell membranes, cause DNA fragmentation, and induce apoptosis and abnormal gene expression which, together, lead to impaired embryonic development [53–56]. It can be concluded that a great part of the oxidative stress suffered by gametes and embryos in vitro is due to their exposure to excessive O_2, and is therefore iatrogenic. Oxidation of zona pellucida glycoproteins also results in zona hardening.

Beyond the obvious functional damage caused by oxidative damage to membranes and DNA, the metabolic effort of the transcription and translation processes involved in unnecessary gene expression (which is also seen in other types of cells when cultured in high pO_2) represents major physiological stress to the embryo. Despite convincing evidence from domesticated species, conclusive evidence of a specific detrimental effect of exposing human embryos to ambient pO_2 in culture was elusive for many years [1, 57, 58], but is now being reported in an increasing number of studies [59–62].

Common antioxidants include glutathione (GSH) and vitamins C and E (ascorbic acid and α-tocopherol), but the reduced forms of GSH and vitamin C are unstable in aqueous solution, and vitamin E is insoluble in water. Cysteamine, which increases intracellular GSH levels by increasing cysteine uptake, is effective as an antioxidant in culture media [56], and taurine also has antioxidant effects [39]. Lipoate, a high efficiency antioxidant, is used in Vitrolife's G5 media; its effectiveness has been attributed to unique antioxidant properties of the lipoate/dihydrolipoate system, its ROS scavenging ability, and a significant beneficial effect on the reduced forms of other antioxidants including GSH [63].

Buffering and pH

Bicarbonate is the standard means of buffering biological systems, and is an essential component for successful IVF [2]. Bicarbonate ions are balanced against the *partial pressure* of CO_2 (pCO_2) via the Henderson–Hasselbalch equation (see Figure 5.2) [27, 64], most often at a concentration of 25 mEq/L based on 25 mM sodium bicarbonate in the medium formulation. Some sequential media systems modify the bicarbonate concentration to achieve different pH values under the same pCO_2.

Equilibrating 25 mEq/L bicarbonate ions at 37 °C at sea level (i.e., at an atmospheric pressure of 101.325 kPa or 760 mm Hg) requires a partial pressure of 44 mm Hg of CO_2, yielding an expected pH of 7.4. At different pCO_2 values the medium will still equilibrate, but with either a different pH or a different balance between bicarbonate ions and protons buffered by other medium components. The final pH of any culture medium is not dependent solely upon the CO_2–bicarbonate system, but is a "bulk-effect" resulting from the interaction of all the components of the medium. A pCO_2 of 44 mm Hg equates to 5.8% v/v at 760 mm Hg atmospheric pressure, but since the ambient atmospheric pressure is more often "low" than "high," many labs use 6% CO_2 either as a setting for their CO_2-in-air or tri-gas incubators or in the formulation of a premixed gas supply. At higher altitudes, where the atmospheric pressure is lower, the %CO_2 must clearly be increased to maintain the necessary pCO_2. Knowing the altitude in meters above sea level, find the average atmospheric pressure (e.g., using the online calculator at http://www.altitude.org/air_pressure.php) and then calculate the required CO_2 proportion as:

$$\%CO_2 = (\text{required } pCO_2/\text{new atmospheric pressure}) \times 100$$

Issues regarding what is the correct pH for a culture medium, and how to measure medium pH are considered later in this chapter.

Phosphate is detrimental to embryo development in vitro [1] and induces abnormal gene expression patterns in bovine embryos [66]. Consequently all modern media have low phosphate levels, and any use of phosphate buffered saline (PBS) with embryos should be eschewed. Although PBS was used as the base medium in early work on the cryopreservation of mammalian embryos [60] such cryomedia included 20% (v/v) human serum, which also contributed to their buffering capacity. Because the dibasic (alkaline) phosphate salt has low solubility in cold water, without any other buffers present – such as in formulations using just HSA – a PBS-based cryomedium becomes highly acidic as it cools towards the freezing point. This acidic extracellular pH (i.e., a pH_e of ~4.0) was found to be highly detrimental to embryo competence post-thaw [67], presumably via deleterious effects upon intracellular pH (pH_i) during the immediate post-thaw period when the ability to regulate pH_i is slow to be reactivated. Consequently, embryo cryomedia should always be buffered using a zwitterion such as HEPES or MOPS.

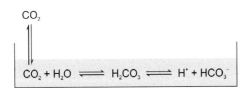

Figure 5.2 Illustration of the equilibration of atmospheric CO_2 against culture medium bicarbonate ions as per the Henderson–Hasselbalch equation. See text and also Mortimer and Quinn [27] and Umbreit [64] for more details.

Zwitterion buffers are neutral molecules having a positive and a negative electrical charge at different locations within the molecule. Common examples in biological media are HEPES (pK_a at 25 °C $= 7.5$; useful range $= 6.8$–8.2) and MOPS (pK_a at 25 °C $= 7.2$; useful range $= 6.5$–7.9). Concerns that HEPES might be embryotoxic come from very old work, certainly using a highly impure product, and there would appear to be no real concern over exposing human embryos to HEPES during handling or cryopreservation [68, 69]. Moreover, so long as the medium was not devoid of bicarbonate, mouse embryos grown in HEPES-buffered T6 medium under air produced the same numbers of live offspring as those grown in bicarbonate-buffered T6 medium under CO_2 [70]. Therefore, using a "handling medium" buffered by HEPES (usually 20 mM) should not be seen as hazardous and, indeed, exposing embryos in a bicarbonate-buffered medium to air for more than 2 minutes will surely be more deleterious due to shifts in pH_e that can adversely affect pH_i [71]. When using HEPES to buffer a culture medium under air, the bicarbonate content must be reduced so as not to stress the buffering system due to shifts in medium formulation caused by loss of bicarbonate from the imbalanced bicarbonate–CO_2 system – but the medium cannot be devoid of bicarbonate as it is an essential cofactor for intracellular processes, for example adenylate cyclase. Consequently, a HEPES-buffered medium, either for embryo handling or for sperm washing, should have its bicarbonate content reduced to around 10 mEq/L, and the final osmolarity of the medium maintained by adjusting the sodium chloride content. In addition, although historically the pH of a HEPES-containing medium was adjusted using sodium hydroxide, modern media are adjusted using the sodium salt of HEPES; the relationship of HEPES and HEPES-Na needs to be titrated for each chemical lot, but will remain constant within a lot for a given medium formulation.

EDTA

Ethylenediaminetetraacetic acid is beneficial to overcoming the 2-cell block in mouse embryos, but if present during the second 48 hours of culture it can inhibit blastocyst development [72]. Its beneficial effect, which requires only 0.01 mM, is mediated by preventing abnormal increases in glycolysis during the early cleavage stages (during which metabolism is primarily based on pyruvate via oxidative phosphorylation) via chelation of divalent cations, such as magnesium, that are essential cofactors of 3-phosphoglycerate kinase [73].

Macromolecules

Most of the original culture media for embryos relied on the addition of heat-inactivated serum to supply many of the organic molecules necessary for embryo function, and some early human IVF media employed fetal calf serum, although this was quite soon replaced by human fetal cord serum and, ultimately, patient serum [1]. As media became more defined, energy substrates, amino acids, vitamins, and even growth factors were included in their complex formulations, allowing their supplementation by serum albumin preparations rather than serum. While bovine serum albumin (BSA) was used quite widely in human IVF and embryo culture media, largely due to the cost of HSA products (typically Cohn fraction V preparations), grave safety concerns over "mad cow" disease and variant Creutzfeldt–Jakob disease led to all commercial media for human ART use employing pharmaceutical grade HSA instead of BSA.

Using HSA eliminated many of the low-molecular-weight components that were responsible for the embryotoxicity of many serum preparations. Major roles of serum albumin in vivo include scavenging ions such as calcium and serving as a low affinity, but high capacity, reservoir for small molecules such as steroids, cholesterol, fatty acids, and vitamins. Indeed, serum albumin is the primary acceptor for the cholesterol that is removed from sperm plasma membrane as a major component of the capacitation process [1, 74, 75]. Since HSA is therefore an essential component of any culture medium intended for human sperm capacitation and fertilization in vitro, its concentration should reflect that seen in oviduct fluid in vivo to support optimally sperm function: 30 mg/mL [17, 76] – but typically only 10 mg/mL is used and there is a trend towards reducing this further, to 5 mg/mL. However, these presumably financially driven reductions in HSA content of commercial ART media are of great concern, in some cases having led to unacceptably high rates of low and failed IVF fertilization. A suboptimal HSA content of IVF media can exacerbate impaired sperm function in many subfertile couples, contributing to a perceived, but erroneous, need for intracytoplasmic sperm injection (ICSI) to achieve higher fertilization rates [77].

Organic macromolecules appear to be essential for embryo culture in vitro, serving roles as a surfactant and a microscale metabolite [1, 78, 79], and while polyvinyl alcohol (PVA) can fulfill the surfactant role [1] under certain experimental conditions, it does not support embryo development as well as serum albumin [79], and is not used in human ART media.

Metabolism and metabolic substrates

Over the past decade Leese has elaborated the intriguing and insightful "quiet embryo hypothesis" [80–82], which proposes that viable preimplantation embryos operate at generally lower metabolic rates than their less viable siblings. Loss of this "quieter" metabolism (for example in response to environmental stress caused by suboptimal temperature, toxins such as ammonium ions, a dysfunctional "active" metabolism, or ROS generation) induces cellular changes that lead to cell death through apoptotic mechanisms. Metabolic up-regulation is often associated with accelerated or precocious development, and can be induced by culture at supraphysiological O_2 concentrations.

Glucose metabolism by precompaction eutherian embryos is a major element in causing developmental blocks, and the need for glucose during early cleavage has been the subject of extensive discussion [1, 3, 6–10]. Even in species without a specific developmental block (e.g., human) the presence of glucose during cleavage inhibits blastocyst development [83–85]. Then, as the embryo's metabolism diversifies following activation of the embryonic genome, glucose becomes an essential substrate for continued development to the blastocyst. While the primary metabolic substrate for human spermatozoa in semen is fructose, once within the female reproductive tract only glucose is available. Traditional IVF media have glucose concentrations similar to serum (2.7–5.6 mM) and whereas glucose is essential for efficient sperm capacitation and hyperactivation, and hence optimal fertilization in vitro, it causes a diversion of the early embryo's metabolism towards glycolysis at a time when the embryo should be relying upon pyruvate metabolism to sustain its energy requirements. For this reason early sequential media system cleavage media were glucose-free, although the presence of glucose in more modern sequential media systems at a concentration similar to midcycle oviduct fluid (c. 0.5 mM) does not appear to inhibit early human embryo development [86].

Lactate was often added to culture media as sodium lactate syrup, which is a racemic mixture of D- and L-isomers. The D-isomer cannot be metabolized and hence is not just a useless component of culture media in that it "wastes space" in the formulation, but it will also exert an adverse effect on cellular homeostasis via reducing pH_i [87]. For example, HTF contains 21.4 mM sodium lactate syrup, giving a concentration of "useful" lactate at ~10.7 mM. While this is essentially the same as the midcycle L(+)lactate concentration of 10.5 mM in human oviduct fluid [7, 86], it is higher than that seen in many current IVF and embryo culture media (4–6 mM). Since human spermatozoa generate energy primarily via fructolysis (glycolysis once removed from seminal plasma), with lactic acid accumulating as a metabolic by-product, adding lactate to sperm media might seem unnecessary. However, admitting air into an anaerobically glycolysing sperm population decreases the rate of sugar utilization (the "Pasteur effect"), and lactic acid undergoes oxidation as a substrate for exogenous respiration. Because human spermatozoa are exposed to an ambient air atmosphere during handling, processing, and analysis, some lactate is usually included in sperm media.

Pyruvate is an essential metabolic substrate during early embryonic development in many eutherian species, including human [84], and likely plays additional roles in regulating pH_i, scavenging free radicals, and disposing of ammonium ions [7]. The pyruvate concentration in midcycle human oviduct fluid has been reported as 0.32 mM [86], which is the same as the 0.33 mM seen in many fertilization and cleavage media. Because the uterine fluid content of pyruvate is around 0.1 mM, more modern blastocyst media mimic this change [7, 86]. However, pyruvate's poor stability in solution is one of the main reasons for the limited shelf life of ready-to-use ART media. Pyruvate in seminal plasma likely derives from it being the immediate precursor to lactic acid during fructolysis, and since human spermatozoa do not need to metabolize pyruvate (B. T. Storey, personal communication, 2006) it could probably be omitted from sperm media intended solely for andrology applications.

Osmolytes

Osmolytes are soluble compounds that affect cellular osmoregulation and hence have essential roles in maintaining cell volume and fluid balance. They are present both inside cells and in their environment. When a cell swells due to external hypotonicity, osmolytes move across the plasma membrane facilitating the efflux of water, thereby restoring normal cell volume. Various amino acids and their derivatives function as organic osmolytes in eutherian oocytes and early embryos, notably substrates of the Gly and β transport systems such as glycine, glutamine, betaine, proline, β-alanine, taurine, and hypotaurine, with their osmoprotectant abilities showing degrees of species- and stage-specificity and in the regulation of hypo- and hypertonic stresses [37, 88–92].

ART media: some physicochemical characteristics
Density

The *density* of a material is defined as its *mass per unit volume*, although it is sometimes expressed as specific gravity (sp.gr.), a dimensionless quantity where density is expressed as multiples of the density of some other standard material, usually water: hence a specific gravity <1.0 means that the substance will float in water.

The vast majority of ART labs nowadays use a 2-step (2-layer) discontinuous density gradient for separating mature, motile human spermatozoa from semen [50, 51]. The upper layer, which typically has half the colloid concentration of the lower layer, serves to hold back the seminal plasma and many of the non-reproductive cells at its upper interface, and the immature spermatozoa accumulate at its lower interface. Since mature human spermatozoa have a density of $>1.12\,g/mL$ the lower layer must have a density close to this (usually 1.1 g/mL). If the density of the lower layer is lower then less mature spermatozoa will reach the pellet. Such spermatozoa typically have retained cytoplasm that contains the biochemical machinery to generate ROS, and hence these spermatozoa are not only less functional themselves, but can also adversely affect the mature spermatozoa alongside them in the pellet [46].

The first widely successful density gradient material for human spermatozoa was *Percoll*, based on polyvinylpyrrolidone (PVP)-coated colloidal silica [50]. Because the Percoll colloid was suspended in only a very weak buffer (~17 mOsm) it was diluted 9+1 with a 10× strength buffer to create an "isotonic stock" preparation that had, ergo, 90% of the colloid concentration. Optimum performance with Percoll was discovered empirically to be achieved using a lower layer that was a further 9+1 dilution of this isotonic stock solution, that is, 81% of the original colloid concentration, having a density of ~1.1 g/mL.

When Percoll was withdrawn from clinical use by its manufacturer, Pharmacia Biotech, two alternative density gradient products based on silane-coated colloidal silica appeared on the market that were essentially isotonic and hence did not require the use of a 10× buffer. *PureSperm* (Nidacon International AB, Göteborg, Sweden) was formulated to contain the same amount of colloid as the original pure (100%) Percoll product. Consequently, its proper use involves a lower layer of 80% (v/v) colloid, typically with a 40% (v/v) upper layer. But the other original Percoll replacement, *ISolate* (Irvine Scientific, Santa Ana, CA, USA), was formulated to be equivalent to the 90% "isotonic stock" Percoll and was therefore used at 90% (v/v) to achieve separation of mature spermatozoa. Unfortunately this distinction was not apparent to many users and gradients of 40% and 80% ISolate have been reported. Because an 80% ISolate lower layer is only equivalent to 72% Percoll colloid higher yields can be obtained – but only by allowing less mature spermatozoa through into the pellet. Workers need to be aware of the continuing confusion regarding density gradient media formulations and their potentially adverse effects on practice [93].

Osmolarity

Osmolarity is the measure of solute concentration in terms of the number of osmoles (Osm) of solute per liter (L) of *solution* (Osm/L); *osmolality*, however, is the measure of the osmoles of solute per kilogram of *solvent* (Osm/kg). When a biologist makes a culture medium in the lab the solutes (salts, glucose, etc.) are dissolved in water in a volumetric flask, giving a final volume of 1000 mL of solution, hence the values would be *osmolarity*; but manufacturing processes usually operate by weight, adding the solutes to a measured volume of water (e.g., $100\,L \equiv 100\,kg$), hence values should be expressed in terms of *osmolality*. For culture media, the practical difference between the two measures is trivial, and values are often (as herein) expressed in terms of mOsm, with the reference range for human blood being 285 to 295 mOsm.

Pioneering work by Brinster and Whitten in the 1960s and 1970s demonstrated that osmolarity was not an important epigenetic regulator, with little difference in embryo development over the range 250 to 300 mOsm [1]. Higher osmolarities impair development, raising doubt over suggestions that oviduct fluid might be 360 mOsm or even higher [88, 89], although the samples upon which such estimates of osmolarity have been based could well have been contaminated during aspiration of the oviduct fluid by cytoplasm from ruptured cells, which could have artificially elevated the potassium ion levels.

Today there are two schools of thought regarding the osmolarity of embryo culture media, one continuing to employ 265–280 mOsm, the other making them isotonic (285–295 mOsm). Most sequential media series maintain consistent osmolarity across the product range, although based on published formulations the original G2 medium was ~16 mOsm lower than G1 [22].

Sperm washing media are typically isotonic with blood serum, hence andrology media are usually 280–295 mOsm. However, the osmolarity of human seminal plasma is higher, and increases with time after ejaculation due to liquefaction, so that after 30–60 minutes at 37 °C the reported range is 340–380 mOsm. Therefore, while sperm washing media should be in the range 280–300 mOsm, density gradient layers should ideally be formulated to ease the 60–100 mOsm osmotic shock that can be caused by transferring spermatozoa directly from seminal plasma to density gradient or culture medium.

pH

The intracellular pH (pH_i) is a critically important regulator of metabolism and other cell functions [1, 94]. However, the relationship between oocyte and embryo pH_i and the pH of the culture environment (pH_e) is complex, and a full understanding of the homeostatic regulation of pH_i and its perturbations during culture in vitro remains elusive. The recommended pH values for commercial fertilization, cleavage, and blastocyst media vary [68, 69], although there is a growing consensus that fertilization is optimized within the range 7.3–7.5, early cleavage proceeds better at 7.2, and blastocyst development is improved at 7.3. But how the pH_e in different commercial media systems affects pH_i regulation could well differ according to their formulations, with at least one manufacturer continuing to employ 7.3–7.5 for all three stage-specific media variants.

While oocytes seem to have limited ability to regulate pH_i and pH_i follows pH_e quite closely, embryos maintain a pH_i of 7.1–7.2 even when pH_e is ~7.4 or even higher [95]. Early human preimplantation embryos regulate pH_i through opposing mechanisms: a HCO_3^-/Cl^- exchanger that relieves alkalosis, and a Na^+/K^+ antiporter that relieves acidosis. Between them, these mechanisms maintain pH_i in a narrow range from ~6.8–6.9 to 7.1 [96]. Human preimplantation embryos, at all stages from zygote to blastocyst, have the ability to recover from intracellular alkalosis (which was not increased by elevated pH_e), but cannot recover from mild acidosis induced by decreased pH_e until the blastocyst stage [97]. Acidification of pH_i affects metabolism and disrupts cellular organization, and hence affects development, being expressed through fragmentation, irregular cleavage, and impaired blastocyst development [68, 69, 98, 99]. Further downstream effects on gene expression and imprinting should not be surprising.

As noted already (see "Bicarbonate," above), the pH of a culture medium is not due simply to the equilibration of the sodium bicarbonate in the medium formulation against the CO_2 content of the incubator atmosphere; it is the result of complex interactions between numerous compounds in the medium as a whole that affects its final pH and buffering capacity. But since these interactions are constrained by the basic laws of chemistry and physics, if a medium that has a constant, defined formulation is equilibrated against the known, required pCO_2 at 37 °C then the result will always be the same. Variations in measurements of medium pH will therefore be due to one of only a few possible errors:

1. Incorrect pCO_2: either due to failing to adjust properly the $\%CO_2$ for altitude, continuous variations in atmospheric pressure (and hence variable pCO_2 at a constant $\%CO_2$) due to the weather, or unfounded or even erroneous assumptions that measurements of $\%CO_2$ are accurate and reliable, for example the long-known inaccuracy of Fyrite measurements [94].

2. Inadequate medium equilibration as a result of inadequate advance dish preparation or prior access to the incubator. Even a modern "big-box" incubator with an infrared controller takes several minutes to re-equilibrate its $\%CO_2$ after opening, and until the CO_2 level has been reestablished *all* media inside the incubator will be subjected to disequilibrium and hence fluctuations in the bicarbonate–CO_2 buffering system. Full re-equilibration requires a certain period of time *after* the CO_2 level has been reestablished [100].

3. Drift in medium formulation, which typically – and surprisingly often – arises due to leaving culture medium under a large air dead space, such as in a part bottle. Considerations here are whether the manufacturer purged the bottle with the correct pCO_2 after filling, and whether embryologists are aware of the risk of loss of bicarbonate within part, sometimes even mostly, empty bottles of medium. As an extension of this, should the air be purged from opened media bottles after each accession and replaced by mixed gas?

4. Error(s) in medium manufacture – which hopefully will not arise with effective manufacturers' QC and QA systems.

5. Errors of measurement, which are potentially substantial and highly prevalent:

   • Measurements must be made without allowing the temperature or pCO_2 to change and hence affect the medium's pH (which can occur within 30 seconds). Also since altitude above sea level will change the actual pCO_2 for any given $\%CO_2$, and because the atmospheric pressure changes continuously with the weather, converting $\%CO_2$ into pCO_2 requires that the atmospheric pressure be known at the time of making the measurement.

   • The type of pH probe can affect the results by as much as 0.2 pH units.

   • Not using a probe correctly, especially ensuring the proper level of immersion, not just in the often micro-volume specimen but also in the calibration buffers.

   • Difficulties in properly calibrating a pH probe for use at 37 °C, including the lack of any calibration buffers certified for 37 °C. Includes the issue of regular validation of the probe's "efficiency" over a 2- or 3-point calibration span.

   • Unreliability of automatic temperature correction over the 12–18 °C differential between "ambient temperature" and 37 °C. A pH probe calibrated at "ambient" temperature (20–22 °C) and used at 37 °C could read up to 0.1 pH units low.

   • Improper maintenance of pH probes, a common cause of probe deterioration, including improper storage (e.g., in water, saline, or air rather than storage solution), not re-filling with KCl solution as/when required, not cleaning off the adsorbed protein which accumulates with exposure to culture medium, and partial drying out.

Given all these difficulties, it is probable that many – perhaps even a great majority – of the pH measurements made on bicarbonate-buffered culture media at 37 °C are heavily affected by artifact. Yet some embryologists measure medium pH and then attempt to titrate the % CO_2 to adjust medium pH into a desired narrow range. Regardless of the accuracy and calibration of the analytical device being used to measure pH, such attempts are largely futile as they ignore the impact of the weather, which can induce changes as large or larger than their careful adjustments, even from one hour to the next. Incubators only measure % CO_2, and not atmospheric pressure, so medium pH will fluctuate continuously due to variations in pCO_2 – even if the %CO_2 is maintained perfectly, which it rarely is in a busy IVF lab using big-box incubators [94]. Striving to adjust an incubator's %CO_2 setting to maintain culture medium pH can only be an exercise in frustration – and it will have no significant impact upon embryo developmental potential [95]. It has also been suggested that if a medium's pH changes rapidly in response to a small alteration in %CO_2 then perhaps one should be more concerned that the medium's intrinsic buffering is inherently unstable, since the other sources of pH buffering within a modern formulation should dampen, or even eliminate, such small fluctuations.

Finally, it should be noted that the required pCO_2 does depend on the medium being used. While Quinn's Advantage media have been formulated to equilibrate against 5% CO_2 at sea level, most other commercial media require 5.8–6% CO_2, for example the Cook Sydney IVF sequential culture medium system contains 25 mM bicarbonate and was formulated to equilibrate against 6% CO_2 ($pCO_2 = 45.6$ mm Hg) for a pH of 7.3 [15, 27].

Our approach has been to control the system, through knowing the bicarbonate content of the medium and maintaining the manufacturer's stated pCO_2 requirement for their medium's proper equilibration at 37 °C. Using Cook MINC or, more recently, Planer/Origio BT37 ("PLINC") benchtop incubators, we specify the required composition of the premixed gas (with appropriate adjustments for altitude) and verify that the gas mixture is within the acceptable tolerance range based on its certificate of assay. With the sole exception of a situation where a gas manufacturer fails to provide the defined composition, medium pH has not been measured in laboratories for which the authors have been responsible since 1996, when the original MINC system validation was completed. Using the Cook sequential media system these laboratories have achieved, and continue to achieve, world-class results in terms of embryo quality and clinical outcomes, which can be generally summarized as >50% of day 3 embryos with <10% (and often 0%) fragments and excellent blastocyst development rates – usually on day 5 (although this is subject to variations in clinical protocols, notably stimulations and hCG trigger timing) – allowing at least two-thirds of all patients where the female partner is <40 years to have day-5 transfers (increasingly of just single blastocysts) resulting in ongoing pregnancy rates of over 50%. Our opinion is that with thorough systems and quality control, measuring medium pH – and especially attempting to adjust it via altering the pCO_2 – is of no practical value.

Sequential versus "one-step" media

The question of whether sequential culture media systems perform better than a "one-step" medium remains highly contentious in the human ART field and eloquent arguments based on critical analyses of studies of embryo development during in vitro culture have been made to question the need for sequential media [9, 11]. But is the apparently morphologically normal development of embryos sufficient in this century of the "-omics"? Genomic, proteomic, and metabolomic analyses of embryos are increasingly common research tools [101], and substantial research effort is being invested in non-invasive methods for identifying the most competent embryos. Given the already available evidence that in vitro culture conditions can affect gene imprinting and expression as well as behavior in resultant adults [40, 41, 53] it is not surprising that clinical concern is being expressed regarding the epigenetic effects of ART [102]. Extrapolating from the risk management principles employed in public health, it is clear that endpoints such as "good blastocyst development" – or even "birth of live young" – will not remain adequate for much longer when making critical decisions regarding embryo culture systems that can affect future generations.

Adopting a best practice approach to human ART requires critical rethinking of not just embryo culture media but the entire culture system, and at least for now it would seem wisest to strive to emulate nature as far as possible, mimicking the changing microenvironments that exist in the female reproductive tract and supporting, not stressing through requiring adaptation, embryo metabolism.

Conclusions

It is increasingly clear that the real endpoint for the production of embryos with maximum developmental competence does not stop with implantation, or even the birth of a healthy baby. Success over the entire IVF process depends entirely upon respecting the physiology of the gametes and embryos, and the laboratory systems must be optimized using all available technology to ensure that the chemistry and physics of the culture system, as well as the operational and technical procedures, support the physiology [100]. While embryos might be highly adaptable, any adaptation will have a metabolic cost, and that cost will equate to stress to the embryo. Any failure, no matter how small, to support optimally the physiology of the gametes and embryos during their sojourn in vitro will constitute potential stress that – especially in combination with other failures which could act not just additively but synergistically – will risk diminished outcomes.

It is not sufficient for an embryologist to use any particular products because someone has told them they are the best, or because "that's what we have used for years," or they are what someone used somewhere else and they "got good results." Embryologists should understand the science of their profession so they can make their own informed decisions. It is hoped that this chapter will have helped increase understanding of where the current generation of human ART media came from, how/why they were formulated as they are, where some limitations might exist, and where opportunities for improvement might be found.

References

1. Bavister BD. Culture of preimplantation embryos: facts and artifacts. *Hum Reprod Update* 1995;1:91–148.

2. Harrison RAP. Capacitation mechanisms, and the role of capacitation as seen in Eutherian mammals. *Reprod Fertil Dev* 1996;8:581–94.

3. Scott LA. Oocyte and embryo culture. In: Keel BA, May JV, De Jonge CJ, eds. *Handbook of the Assisted Reproduction Laboratory*. Boca Raton, CRC Press. 2000;197–219.

4. Bavister BD. How animal embryo research led to the first documented human IVF. *Reprod BioMed Online* 2002; 4(Suppl 1):24–9.

5. Biggers JD. Thoughts on embryo culture condition. *Reprod BioMed Online* 2001;4:30–8.

6. Leese HJ. What does an embryo need? *Hum Fertil* 2003;6:180–5.

7. Quinn P. Media used in assisted reproductive technologies laboratories. In: Patrizio P, Guelman V, Tucker M., eds. *A Color Atlas for Human Assisted Reproduction: Laboratory and Clinical Insights*. Philadelphia, Williams & Wilkins. 2003;241–56.

8. Pool TB. An update on embryo culture for human assisted reproductive technology: media, performance, and safety. *Semin Reprod Med* 2005;**23**:309–18.

9. Biggers JD, Summers MC. Choosing a culture medium: making informed choices. *Fertil Steril* 2008;**90**:473–83.

10. Gardner DK. Dissection of culture media for embryos: the most important and less important components and characteristics. *Reprod Fertil Dev* 2008;**20**:9–18.

11. Vajta G, Rienzi L, Cobo A, Yovich J. Embryo culture: can we perform better than nature? *Reprod Biomed Online* 2010;**20**:453–69.

12. FDA. *PHS Guideline on Infectious Disease Issues in Xenotransplantation*, January 29, 2001. www.fda.gov/ BiologicsBloodVaccines/SafetyAvailability/ ucm136703.htm (accessed September 14, 2011).

13. FDA. *Information and Recommendations for Physicians Involved in the Co-Culture of Human Embryos with Non-Human Animal Cells*. www.fda.gov/ BiologicsBloodVaccines/ Xenotransplantation/ucm136532.htm (accessed September 14, 2011).

14. Gardner DK, Lane M. Alleviation of the '2-cell block' and development to the blastocyst of CF1 mouse embryos: role of amino acids, EDTA and physical parameters. *Hum Reprod* 1996;**11**:2703–12.

15. Mortimer D, Henman MJ, Jansen RPS. *Development of an Improved Embryo Culture System for Clinical Human IVF*. Eight Mile Plains, Australia, William A. Cook, 2002.

16. Lawitts JA, Biggers JD. Optimization of mouse embryo culture media using simplex methods. *J Reprod Fertil* 1991;**91**:543–56.

17. Mortimer D. Elaboration of a new culture medium for physiological studies on human sperm motility and capacitation. *Hum Reprod* 1986;**1**:247–50.

18. Leese HJ. The formation and function of oviduct fluid. *J Reprod Fertil* 1988;**82**:843–56.

19. Menezo Y. Milieu synthétique pour la survie et la maturation des gamètes et pour la culture de l'oeuf fécondé. *CR Acad Sci Paris Série D* 1976;**282**:1967–70.

20. Tervit HR, Whittingham DG, Rowson LE. Successful culture in vitro of sheep and cattle ova. *J Reprod Fertil* 1972;**30**:493–7.

21. Quinn P, Kerin JF, Warnes GM. Improved pregnancy rate in human in vitro fertilization with the use of a medium based on the composition of human tubal fluid. *Fertil Steril* 1985;**44**:493–8.

22. Barnes FL, Crombie A, Gardner DK, *et al.* Blastocyst development and birth after in-vitro maturation of human primary oocytes, intracytoplasmic sperm injection and assisted hatching. *Hum Reprod* 1995;**10**:3243–7.

23. Gardner DK, Lane M. Culture and selection of viable blastocysts: a feasible proposition for human IVF? *Hum Reprod Update* 1997;**3**:367–82.

24. Gardner DK, Lane M, Schoolcraft WB. Physiology and culture of the human blastocyst. *J Reprod Immunol* 2002;**55**:85–100.

25. Eagle H. Amino acid metabolism in mammalian cell cultures. *Science* 1959;**130**:432–7.

26. Australian Institute of Health and Welfare National Perinatal Statistics Unit. *Assisted Conception Australia and New Zealand 1991*. Sydney, 1993. ISSN 1038-7234.

27. Mortimer D, Quinn P. Bicarbonate-buffered media and CO_2. *Alpha Newsletter* 1996;**5**:10.

28. Mortimer D. Human blastocyst development media. *Hum Reprod* 2001;**16**:2725–6.

29. Lane M, Gardner DK. Differential regulation of mouse embryo development and viability by amino acids. *J Reprod Fertil* 1997;**109**:153–64.

30. Ho Y, Wigglesworth K, Eppig JJ, Schultz RM. Preimplantation development of

mouse embryos in KSOM: augmentation by amino acids and analysis of gene expression. *Mol Reprod Dev* 1995;**41**:232–8.

31. Walker SK, Hill JL, Kleemann DO, Nancarrow CD. Development of ovine embryos in synthetic oviductal fluid containing amino acids at oviductal fluid concentrations. *Biol Reprod* 1996;**55**:703–8.

32. Biggers JD, Racowsky C. The development of fertilized human ova to the blastocyst stage in KSOM(AA) medium: is a two-step protocol necessary? *Reprod Biomed Online* 2002;**5**:133–40.

33. Ali J, Whitten WK, Shelton JN. Effect of culture systems on mouse early embryo development. *Hum Reprod* 1993;**8**: 1110–14.

34. Lawitts JA, Biggers JD. Joint effects of sodium chloride, glutamine, and glucose in mouse preimplantation embryo culture media. *Mol Reprod Dev* 1992;**31**:189–94.

35. Chatot CL, Ziomek CA, Bavister BD, *et al.* An improved culture medium supports development of random-bred 1-cell mouse embryos in vitro. *J Reprod Fertil* 1989;**86**:679–88.

36. Van Winkle LJ, Haghighat N, Campione AL. Glycine protects preimplantation mouse conceptuses from a detrimental effect on development of the inorganic ions in oviductal fluid. *J Exp Zool* 1990;**253**:215–19.

37. Lee ES, Fukui Y. Synergistic effect of alanine and glycine on bovine embryos cultured in a chemically defined medium and amino acid uptake by vitro-produced bovine morulae and blastocysts. *Biol Reprod* 1996;**55**:1383–9.

38. Spindle A. Beneficial effects of taurine on mouse zygotes developing in protein-free culture medium. *Theriogenology* 1995;**44**:761–72.

39. Liu Z, Foote RH, Yang X. Development of early bovine embryos in co-culture with KSOM and taurine, superoxide dismutase or insulin. *Theriogenology* 1995;**44**:741–50.

40. Ecker DJ, Stein P, Xu Z, *et al.* Long-term effects of culture of preimplantation mouse embryos on behavior. *Proc Natl Acad Sci U S A* 2004;**101**:1595–600.

41. Rinaudo P, Schultz RM. Effects of embryo culture on global pattern of gene expression in preimplantation mouse embryos. *Reproduction* 2004;**128**:301–11.

42. Lane M, Gardner DK. Increase in postimplantation development of cultured mouse embryos by amino acids and induction of fetal retardation and exencephaly by ammonium ions. *J Reprod Fertil* 1994;**102**:305–12.

43. Thompson J, Lane M, Robertson S. Adaptive responses of early embryos to the microenvironment and consequences for post-implantation development. In: Wintour EM, Owens JA, eds. *Early Life Origins of Health and Disease* (*Adv Exp Biol Med* 573). New York, Springer Science+Business Media. 2006;58–69.

44. Guérin P, El Mouatassim S, Ménézo Y. Oxidative stress and protection against reactive oxygen species in the pre-implantation embryo and its surroundings. *Hum Reprod Update* 2001;**7**:175–89.

45. Agarwal A, Gupta S, Sharma RK. Role of oxidative stress in female reproduction. *Reprod Biol Endocrinol* 2005;**3**:28, doi:10.1186/1477–7827–3–28.

46. Mortimer D. Sperm preparation techniques and iatrogenic failures of in-vitro fertilization. *Hum Reprod* 1991;**6**:173–6.

47. Aitken RJ, Gordon E, Harkiss D, *et al.* Relative impact of oxidative stress on the functional competence and genomic integrity of human spermatozoa. *Biol Reprod* 1998;**59**:1037–46.

48. Aitken RJ, De Iuliis GN. On the possible origins of DNA damage in human spermatozoa. *Mol Hum Reprod* 2010;**16**:3–13.

49. Aitken RJ, Baker MA, De Iuliis GN, Nixon B. New insights into sperm physiology and pathology. *Handbook Exp Pharmacol* 2010;**198**:99–115.

50. Mortimer D. Sperm preparation methods. *J Androl* 2000;**21**:357–66.

51. Björndahl L, Mortimer D, Barratt CLR, *et al. A Practical Guide to Basic Laboratory Andrology.* Cambridge, Cambridge University Press, 2010.

52. Fischer B, Bavister BD. Oxygen tension in the oviduct and uterus of rhesus monkeys, hamsters and rabbits. *J Reprod Fertil* 1993;**99**:673–9.

53. Rinaudo PF, Giritharan G, Talbi S, *et al.* Effects of oxygen tension on gene expression in preimplantation mouse embryos. *Fertil Steril* 2006;**86**:1252–65.

54. Bain NT, Madan P, Betts DH. The early embryo response to intracellular reactive oxygen species is developmentally regulated. *Reprod Fertil Dev* 2011;**23**:561–75.

55. Arias ME, Sanchez R, Felmer R. Evaluation of different culture systems with low oxygen tension on the development, quality and oxidative stress-related genes of bovine embryos produced in vitro. *Zygote* 2012;**20**:209–17.

56. Deleuze S, Goudet G. Cysteamine supplementation of in vitro maturation media: a review. *Reprod Domest Anim* 2010;**45**:e476–82.

57. Bavister B. Oxygen concentration and preimplantation development. *Reprod Biomed Online* 2004;**9**:484–6.

58. Thompson JG, Simpson AC, Pugh PA, *et al.* Effect of oxygen concentration on in-vitro development of preimplantation sheep and cattle embryos. *J Reprod Fertil* 1990;**89**:573–8.

59. Petersen A, Mikkelsen AL, Lindenberg S. The impact of oxygen tension on developmental competence of post-thaw human embryos. *Acta Obstet Gynecol Scand* 2005;**84**:1181–4.

60. Kovacic B, Vlaisavljevic V. Influence of atmospheric versus reduced oxygen concentration on development of human blastocysts in vitro: a prospective study on sibling oocytes. *Reprod Biomed Online* 2008;**17**:229–36.

61. Waldenström U, Engström AB, Hellberg D, Nilsson S. Low-oxygen compared with high-oxygen atmosphere in blastocyst culture, a prospective randomized study. *Fertil Steril* 2009;**91**:2461–5.

62. Meintjes M, Chantilis SJ, Douglas JD, *et al.* A controlled randomized trial evaluating the effect of lowered incubator oxygen tension on live births in a predominantly blastocyst transfer program. *Hum Reprod* 2009;**24**:300–7.

63. Bilska A, Wlodek L. Lipoic acid – the drug of the future? *Pharmacol Rep* 2005;**57**:570–7.

64. Umbreit WW. Carbon dioxide and bicarbonate. In: Umbreit WW, Burris RH, Stauffer JF, eds. *Manometric Techniques.* Minneapolis, Burgess Publishing Co. 1957;18–27.

65. Lassalle B, Testart J, Renard JP. Human embryo features that influence the success of cryopreservation with the use of 1,2 propanediol. *Fertil Steril*, 1985;**44**:645–51.

66. Palasz AT, Breña PB, De la Fuente J, Gutiérrez-Adán A. The effect of different zwitterionic buffers and PBS used for out-of-incubator procedures during standard in vitro embryo production on development, morphology and gene expression of bovine embryos. *Theriogenology* 2008;**70**:1461–70.

67. Cullinan RT, Catt JW, Fussell S, Henman M, Mortimer D. Improved implantation rates of cryopreserved human embryos thawed in a phosphate-free medium. *Hum Reprod* 1998;**13**(Abstract Book 1):59–60.

68. Swain JE. Back to basics: pH for the ARTisan. *J Clin Embryol* 2010;**13**(2):9–28.

69. Swain JE. Optimizing the culture environment in the IVF laboratory: impact of pH and buffer capacity on gamete and embryo quality. *Reprod Biomed Online* 2010;**21**:6–16.

70. Mahadevan MM, Fleetham J, Church RB, Taylor PJ. Growth of mouse embryos in bicarbonate media buffered by carbon dioxide, hepes, or phosphate. *J In Vitro Fert Embryo Transf* 1986;**3**:304–8.

71. Swain JE, Pool TB. New pH-buffering system for media utilized during gamete and embryo manipulations for assisted reproduction. *Reprod Biomed Online* 2009;**18**:799–810.

72. Abramczuk J, Solter D, Koprowski H. The beneficial effect of EDTA on development of mouse one-cell embryos in chemically defined medium. *Dev Biol* 1977;**61**:378–83.

73. Lane M, Gardner DK. Inhibiting 3-phosphoglycerate kinase by EDTA stimulates the development of the cleavage stage mouse embryo. *Mol Reprod Dev* 2001;**60**:233–40.

74. Davis BK. Timing of fertilization in mammals: sperm cholesterol/phospholipid ratio as a determinant of the capacitation interval. *Proc Natl Acad Sci U S A* 1981;**78**:7560–4.

75. Langlais J, Kan FW, Granger L, *et al* Identification of sterol acceptors that stimulate cholesterol efflux from human spermatozoa during in vitro capacitation. *Gamete Res* 1988;**20**:185–201.

76. Lippes J, Krasner J, Alfonso LA, *et al.* Human oviductal fluid proteins. *Fertil Steril* 1981;**36**:623–9.

77. Mortimer D, Mortimer ST. ICSI for all? In: Kovacs G, ed. *How to Improve your ART Success Rates: An Evidence-Based Review of Adjuncts to IVF*. Cambridge, Cambridge University Press. 2011;135–40.

78. Pemble LB, Kaye PL. Whole protein uptake and metabolism by mouse blastocysts. *J Reprod Fertil* 1986;**78**:149–57.

79. Thompson JG. In vitro culture and embryo metabolism of cattle and sheep embryos – a decade of achievement. *Anim Reprod Sci* 2000;**60**–61:263–75.

80. Leese HJ. Quiet please, do not disturb: a hypothesis of embryo metabolism and viability. *Bioessays* 2002;**24**:845–9.

81. Leese HJ, Sturmey RG, Baumann CG, McEvoy TG. Embryo viability and metabolism: obeying the quiet rules. *Hum Reprod* 2007;**22**:3047–50.

82. Leese HJ, Baumann CG, Brison DR, McEvoy TG, Sturmey RG. Metabolism of the viable mammalian embryo: quietness revisited. *Mol Hum Reprod* 2008;**14**:667–72.

83. Quinn P. Enhanced results in mouse and human embryo culture using a modified human tubal fluid medium lacking glucose and phosphate. *J Assist Reprod Genet* 1995;**12**:97–105.

84. Conaghan J, Handyside AH, Winston RM, Leese HJ. Effects of pyruvate and glucose on the development of human preimplantation embryos *in vitro*. *J Reprod Fertil* 1993;**99**:87–95.

85. Barnett DK, Clayton MK, Kimura J, Bavister BD. Glucose and phosphate toxicity in hamster preimplantation embryos involves disruption of cellular organization, including distribution of active mitochondria. *Mol Reprod Dev* 1997;**48**:227–37.

86. Gardner DK, Lane M, Calderon I, Leeton J. Environment of the preimplantation human embryo in vivo: metabolite analysis of oviduct and uterine fluids and metabolism of cumulus cells. *Fertil Steril* 1996;**65**:349–53.

87. Lane M, Gardner DK. Blastomere homeostasis. In: Gardner DK, Lane M, eds. *ART and the Human Blastocyst*. New York, Springer-Verlag. 2001;69–90.

88. Van Winkle LJ, Haghighat N, Campione AL. Glycine protects preimplantation mouse conceptuses from a detrimental effect on development of the inorganic ions in oviductal fluid. *J Exp Zool* 1990;**253**:215–19.

89. Dawson KM, Baltz JM. Organic osmolytes and embryos: substrates of the Gly and beta transport systems protect mouse zygotes against the effects of raised osmolarity. *Biol Reprod* 1997;**56**:1550–8.

90. Dumoulin JCM, van Wissen LCP, Menheere PPCA, *et al.* Taurine acts as an osmolyte in human and mouse oocytes and embryos. *Biol Reprod* 1997;**56**:739–44.

91. Richards T, Wang F, Liu L, *et al.* Rescue of postcompaction-stage mouse embryo development from hypertonicity by amino acid transporter substrates that may function as organic osmolytes. *Biol Reprod* 2010;**82**:769–77.

92. Baltz JM, Tartia AP. Cell volume regulation in oocytes and early embryos: connecting physiology to successful culture media. *Hum Reprod Update* 2010;**16**:166–76.

93. Barratt CL, Björndahl L, Menkveld R, Mortimer D. ESHRE special interest group for andrology basic semen analysis course: a continued focus on accuracy, quality,

efficiency and clinical relevance. *Hum Reprod* 2011;**26**:3207–12.

94. Pool TB. Optimizing pH in clinical embryology. *Clin Embryologist* 2004;7 (3):1–17.

95. Barnett DK, Bavister BD. What is the relationship between the metabolism of preimplantation embryos and their developmental competence? *Mol Reprod Dev* 1996;**43**:105–33.

96. Phillips KP, Léveillé MC, Claman P, Baltz JM. Intracellular pH regulation in human preimplantation embryos. *Hum Reprod* 2000;**15**:896–904.

97. Dale B, Menezo Y, Cohen J, *et al.* Intracellular pH regulation in the human oocyte. *Hum Reprod* 1998;**13**:964–70.

98. Squirrell JM, Lane M, Bavister BD. Altering intracellular pH disrupts development and cellular organization in preimplantation hamster embryos. *Biol Reprod* 2001;**64**:1845–54.

99. Zander-Fox DL, Mitchell M, Thompson JG, Lane M. Alterations in mouse embryo intracellular pH by DMO during culture impair implantation and fetal growth. *Reprod Biomed Online* 2010;**21**:219–29.

100. Mortimer D, Mortimer ST. *Quality and Risk Management in the IVF Laboratory.* Cambridge, Cambridge University Press, 2005.

101. Katz-Jaffe MG, Gardner DK. Embryology in the era of proteomics. *Theriogenology* 2007;**68**(1):S125–30.

102. Iliadou AN, Janson PC, Cnattingius S. Epigenetics and assisted reproductive technology. *J Intern Med* 2011;**270**: 414–20.

Chapter

6

Macromolecular supplementation of embryo culture media

Thomas B. Pool

Introduction

The propagation of human embryos in vitro followed by uterine transfer facilitates pregnancy and delivery at rates never envisioned at the dawn of clinical in vitro fertilization (IVF). The most recent data reported by the Society of Assisted Reproductive Technology (SART) confirm this in their annual (2009) analysis of over 39 000 IVF cycles from women, < 35 years of age, using their own eggs [1]. The live birth rate in this group was 41.4% per cycle, 44.6% per oocyte retrieval, and 47.5% per embryo transfer. But consider the environment in which these viable embryos were produced. Oocytes and resulting embryos were placed upon a two-dimensional surface of irradiated polystyrene and covered with a dilute aqueous solution of monovalent and divalent anions and cations, amino acids, metabolic substrates, protein, and antibiotics. For some, the environment included vitamins, fatty acids, nucleic acid precursors, and, perhaps, even bioactive polypeptides. The osmotic pressure was in the range of 280–285 milliosmoles and the maximum concentration of any of the components was determined not by biological need, but rather by the solubility of the ingredient at ambient temperature in water. This solution, approaching thermodynamic ideality, was then covered by oil, a layer that provided protection from contamination, dehydration, and an excessive rate of gas loss when out of the incubator but one that also partitions any lipid-soluble component of the medium, either included at formulation or produced by embryos upon incubation. The cultured embryos could modify the composition of the medium by taking up specific components, metabolizing them, and releasing by-products of metabolism back into the medium. They may also have even released their own growth-promoting factors as well but these types of embryo-generated modifications to the composition of the culture medium occur at rates requiring heroic analytical measures to detect. Contemporary culture media, therefore, provide to the oocyte/embryo a fixed set of chemical conditions that changes forms largely by degradative oxidative processes or by alterations in carbonic acid concentration as dishes are moved in and out of the incubator.

For contrast, consider the conditions encountered in vivo by the oocyte and developing embryo. The environment is a dynamic one in which development occurs on a moist surface under healthy conditions, likely not one in which the embryo is totally submersed in fluid as in tubal blockage or partial blockage. The matrix upon which the embryo develops is three-dimensional and includes large glycosylated, polydisperse molecules, rendering it foreign to the near ideal solution the embryo encounters in vitro. The underlying

Culture Media, Solutions, and Systems in Human ART, ed. Patrick Quinn. Published by Cambridge University Press. © Cambridge University Press 2014.

epithelium modulates and can change the composition and concentration of ingredients in the immediate chemical environment of the embryo. By contrast, the embryo in vitro, if it is to retain viability, is left to adjust its metabolism to relatively fixed conditions, if need be, as alternative metabolic pathways within the embryo constitute the only flexible members of the culture system. Or do they?

Consider historically the breadth of culture medium composition used in human IVF, all of which have resulted in the generation of viable human embryos, albeit at differing levels of efficacy. Is it likely that the capacity of an embryo to employ alternative pathways is the sole mechanism that provides viability or is there some additional component of the culture system that modulates an embryo's interaction with the in vitro chemical environment? Macromolecular supplementation of culture media, in the form of whole serum, isolated serum proteins, recombinant serum proteins, or alternative polymers provides both chemical and physical interface of embryos with their microenvironment and are crucial for maximizing embryonic viability. It is the intent of this chapter to explore macromolecular supplements in both historical and contemporary usage, focusing upon the possible mechanisms employed in delivering viability, both in vivo and in vitro.

The use of whole serum

As summarized in earlier reviews [2, 3], the use of whole serum as a source of macromolecular supplementation for human embryo culture was likely related to the manner in which many programs acquired culture technology at the dawn of clinical IVF. Rather than adapting the methods, systems, and media developed over a number of years for embryo culture of laboratory species such as the mouse and rabbit (see the review of Biggers [4]), many centers simply used those in common use for somatic cell culture. Only within the past five or so years has the medium developed in Professor Biggers' laboratory been introduced commercially as a successful single medium for extended culture of human embryos. But in the late 1970s and into the 1980s, both simple salt solutions such as Earle's as well as complex media such as Ham's F-10 became mainstays of the clinical IVF laboratory and the common approach was to supplement both with heat-inactivated whole serum. Of particular importance, however, was the demonstration in 1986 by Caro and Trounson [5] that fertilization of human oocytes, followed by their subsequent development in vitro into viable embryos, could occur in medium containing no protein. This established the principle that macromolecules in the culture environment in vitro may modulate the efficiency of embryo production but are not obligate components of the culture system. More recently, Ali et al. have published studies using protein-free, chemically defined media for clinical IVF that describe high pregnancy rates [6]. Unfortunately, the composition of the successful medium was not given and, thus, this work cannot be repeated by other laboratories. To date, no commercial form of protein-free media exists for clinical IVF.

Table 6.1 describes the chronological introduction of serum and serum fractions as macromolecular supplements into clinical IVF. As can be seen, the movement away from whole serum supplementation began in the mid 1980s and the use of serum, even from autologous sources, has been all but abandoned. This stems from a number of reports that the use of whole serum can be deleterious upon embryogenesis in vitro. Gardner et al. reported that whole serum introduced a darkness and granularity to the blastocyst, produced granular vesicles in cells of the trophectoderm, and induced an excess production of

Table 6.1. Serum and serum fractions used for human embryo culture

Supplement	Year	Investigator	Reference
Fetal calf serum	1965	Edwards	[23]
Maternal serum	1980	Edwards *et al.*	[24]
Fetal cord serum, high- and low-molecular-weight fractions; albumin	1983	Saito *et al.*	[25]
Fetal cord serum, maternal serum	1984	Leung *et al.*	[26]
Bovine serum albumin	1969	Edwards *et al.*	[15]
Human serum albumin (HSA)	1984	Menezo *et al.*	[16]
HSA; Albuminar-5	1989	Ashwood-Smith *et al.*	[17]
HSA; Albuminar-20	1990	Staessen *et al.*	[18]
HSA; Plasmanate*	1993	Adler *et al.*	[27]
HSA/globulins; Plasmatein	1994	Pool and Martin	[28]
HSA/globulins; SSS	1995	Weathersbee *et al.*	[29]

* Plasmanate contains globulins at a concentration lower than Plasmatein. The authors used it as a source of albumin with no mention of globulins.

lactate by blastocysts as well [7]. Dorland *et al.* [8] used transmission electron microscopy to describe mitochondrial degeneration in blastocysts propagated in the presence of whole serum but it was the disturbing report by Walker *et al* [9] that garnered the most attention. Their group was the first to describe the birth of abnormally large offspring following the transfer of embryos grown in the presence of whole serum, an observation made originally in sheep and later extended to cattle. The phenomenon then gained the common name of large calf syndrome. Jeremy Thompson and colleagues showed that the trophectoderm vesicles were actually lipid, that the gestational period of animals receiving transferred embryos produced in whole serum was extended, and that the use of bovine serum albumin as a protein supplement, instead of whole serum, alleviated large calf syndrome [10].

While large offspring syndrome does not occur in humans, there are a number of other reasons to avoid the use of whole serum as a macromolecular source for embryo culture. Serum has been described as a "pathological fluid" [7] because it results only after clotting. It contains a number of ill-defined components and differs in composition from batch to batch, rendering every lot of culture medium supplemented with serum as unique. Clearly, there are infectious disease concerns, particularly when one considers the spongiform encephalopathies that may take years to develop and detect in offspring. Even the use of autologous maternal serum has significant drawbacks. While it is well known that maternal sera can differ significantly in their ability to support embryogenesis, there is no useful bioassay that can identify inferior lots. Clarke *et al.* examined 22 lots of maternal sera used for IVF patients using a 1-cell mouse embryo assay [11]. Mouse embryos grown in Ham's F-10 supplemented with 7.5% maternal serum were evaluated for blastocyst formation and compared with the respective growth of human embryos in the same media. No correlation was seen between the performance in mouse cultures and that in human cultures. Additionally, there was no correlation with clinical pregnancy in humans. Another concern is that serum from women experiencing certain forms of infertility may present growth inhibitory substances to the culture environment. This was demonstrated to be the case for sera from women with idiopathic infertility by Dokras *et al.* [12] both in mouse and human embryo culture.

Albumin and plasma protein fractions
Serum albumin

The total protein concentration of serum ranges from 60 to 80 g/L, approximately 60% being the single protein albumin. A wide range of putative functions have been ascribed to albumin including being both a pH and osmotic buffer, a membrane stabilizer, a carrier of growth-promoting substances (amino acids, vitamins, fatty acids, hormones, growth factors), a surfactant, a scavenger of heavy metals and toxins, as well as a nitrogen source upon breakdown [13]. In fact, the role it can serve as a carrier was demonstrated clearly by Gray *et al.* [14], who showed that sodium citrate associated with albumin, not albumin per se, was growth promoting to rabbit embryos. The use of bovine serum albumin (BSA) in human IVF dates back to 1969 in the experimental setting [15] but it was Menezo *et al.* that included it in media intended for clinical IVF in the form of medium B-2 [16]. Concerns were expressed by Ashwood-Smith *et al.* that the use of animal products may introduce viruses plus, if introduced into a patient, might sensitize them to a foreign protein [17]. His group used, instead, a commercial source of human serum albumin, Albuminar-5 (see Table 6.1), a preparation marketed as a plasma volume expander for human use. In a trial comparison, they demonstrated that the fertilization rates in Albuminar were equivalent to those obtained in whole patient serum. Staessen *et al.* subsequently showed that both the percent of cleaved embryos and pregnancy rates were significantly increased when Albuminar was used as the protein supplement compared to whole serum in human IVF [18].

One concern arose regarding the substitution of serum albumin for whole serum and that was as a supplement for embryo cryopreservation media. Warnes *et al.* found normal serum albumin to be equivalent to patient serum as a medium supplement with respect to fertilization, embryo quality, and pregnancy in fresh IVF cycles but saw pregnancy and implantation rates drop significantly when embryos were thawed in media supplemented with albumin [19]. Additionally, inclusion of albumin in culture and freezing media reduced the implantation rate compared to serum supplementation. As noted by the authors, the serum albumin solution used (stock solution of 5% normal serum albumin) is globulin depleted and thus lacking in carbohydrates. Further, the final concentration of protein in the albumin-supplemented medium was 2.5 mg/mL, lower than the total protein concentration of serum-supplemented media (3–4 mg/mL). Whether it was the concentration of protein or lack of carbohydrate is not resolved but the use of supplements at higher protein concentration, particularly when the albumin-based solution contains α and β globulins as well (see work of Kramer [20] discussed below), has subsequently produced excellent outcomes in freeze/thaw solutions and is now the industry standard in the USA and Japan.

Recombinant human albumin

As noted earlier, one concern for using natural products is the possibility of transmitting diseases, such as Creutzfeldt–Jakob disease (CJD) and new variant CJD (nvCJD), spongiform encephalopathies that are caused by prions. Additionally, natural products can vary batch to batch due to variations in donors and preparative methods [13]. To circumvent these issues, human albumin produced through recombinant technology has been introduced to the human culture environment. Bungum conducted a prospective, randomized trial comparing sequential culture media supplemented with either human serum albumin (HSA) or recombinant human albumin (rHA) [21]. In this study, which enrolled 85 women, equivalent rates of fertilization, cleavage, blastocyst formation, implantation, pregnancy, and pregnancy loss were seen in both groups. This is an important study considering the role albumin can play as a carrier molecule. One would predict a totally different profile of lipids would be associated with albumin produced in CHO cells compared to the human liver. A phase I clinical trial later compared the tolerability, safety, and pharmacokinetics/pharmacodynamics directly in human patients [22]. No immunological issues were identified and there was no difference in safety or efficacy measured in the comparison. rHA is now included as the sole protein source in a wide array of commercially available human embryo culture media.

α and β globulins

Plasma volume expanders such as Albuminar and Plasmanate (see Table 6.1) are prepared by precipitating whole, pooled plasma with cold ethanol. The predominate protein resulting from this is albumin but it is also accompanied by serum glycoproteins, the α and β globulins. These globulins, so named by their electrophoretic mobility under non-denaturing conditions, constitute collectively 24–27 grams of serum protein per liter. Pool and Martin first noted that various commercial plasma volume expanders, also known as plasma protein fractions (PPFs), differed in the amount of α and β globulins that accompanied albumin, further realizing that the one performing best as a culture supplement was one with the highest concentrations of globulins [28]. This product, Plasmatein, produced high continuing pregnancy rates when used as a macromolecular supplement for human embryo culture medium and produced shortened intermitotic intervals in cleaving embryos when compared with serum albumin [28, 29]. A list of various members of the α and β globulin families are given in Table 6.2. There are drawbacks to using commercial plasma volume expanders as they contain preservatives and also vary lot to lot in the concentrations of globulins. As a result, Weathersbee et al. constructed a human serum albumin-based protein supplement to which α and β globulins were added at precise and repeatable concentrations [29]. The marketed form of this supplement was named Synthetic Serum Substitute (SSS), reflecting that the process of producing it was a synthesis of individual components rather than a precipitate of a more complex initial solution. Some felt the name was inappropriate since the materials themselves were not "synthetic" [13] and the product was renamed serum substitute solution (still SSS) to alleviate this concern. When used at a

Table 6.2. Alpha and beta globulins

Glycoprotein	Molecular weight (kDa)
Alpha 1 globulins	
α1-antitrypsin	45
α1-antichymotrypsin	68
orosomucoid (acid glycoprotein)	44
serum amyloid A	15
α1-lipoprotein	65–71
retinol-binding protein 21–22	21–22
transcortin	66
Alpha 2 globulins	
haptoglobin	89–100
α-2u globulin	20
α2-macroglobulin	720
ceruloplasmin	151
thyroxine-binding globulin	46.3
α2-antiplasmin	70
protein C	62
α2-lipoprotein	~80
Beta globulins	
sex hormone-binding	
globulin	52; 95–115
transferrin	80
angiostatin	38
hemopexin	57
β2-microglobulin	11.8
factor H	150
plasminogen	88
properdin	223

concentration (volume/volume) of 10%, equivalent to 6 mg/mL total protein, it produces rapid cleavage rates in mouse and human embryos [29] and results in pregnancy rates fully equivalent to Plasmatein.

That α and β globulins significantly increase both blastocyst formation and hatching in a dose-dependent manner was shown by Tanikawa *et al.* using a mouse 1-cell assay [30]. Increases at all concentrations of globulins, beginning at 0.2 mg/mL, added to a base medium of 4 mg/mL of albumin in Human Tubal Fluid medium (HTF; Irvine Scientific, Santa Ana, CA) were significantly different from blastocyst formation and hatching in HTF/albumin alone. In another investigation, Tucker *et al.* compared embryogenesis of B6D2F1 1-cell mouse embryos cultured in HTF alone or HTF supplemented with 15% maternal serum from patients with tubal infertility, with 15% maternal serum from endometriosis patients, with 15% donor serum, or with 15% SSS [31]. By 48 hours, 64.9% of embryos were morulae in the SSS group compared to 5.4%, 0, 8.2%, and 6.1% for the other groups, respectively. In addition, blastocyst formation at both 72 and 96 hours was significantly higher in the SSS group compared to all others. A trial of SSS in humans compared to maternal or donor serum was also included in this same report. No difference in embryogenesis or embryo quality was noted between the two groups but fertilization was improved in the SSS group. That same year, Desai *et al.* performed a retrospective comparison of 68 patients whose embryos were grown in HTF with 10% SSS versus embryos from 263 similar cycles where embryos were cultured either in HTF with 10% maternal serum or 6% Plasmanate [32]. The pregnancy rate was higher in the SSS group (38.2%) compared to either the maternal serum group (28%) or Plasmanate group (24.9%) but it did not reach statistical significance. The implantation rate, however, was significantly increased in the SSS group (17.8%) compared to the maternal serum group (10.4%) or Plasmanate group (10.3%). The most thorough analysis of the effects of using globulin-supplemented media compared to HSA alone in human IVF was performed by Meintjes *et al.* in 2009 [33]. In this randomized, controlled trial, 528 patients were randomized to embryo culture with media G1/G2 (Vitrolife, Gothenburg, Sweden) supplemented with either HSA alone (5 mg/mL) or HSA (5 mg/mL) with an additional 10% SSS. Embryos were separated to these two groups at the 2 pronuclear stage and clinical endpoints included implantation (1151 embryos) and live birth rates (528 patients). All of the following measures were increased significantly with the addition of protein containing globulins: implantation rate from day-5 transfers, implantation rates overall, live birth implantation rates from day-5 transfers, live birth rates from day-5 transfers, and live birth rates overall. It should be noted that total protein concentration in the SSS group was 11 mg/mL whereas it was 5 mg/mL for the HSA group. To my knowledge, there are no reports showing a statistically significant improvement in pregnancy and implantation rates in human IVF simply by increasing the concentration of albumin. Ben-Yosef *et al.* reported an increase in both of these parameters by increasing the concentration of SSS from 10% to 20% in a large series of IVF patients [34]. This is consistent with the findings of Tanikawa *et al.* [30] on the dose–response relationship of α and β globulins to enhanced embryogenesis in the mouse. There are now multiple commercial medium companies offering albumin solutions containing α and β globulins for use as a macromolecular supplement for human embryo culture. It should be noted that not all attempts to amalgamate an effective combination of proteins intended to replace serum as a medium supplement have been successful. Psalti *et al.* demonstrated adverse effects upon fertilization and embryo development when UltraSerG, a mixture of albumin, adhesion factors, and purified growth factors, was used as a serum replacement [35].

As mentioned earlier, the use of protein supplements containing globulins has significantly improved outcomes from embryo cryopreservation. Kramer compared the effects of using a globulin-rich protein source (SSS) versus human serum albumin in freeze, thaw, and post-thaw solutions during control-rate blastocyst cryopreservation in both the mouse and the human [20]. Blastocyst re-expansion was significantly higher when embryos were frozen, thawed, and cultured post-thaw in medium containing SSS compared to HSA. Total cell number of re-expanded blastocysts was moderately greater for the SSS group as well. A retrospective analysis of human blastocysts cryopreserved initially in freezing solution containing HSA was conducted with either HSA or SSS in the thaw solution. Embryo survival (83.3% versus 43.9%), expansion (66.7% versus 15.8%), clinical pregnancy rate per thaw (55.6% versus 10.5%), and implantation rates (53.8% versus 13.3%) were all significantly higher when blastocysts were thawed and cultured post-thaw in the presence of SSS compared to HSA, respectively.

The future: alternatives to human-derived products

One important reason to find alternatives to human-derived products, such as the globulins, is to render macromolecular supplementation of human embryo culture media safe, standardized, pyrogen-free, and acceptable worldwide; as it is currently, supplementation with human globulins is prohibited in a number of countries due to potential contamination with prions. Utilizing recombinant technology to produce the myriad of glycosylated species represented in the α and β globulins is not the realistic option it was for the single protein albumin. Yet engineering an effective alternative hinges upon our understanding of the explicit functions macromolecules play in the embryonic microenvironment, something of which we remain woefully ignorant. There are reasons to believe that macromolecules function in multiple ways through general chemical mechanisms, as noted earlier for albumin, through specific chemical mechanisms, such as growth factors, as well as through non-specific physical means. An equally important consideration is the manner in which macromolecules are presented to the preimplantation embryo. Is the presence of macromolecules as soluble components of a dilute aqueous solution the appropriate form? Certainly, it is for albumin and embryotrophic ligands such as growth factors but what about polydisperse, glycosylated entities such as glycosaminoglycans and mucins? Can such macromolecules be presented in the in vitro environment which employs a two-dimensional matrix of polystyrene as effectively as they are in a three-dimensional matrix as is seen in vivo?

Do macromolecules penetrate the zona pellucida? Without a doubt, supplementation with whole serum and, perhaps, with globulin-containing plasma protein fractions delivers blood-borne, low-molecular-weight growth-promoting polypeptides to the embryonic microenvironment. Not only do these cross the zona pellucida, but also a consideration of zona permeability becomes irrelevant to some proteins as they are produced inside of the zona by the embryo in an autocrine process. The nature and activity of these factors are not the subject of this chapter but the reader is referred to the work of Kane et al. [36] and more recently to that of O'Neill [37] for authoritative reviews on potential embryotrophic ligands, their embryo stage-specific relevance, and their mechanism of action. But what about the larger members of the macromolecular complex seen in PPFs? There is little published information on the permeability of the human zona pellucida as established by extensive experimentation but it has been measured in the mouse. Legge traced the permeability of mouse zonae using graded neutral fluorescein isothiocyanate (FITC)-labeled dextrans and galactose lectins [38]. The dextrans covered molecular weights from 3.84 to 170 kDa whereas the lectins ranged from 40 to 247 kDa. From these studies it was concluded that zona intact pre- and post-ovulatory oocytes are permeable to markers up to a molecular weight range of 170 kDa. Movement was diminished at 150 kDa and there was no detected permeability at 170 kDa. Fertilization reduces permeability and a decrease was measured at 110 kDa. As can be seen in Table 6.2, all but just a few of the members of the α and β globulins would penetrate the zona, assuming that permeability characteristics of the human resemble those of the mouse. Clearly, albumin can cross the zona with ease at 66 kDa and many of the functions ascribed to this protein can occur within direct proximity to the oocyte/blastomere plasma membrane. A caveat exists, however, given the fact that many members of the macromolecular complex encountered by embryos in the in vivo milieu emanate from fixed sites or exist in colloidal form, and thus are not truly in solution. How can entities such as these exert any effect upon preimplantation embryogenesis?

Additionally, there are estrogen-dependent oviductal glycoproteins synthesized in humans [39] that are of a molecular weight, 120–130 kDa, that would be excluded with a zonal cut-off of 110 kDa. What influence might these have upon embryogenesis as well?

Hunter has suggested that these glycoproteins may be contributing to the "economy" of early development by affecting the concentrations of cations, sugars, and other substrates presented to embryos [40]. Thus, they function as entities that modulate the embryonic microenvironment by binding and releasing elements essential to embryo metabolism. An expanded consideration of this has been reviewed by Pool *et al.* [2, 28] and Pool [3]. What about carbohydrate-containing proteins that are not in solution – does their structure allow for such potential binding and release? A consideration of the structure of the one mucin, MUC1, synthesized in the Fallopian tube yields some insight into this possibility. Meseguer *et al.* have shown that MUC1 is a heavily glycosylated transmembrane mucin present on the apical surface of upper reproductive tract epithelial cells [41]. As described by Al-Azemi *et al.* [42], the extracellular domain of MUC1 contains up to 125 tandem repeats of amino acids enriched for the presence of serine, threonine, and proline residues. These residues are then O-linked to oligosaccharides that project into the aqueous environment from fixed sites. The concentration of oligosaccharides is sufficiently high to protect the polypeptide backbone from proteolysis and it is not rate-limited by solubility; rather, the concentration of oligosaccharides is determined genetically, as stipulated by the coding region that produces the amino acid repeats. A stylized depiction of this structure is given in Figure 6.1. The resemblance of the organization of the oligosaccharides in MUC1, being fixed at one end yet free at the other, is strikingly similar to that of ion exchange resins used in biochemical purification strategies. In this, proteins, as well as other entities, are bound then reversibly released upon a shift in either ionic strength or pH. Although mucins are most often thought of as lubricants and biochemical colloids that prevent implantation [41, 42], they may well function as direct mediators of the embryonic microenvironment in the Fallopian tube as well as the uterus.

Another possible mechanism that would allow for oviductal glycoproteins to modulate the embryonic microenvironment in a non-specific, physical manner relates to the interactions of carbohydrate hydroxyl groups with water. Details of this possibility have been reviewed in earlier work [2, 3, 28] but relate to the density of hydroxyl groups in the carbohydrate moieties of glycoproteins, their steric hindrance, and how this affects hydrogen bonding with water. Franks details this interaction, noting that the hydrogen bond between a water molecule and a hydroxyl group of a polyhydroxylated compound, although

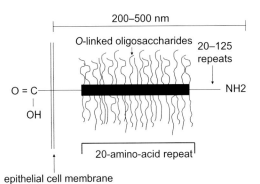

Figure 6.1 A stylized representation of mucin MUC1 found in the human uterus and oviduct. Oligosaccharides are O-linked to serine, threonine, and proline residues in a 20-amino-acid repeat that recurs from 20 to 125 times on the molecule. The C-terminus is anchored in the cytoplasm of epithelial cells whereas the N-terminus projects towards the lumen of the reproductive tract. For a comprehensive description of MUC1 see Gum [43], Meseguer *et al.* [41], and Al-Azemi *et al.* [42].

similar to a water–water interaction, is slightly altered [44]. The effect, however, is amplified by the number of such altered interactions that occur over a large molecule, altering some of the basic properties of water. Such altered interactions can produce profound biological effects and may effectively gate how an embryo "sees" the immediate microenvironment, perhaps through alterations in exchange dynamics of water, etc. Serum albumin, as indicated earlier, plays multiple roles but is a molecule designed to interact with water, functioning to retain water in the vasculature in order to prevent tissue edema in vivo. The increase in measurable oncotic efficiency of glycoproteins compared to albumin is verification that polyhydroxylation intensifies this interaction. This coupled with the water:macromolecular ratio in the reproductive tract is indicative that the conditions an embryo encounters in vivo are far from the near ideal, dilute solution provided by contemporary embryo culture technology.

It is clear that macromolecules modulate the embryonic microenvironment in a number of different ways, on multiple levels of cellular and biochemical organization, and through a variety of specific mechanisms, many currently unknown. It is not surprising, therefore, that previous attempts to substitute compounds such as polyvinyl alcohol [45], dextran [2, 3, 28], and hyaluronan [46] for proteinaceous/glycoproteinaceous macromolecules have met with varying degrees of success. Certainly, they have not been accepted as a universal replacement and there is much room for innovation. One final consideration is the nature of the culture platform from a design perspective, namely, can any form of macromolecular supplementation offered as a soluble component in a microdrop present to the cultured embryo the same physical and chemical conditions encountered in the three-dimensional confines of the reproductive tract? Is there a way to present macromolecules from fixed sites as well as in solution and to provide simultaneously one form of mechanical stimulation currently not given in contemporary static microdrop culture – namely, movement? An excellent recent review on the potential ways to offer movement to embryos in culture has been written by Swain and Smith [47] and suggests that gentle mechanical stimulation of embryos, as encountered in vivo, may stimulate signaling pathways that heretofore may be bypassed by current static platforms. Further is the intriguing possibility that macromolecules are mechanistically involved in this process as is known for somatic cell–extracellular matrix interactions elsewhere in the body.

References

1. SART CORS Online. *Clinic Summary Report*. 2009. https://www.sartcorsonline. com/rptCSR_PublicMultYear.aspx? ClinicPKID=0 (accessed September 15, 2011).

2. Pool TB, Atiee SH, Martin JE. Oocyte and embryo culture: basic concepts and recent advances. In: May J, ed. *Assisted Reproduction: Laboratory Considerations. Infertility and Reproductive Medicine Clinics of North America*. 1998;**9**:181–203.

3. Pool TB. Blastocyst development in culture: the role of macromolecules. In: Gardner DK, Lane M, eds. *ART and the Human Blastocyst*. New York, Springer. 2001;105–17.

4. Biggers, JD. Pioneering mammalian embryo culture. In: Bavister BD, ed. *The Mammalian Preimplantation Embryo*. New York, Plenum Press. 1987;1–22.

5. Caro CM, Trounson AO. Successful fertilization, embryo development and pregnancy in humans in in vitro fertilization (IVF) using a chemically defined culture medium containing no protein. *J In Vitro Fert Embryo Transf* 1986;**3**:215–17.

6. Ali J, Shahata MAM, Al-Natsha SD. Formulation of a protein-free medium for

human assisted reproduction. *Hum Reprod* 2000;**15**:145–56.

7. Gardner DK. Mammalian embryo culture in the absence of serum or somatic cell support. *Cell Biol Int* 1994;**18**;1163–79.

8. Dorland M, Gardner DK, Trounson AO. Serum in synthetic oviduct fluid causes mitochondrial degeneration in ovine embryos. *J Reprod Fertil Abstract Series* 1994;**13**:70.

9. Walker SK, Heard TM, Seamark RF. In vitro culture of sheep embryos without co-culture: successes and perspectives. *Theriogenology* 1992;**37**:111–26.

10. Thompson JG, Gardner DK, Pugh PA, *et al.* Lamb birth weight following transfer is affected by the culture system used for pre-elongation development of embryos. *J Reprod Fertil Abstract Series* 1994;**13**:69.

11. Clarke RN, Griffin PM, Biggers JD. Screening of maternal sera using a mouse embryo culture assay is not predictive of human embryo development or IVF outcome. *J Assist Reprod Genet* 1995;**12**:20–5.

12. Dokras A, Sargent IL, Redman CWG, *et al.* Sera from women with unexplained infertility inhibit both mouse and human embryo growth in vitro. *Fertil Steril* 1993;**60**:285–92.

13. Blake D, Svalander P, Jin M, *et al.* Protein supplementation of human IVF culture media. *J Assist Reprod Genet* 2002;**19**:137–43.

14. Gray CW, Morgan PM, Kane MT. Purification of an embryotrophic factor from commercial bovine serum albumin and its identification as citrate. *J Reprod Fertil* 1992;**94**:471–80.

15. Edwards RG, Bavister BD, Steptoe PC. Early stages of fertilization in vitro of human oocytes matured in vitro. *Nature* 1969;**221**:632–5.

16. Menezo Y, Testart J, Perone D. Serum is not necessary in human in vitro fertilization and embryo development. *Fertil Steril* 1984;**42**:750–5.

17. Ashwood-Smith MJ, Hollands P, Edwards RG. The use of Albuminar (TM) as a medium supplement in clinical IVF. *Hum Reprod* 1989;**4**:702–5.

18. Staessen C, Van den Abbeel E, Carle M, *et al.* Comparison between human serum and Albuminar-20 (TM) supplement for in vitro fertilization. *Hum Reprod* 1990;**5**:336–41.

19. Warnes GM, Payne D, Jeffrey R, *et al.* Reduced pregnancy rates following the transfer of human embryos frozen or thawed in culture media supplemented with normal serum albumin. *Hum Reprod* 1997;**12**:1525–30.

20. Kramer JM. Supplementation of freeze and thaw solutions with a globulin-rich protein source improves post-thaw survival and implantation of control-rate cryopreserved blastocysts. *J Clin Embryol* 2010;**13**:41–9.

21. Bungum M. Recombinant human albumin as a protein source in culture media used for IVF: a prospective randomized study. *Reprod Biomed Online* 2002;**4**:233–6.

22. Bosse D, Praus M, Kiessling P, *et al.* Phase I comparability of recombinant human albumin and human serum albumin. *J Clin Pharmacol* 2005;**45**:57–67.

23. Edwards RG. Maturation in vitro of mouse, sheep, cow, pig, rhesus monkey and human ovarian oocytes. *Nature* 1965;**208**:349–51.

24. Edwards RG, Steptoe PC, Purdy JM. Establishing full-term human pregnancies using cleaving embryos grown in vitro. *Br J Obstet Gynaecol* 1980;**87**:737–56.

25. Saito H, Marrs RP, Berger T, *et al.* Enhancement of in vitro development by specific serum supplements. *Fertil Steril (Abstr)* 1983;**39**:423.

26. Leung PCS, Gronow MJ, Kellow GN, *et al.* Serum supplement in human in vitro fertilization and embryo development. *Fertil Steril* 1984;**41**:36–9.

27. Adler A, McVicker Reing A, Bedford JM, *et al.* Plasmanate as a medium supplement for in vitro fertilization. *J Assist Reprod Genet* 1993;**10**:67–71.

28. Pool TB, Martin JE. High continuing pregnancy rates after in vitro fertilization-embryo transfer using medium supplemented with a plasma protein

fraction containing α and β globulins. *Fertil Steril* 1994;**61**:714–19.

29. Weathersbee PS, Pool TB, Ord T. Synthetic serum substitute (SSS): a globulin-enriched protein supplement for human embryo culture. *J Assist Reprod Genet* 1995;**12**:354–60.

30. Tanikawa M, Harada T, Ito M, *et al.* Globulins in protein supplements promote the development of preimplantation embryos. *J Assist Reprod Genet* 1999;**16**:555–7.

31. Tucker K, Hurst BS, Guadagnoli S, *et al.* Evaluation of synthetic serum substitute versus serum as a protein supplementation for mouse and human embryo culture. *J Assist Reprod Genet* 1996;**13**:32–7.

32. Desai N, Sheean LA, Martin D, *et al.* Clinical experience with synthetic serum substitute as a protein supplement in IVF culture media: a retrospective study. *J Assist Reprod Genet* 1996;**13**:23–31.

33. Meintjes M, Chantilis SJ, Ward DC, *et al.* A randomized controlled study of human serum albumin and serum substitute supplement as protein supplements for IVF culture and the effect on live birth rates. *Hum Reprod* 2009;**24**:782–9.

34. Ben-Yosef D, Yovel I, Schwartz T, *et al.* Increasing synthetic serum substitute (SSS) concentrations in P1 glucose/phosphate-free medium improves implantation rate: a comparative study. *J Assist Reprod Genet* 2001;**18**:588–92.

35. Psalti I, Loumaye E, Pensis M, *et al.* Evaluation of a synthetic serum substitute to replace fetal cord serum for human oocyte fertilization and embryo growth in vitro. *Fertil Steril* 1989;**52**:807–11.

36. Kane MT, Morgan PM, Coonan C. Peptide growth factors and preimplantation development. *Hum Reprod Update* 1997;**3**:137–57.

37. O'Neill C. The potential roles for embryotrophic ligands in preimplantation embryo development. *Hum Reprod Update* 2008;**14**:275–85.

38. Legge M. Oocyte and zygote zona pellucida permeability to macromolecules. *J Exp Zool* 1995;**271**:145–50.

39. Verhage HG, Fazbealas AT, Donnelly K. The in vitro synthesis and release of proteins in the human oviduct. *Endocrinology* 1988;**22**:1639–45.

40. Hunter RHF. Modulation of gamete and embryonic microenvironments by oviduct glycoproteins. *Mol Reprod Dev* 1994;**39**:176–81.

41. Meseguer M, Aplin JD, Caballero-Campo P *et al.* Human endometrial mucin MUC1 is up-regulated by progesterone and down-regulated in vitro by the human blastocyst. *Biol Reprod* 2001;**64**:590–601.

42. Al-Azemi M, Refaat B, Ledger W. The expression of MUC1 in human fallopian tube during the menstrual cycle and in ectopic pregnancy. *Hum Reprod* 2009;**24**:2582–7.

43. Gum JR. Human mucin glycoproteins: varied structures predict diverse properties and specific functions. *Biochem Soc Trans* 1995;**23**:795–9.

44. Franks F. Solute-water interactions: do polyhydroxy compounds alter the properties of water? *Cryobiology* 1983;**20**:335–45.

45. Bavister BD. Substitution of a synthetic polymer for protein in a mammalian gamete culture system. *J Exp Zool* 1981;**217**:45–51.

46. Gardner DK, Rodriguez-Martinez H, Lane M. Fetal development after transfer is increased by replacing protein with the glycosaminoglycan hyaluronan for mouse embryo culture and transfer. *Hum Reprod* 1999;**14**:2575–80.

47. Swain JE, Smith GD. Advances in embryo culture platforms: novel approaches to improve preimplantation embryo development through modifications of the microenvironment. *Hum Reprod Update* 2011;**17**:541–57.

Chapter

7

Monozygotic twinning and assisted reproduction. Laboratory or clinical?

Marius Meintjes

Introduction

Assisted reproductive technologies (ART) became known as a major contributor to the worldwide epidemiological increase of twins and higher-order multiple pregnancies since the first live in vitro fertilization (IVF) birth in 1978 [1]. This increase has largely been correlated with the transfer of multiple embryos resulting in more than one dizygous (DZ) implantation. Even though the first monozygotic (MZ) twin after IVF was already reported in 1984 [2], it was not until the introduction of clinical blastocyst transfer that notice was taken of the common occurrence of MZ pregnancies. MZ twins after blastocyst transfer were first reported in the late 1990s [3]. Since then, numerous reports confirmed the observed increase in MZ twin pregnancies after blastocyst transfer [4–6] compared with what is seen after ovulation induction alone [7], cleavage stage embryo transfer, or frozen-thawed embryo transfers [8].

DZ twins are the result from the fertilization of more than one oocyte, with the twins sharing the same genetic relationship as common siblings. MZ twins are the consequence from a single fertilized oocyte splitting at some stage of early development to form two or more identical embryos, which can be considered clones of each other. The implications of unpredicted and unintended MZ pregnancies are twofold: (1) unwanted multiple pregnancies, even with single embryo transfers and (2) placental and amniotic sharing between babies, not necessarily seen with DZ multiple pregnancies. Multiple pregnancies in itself, regardless if DZ or MZ, pose significant risks to the babies such as a 50% increased chance of premature birth and a 4–7 times increase in perinatal mortality [9]. Increased risks to the mother include gestational diabetes and preeclampsia. MZ multiple pregnancies pose significant additional risk to the babies, depending on the type of placental arrangement. MZ twinning or single-zygote twinning can be considered as a pathological event and in itself a malformation [10]. MZ twins are even more likely to be delivered prematurely because of frequently being unequal in size, or to have various developmental abnormalities due to the close proximity of development and the lack of physical separation between the developing twins [11]. Monoamnionic (MA) twins (presence of two babies in the same sac without any separation, Figure 7.1) are even at higher risk for twin–twin transfusion syndrome and umbilical cord entanglement, frequently resulting in fetal demise [12].

The noticeable increase in MZ pregnancies after ART, especially after blastocyst transfer [6, 13], and the potential adverse consequences to the babies and mother as a result of an unanticipated and unsolicited MZ pregnancy, calls for the understanding of the etiology to

Culture Media, Solutions, and Systems in Human ART, ed. Patrick Quinn. Published by Cambridge University Press. © Cambridge University Press 2014.

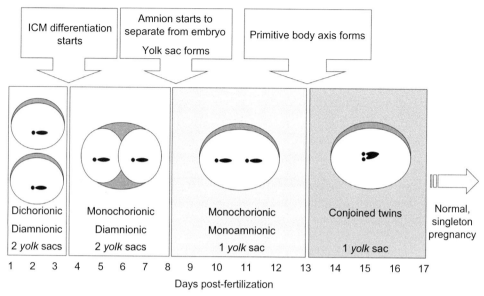

Figure 7.1 The spectrum of possible MZ placentations. The earlier the MZ splitting event, the more separated the twins will be, with less risk for complications beyond that of simple multiple gestation. The later the splitting event, the more closely associated will the placentas and twins be, proportionally increasing the risk for further complications such as twin–twin transfusion syndrome or ultimately conjoined twins – both twins laid down within one ectoderm. ICM = inner cell mass. Adapted from [8, 60].

prevent future iatrogenic MZ twinning. In addition, a better understanding of the underlying causes of MZ twinning will at least enable fertility specialists to counsel patients appropriately regarding the risk factors and consequences of MZ twinning as a consequence of ART.

The standard and most common explanation offered for the cause of observed MZ twins after ART usually centers around zona pellucida manipulation and subsequent interference with in vivo hatching after in vitro-produced embryo transfer [14–16]. Laboratory and clinical observations, for the most part, do not support this commonly held belief. A threefold increase in MZ twinning is noted after ovulation induction alone without any in vitro manipulation [7]. Several larger studies failed to observe any correlation between assisted hatching, intracytoplasmic sperm injection (ICSI), and MZ twinning even though documenting a significant increase in the MZ twinning rate [17, 18]. MZ splitting was observed in 1–2% of zona-free embryo transfers [19]. MZ twinning rates are not different between non-IVF ovulation induction and cleavage stage IVF embryo transfer, but are significantly increased when transferring blastocysts [5] and donor oocytes [8]. Double inner cell masses (ICMs) were observed in mouse blastocysts after IVF [20] and in the human [21] before any in vitro or in vivo hatching, prospectively leading to MZ twins. If zona interference of normal hatching is the cause, one will expect the most common placental type to be dichorionic (DC). On the contrary, the most common MZ placentation type observed after ART is monochorionic, diamnionic (MC-DA) [5, 8]. The different types of MZ placentations observed (dichorionic, monochorionic-diamnionic, monochorionic-monoamnionic [MC-MA], and conjoined twins, Figure 7.1) [8, 22] suggest that more than one mechanism or a combination of mechanisms during the peri-implantation period may be at work [4].

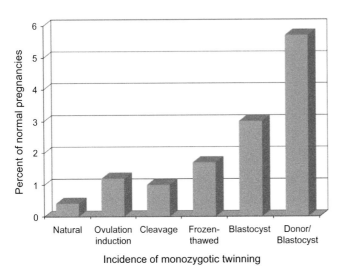

Figure 7.2 The incidence of MZ twinning as a percentage of normal pregnancies. This graph clearly demonstrates that ovulation induction without any ART increases the incidence of MZ pregnancies, and that the transfer of cleavage stage or frozen-thawed embryos does not increase the incidence any further and that blastocyst transfer in itself is responsible for a significant additional increase. Data from program data and [5, 7, 14, 23, 59]

Even though we do not have all the answers yet, certain observations or trends related to MZ twinning and ART are well documented. MZ twinning is increased about three times (from 0.4% to 1.2%) [23] after ovulation induction alone, and especially when using clomiphene citrate [24]. The ovulation induction-related increase in MZ pregnancies occurs clearly before any in vitro gamete culture or micromanipulation procedure. Furthermore, MZ twinning rates are not increased over that of ovulation induction alone when transferring cleavage stage [17, 18] or frozen-thawed embryos [25]. However, the incidence of MZ twinning significantly increases further (~3%) when transferring blastocysts [26, 27], and even more so when transferring embryos from donor oocytes (~5%) (Figure 7.2) [8].

Monochorionic placentations are much higher (>90%) [8] for ART-generated MZ pregnancies than for naturally occurring MZ pregnancies (~69%) [28]. However, based on the full spectrum of MZ placental variations observed after ART, it is clear that the timing of the MZ twinning event and the mechanism leading to the splitting of the embryo varies [4, 29, 30]. The impact of in vitro zona pellucida manipulation such as with ICSI or assisted hatching is inconclusive at best, and likely has no overall impact [17, 18]. Even so, zona-induced atypical hatching may account for the occasional mechanical splitting of a blastocyst [31], giving rise to DC, MZ twins.

MZ twinning events tend to occur in batches, with long periods of no MZ twinning followed by periods with several MZ twin pregnancies in a row [5]. Blastocyst MZ twin rates are higher (13.2%) for some programs [32] than for others (0%) [33], with significant variation in MZ rates between different ART programs [8]. MZ twin rates after blastocyst transfer has been reduced over time to match those seen after cleavage stage embryo transfer, attributed to improvements in blastocyst culture and selection [33, 34]. Blastocysts transferred after co-culture are not as prone to result in MZ pregnancies as blastocysts transferred after culturing in media alone [5, 35]. MZ twinning rates are different when embryos are cultured in different culture media or culture conditions, regardless of the day of transfer [36].

Triplets are a frequent and unwelcome occurrence in the spectrum of ART MZ pregnancies, commonly presented as a MZ twin and a DZ singleton [37]. Although less common; MC, MZ triplets after ART are not unheard of [16, 38, 39]. DZ triplets (MZ twin and one DZ singleton) are more common than MZ twins alone [18, 26, 40]. A blastocyst with two distinctive ICMs on day 5 led to DC, MZ twins when transferred [21], and a blastocyst demonstrating atypical hatching in vitro similarly resulted in DC, MZ twins [31].

Unlike natural DZ twinning rates, which vary significantly between populations (1.3/1000 in Japan; 50/1000 in Nigeria) [41], MZ twinning rates remain remarkably constant between different people groups and countries [1, 4, 42]. However, rare, familial MZ twinning does exist and can be transmitted by the father or the mother [43, 44]. In certain villages in India and Brazil, up to 5% of all births can be MZ twins [45].

In summary, the only convincing risk factors for MZ twinning supported by the literature are: (1) ovulation induction and (2) extended embryo culture. With these publications in mind, we endeavored to examine more closely 73 consecutive MZ multiple pregnancies in our own program. The objective was to identify laboratory or clinical parameters in our program that may be correlated to the increase in observed MZ pregnancies, specifically when transferring blastocysts.

Materials and methods

Data were prospectively collected for this retrospective analysis of 73 MZ pregnancies identified from 3038 consecutive pregnancies over a 5-year period. Patients considered for this study underwent IVF at one of two facilities. During the study time period, these facilities used central supplies of culture disposables, common batches of culture media from the same shipments, identical protocols, and were under the same laboratory management. These 3038 cases were clinically managed and overseen by seven different physicians with no facility or individual crossover. Follicular stimulation and luteal support protocols were not standardized.

Specific laboratory and clinical parameters were evaluated to include the following: any effect of facility (different clinical management and patients, but same supplies, equipment, and laboratory protocols); specific physician effect, regardless of the facility; embryo quality at the time of transfer; day of transfer; frozen blastocysts versus fresh blastocyst transfer; use of ICSI; patient age; the use of donor oocytes; most common as a DZ triplet pregnancy or rather occurring as pure MZ twins; placentation type; fetal gender; duration of ovarian stimulation; and the type of stimulation protocol used. Any differences in these parameters were identified using a chi-square analysis or t-test as appropriate.

Results

The 73 MZ pregnancies out of the 3038 consecutive pregnancies resulted in an overall MZ pregnancy rate of 2.4%. A wide spectrum of MZ twin placentations was observed to include 18/73 (24.7%) DC, 47/73 (64.4%) MC-DA, 7/73 (9.6%) MC-MA, and 1/73 (1.4%) conjoined twin (Table 7.1). Five of seven MC-MA pregnancies resulted in a pregnancy loss before 25 weeks of gestation. The same loss rate was not observed for the other types of placentations.

The average length of ovarian stimulation for patients with MZ IVF pregnancies (10.6 ± 1.5 days) was longer than for patients with non-MZ IVF pregnancies (10.1 ± 1.3 days; $P < 0.005$). Interestingly, there were differences in MZ pregnancy rates between physicians, with a highest rate of 4.2% (8/189) and a lowest rate of 1.8% (12/682) ($P < 0.05$). Incidentally, the patients of the physician with the highest MZ pregnancy rate also had the

Table 7.1. Monozygotic placentation types observed after 3038 consecutive IVF pregnancies

	Monochorionic	Dichorionic
Monoamnionic	8 (11%)	–
Diamnionic	47 (64.4%)	18 (24.7%)

longest duration of ovarian stimulation (10.7 days versus 9.9 days; $P < 0.0001$) compared with the physician with the lowest rate of MZ twinning.

Significantly more MZ pregnancies resulted from day-5 transfers (59/2040; 2.9%; $P < 0.008$) than from day-2/3 transfers (10/769; 1.3%) or from frozen-thawed (4/229; 1.7%) blastocyst transfers. It was more common for a MZ twin pregnancy to be associated with a third DZ singleton, resulting in a more complicated triplet pregnancy, than for twin MZ pregnancies to be present by themselves (58% versus 42%; $P < 0.05$).

No differences were observed in the overall number of MZ pregnancies between the two laboratories (2.6% versus 2.2%). Furthermore, the following had no effect on the rate of MZ multiple pregnancies: ICSI, embryo quality, patient age (33.0 ± 3.7 years), the use of donor oocytes, fetal gender, and frozen-thawed blastocyst transfers. Retrospectively, patients with MC-MA pregnancies all had one of two things in common: Slightly elevated serum progesterone during the period of ovarian stimulation (1–2 ng/mL) and/or poor quality blastocysts/morulae at the time of transfer. This was not true for patients with DC, MZ pregnancies.

Lessons from the armadillo

Armadillos are known for their precarious way of reproducing. A closer look at armadillo reproduction may be helpful to understand the phenomenon of MZ twinning in humans after ART. Armadillo babies are always one of identical quadruplets (one for each of the four teats), meaning that a litter of four is the same sex and, practically, clones of each other [46]. Armadillo identical quadruplets result from the phenomenon of polyembryony in which one sexually produced embryo splits into four [47]. The four identical quadruplets are achieved by two binary fissions along a dominant embryonic axis [48]. Should one or more of these embryos die in utero, the occasional birth of only three or two identical armadillo babies may result, instead of the customary four [49]. The six species in the specific armadillo genus *Dasypus* are the only vertebrates known to be obligatory polyembryonic [46]. However, the human also has the ability to be polyembryonic on occasion, especially after ART and blastocyst transfer.

The armadillo female ovulates and mates in late fall, the single oocyte is fertilized and then develops to the hatched blastocyst stage, before entering embryonic diapause (blastocyst entering into a dormant phase without immediate further development) [50, 51]. Embryonic diapause, unlike polyembryony, is not restricted to armadillos, but is also observed among marsupials, rodents, bears, bats, and the roe deer, among others. The period of embryonic diapause in the armadillo may last up to 2 years, but typically lasts only 3–4 months to result in the identical quadruplets being born the following spring [51].

Studies in the armadillo suggest that maternal signals may be responsible, in part, for terminating the state of blastocyst diapause and inducing polyembryony, resulting in the

100% natural incidence of MZ quadruplets [51, 52]. The four armadillo fetuses share the same MC, quadro-amnionic placenta, which is strikingly similar to that of the most commonly observed MC-DA placental type in human MZ gestations after ART. Based on the MC placental type in the armadillo, it appears that the ICM of the blastocyst is induced to split into four, likely before or shortly after hatching. The splitting event is thought to be initiated by a circulating progesterone stimulus, followed by an endometrial response through paracrine cytokines and growth factors, commencing two binary fissions along a dominant ICM axis [48].

With the armadillo being the only vertebrate with obligatory polyembryony, the striking similarity in the placentation type between armadillo quadruplets and human MZ twins after ART, and the possibility of human embryonic diapause or delayed implantation [53], one cannot ignore possible similarities in the mechanism behind polyembryony in the armadillo and in the human. Clinical observations in the human suggest that the incidence of polyembryony or MZ twinning is significantly increased after ovulation induction alone, without any in vitro exposure or zona manipulation [7]. Furthermore, the most common placentation type observed for ART-related MZ twins (MC-DA) suggests that the ICM splits within an intact trophoblast, rather than the equal division of the whole embryo. Should the whole embryo split in equal parts as expected after zona-induced atypical hatching, one should routinely observe DC, MZ twins instead of MC-DA twins.

With these striking similarities between ART-related human and natural armadillo polyembryony, one has to consider the role of circulating progesterone, subsequent endometrial paracrine signaling, and delayed implantion/dyssynchrony as possible causative factors of the epidemic of human MZ pregnancies after ART.

A proposed model

Overall, the spectrum of placentations observed suggest that the splitting event occurs at various times during embryo development, and that more than one mechanism or combinations of mechanisms may be responsible for MZ pregnancies. The high incidence of MC and even MA placentas observed strongly suggests that the underlying causes of MZ splitting after ART manifest themselves relatively late in embryogenesis, likely after embryo hatching.

In farm animals, the close synchronization of the embryo and the uterus is critical, so much so, that cleavage stage embryos will not survive a uterine transfer. Furthermore, experimental asynchronous embryo transfer in the horse and the cow confirms that there is a low tolerance for embryo–uterine asynchrony, especially if the embryo is younger than the uterus. For some reason, the human appears to be more tolerant to asynchronous uterine embryo transfers, even allowing pregnancies after uterine pronuclear transfer [54]. Hypothetically, it may be possible that the increased 1–3% of iatrogenic ovulation-induced or blastocyst-transfer MZ pregnancies represent a pathological MZ pregnancy as a result of shock brought about by embryo–endometrial dyssynchrony. If that is the case, one may expect to see MZ pregnancies more commonly when the embryos are too far delayed, the uterus too far advanced, or when enhanced by a specific patient with a genetic or physiological propensity towards MZ splitting [44]. If it were true that the pathogenesis of ART-related MZ pregnancies is mostly brought about by similar mechanisms as those documented in the armadillo, one would expect a dominance of MC-DA placentations.

This hypothesis does not exclude other less common and totally unrelated mechanisms of embryo splitting, such as atypical hatching or double ICMs, but predicts that these

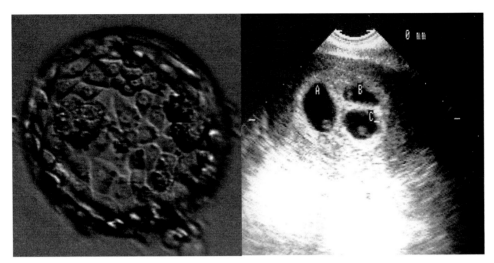

Figure 7.3 Blastocyst at the time of embryo transfer with two distinct ICMs. Mochorionic, diamnionic MZ twins were predicted at the time of transfer. The transfer of this embryo resulted in dichorionic MZ twins and a HZ triplet.

exceptional alternative mechanisms will lead to other placentation types such as DC, MZ pregnancies. Alternatively, it is possible that the same mechanism at work in the armadillo may have its effect over a critical period of several days (Figure 7.1). If so, it may be possible for this one mechanism of action to result in a broader spectrum of MC placentations, but it is still unlikely to be responsible for DC, MZ placentations.

During natural ovulation, there is no hyperstimulation or undue advancement of the endometrium. The newly fertilized embryo develops in an optimum physiological environment and is in continuous two-way communication with the oviduct, and later the uterus (Figure 7.3). During ovulation induction, the endometrium will frequently be advanced, even though continuous embryo–oviduct communication is possible. An advanced endometrium in a genetically predisposed patient may be enough to increase the incidence of MZ pregnancies threefold (~0.4%) as commonly observed in clinical practice.

Since the first successful IVF pregnancy in 1978, we have strived to achieve the same embryo quality in vitro, compared with embryo development in vivo as judged by in vitro morphology, the rate of embryo development, and, most importantly, the embryo's ability to give rise to a healthy baby after transfer. Unfortunately, with culture systems that are not yet perfect, we cannot claim with a clear conscience that we have achieved in vivo equivalency. If we assume then that embryos fertilized and cultured in vitro consistently lag behind their in vivo counterparts (Figure 7.3), it is feasible that these slower embryos may contribute to embryo–endometrial dyssyncrony, especially when faced with an already hyperstimulated endometrium. It is proposed that the transfer of slower embryos, by themselves, may be enough to increase the incidence of MZ pregnancies in susceptible patients, even in the presence of a non-hyperstimulated endometrium as expected in some frozen-thawed embryo transfer cycles.

When embryos are transferred before activation of the embryonic genome (no later than day 3), the embryo and uterine paracrine signals are reset after reestablished embryo–endometrium communication (Figure 7.4), resulting in MZ pregnancy rates no higher than those observed after ovulation induction alone (~1.2%). However, should an embryo be

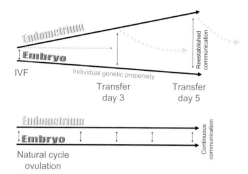

Figure 7.4 A proposed model for continuous normal embryo–endometrium communication compared with disrupted dyssyncronous communication between delayed embryos and an advanced endometrium during ART. The impact of the dyssynchrony is getting worse the longer it takes to reestablish embryo–endometrial communication. Interrupted communication and resultant dyssynchrony then ultimately lead to the pathology of a human MZ pregnancy in 1–3% of patients.

transferred after embryonic genome activation (blastocyst stage), inappropriate epigenetic changes in the embryo may be irreversible, even after reestablishing embryo-endometrial communication at transfer (Figure 7.4). With a delayed blastocyst or morula unable to respond to corrective endometrial signals and/or simply due to the longer time of separation between the blastocyst and the endometrium (increasingly divergent dyssynchronization between slow embryo and fast endometrium, Figure 7.4), an even higher rate (~3%) of MZ pregnancies may be realized.

The mechanism of action that results in ICM splitting and, therefore, MC-DA pregnancies is expected to stay the same, regardless of the day of transfer. However, the day of transfer will proportionally affect the degree of dyssynchronization (Figure 7.3) and, therefore, the expected incidence of MZ splitting. The use of donor oocyte-generated embryos introduces another variable in the quest to synchronize perfectly the in vitro-produced embryo and the recipient uterus: the donor. One would expect a less advanced endometrium than when transferring in a stimulated cycle; nevertheless, the transferred blastocyst, which may be slowed down, and the recipient endometrium are still unable to communicate for at least 5 days. A MZ pregnancy rate at the same or slightly higher level than that for fresh, non-donor blastocyst transfers is not unexpected.

While the genetic contribution of DZ twinning has been well described and varies significantly between population groups, the genetic contribution towards MZ twinning has been identified infrequently [55]. The penetrance for the MZ twinning trait seems to be very low [44]. However, with a natural MZ twin rate of ~0.4% being universal among all population groups and independent of environmental factors [7], a case can be made for a consistent genetic contribution rather than a contribution from the environment. Hereditary MZ twinning can be passed on by the mother, the father, or both [45]. In the absence of a committed gene, it may be that for a splitting event to occur, an embryo–endometrium dyssynchronization threshold must be reached to trigger the splitting signal. The specific threshold level may be subject to significant patient-to-patient variation and subject to a genetic propensity towards ICM splitting of a participating oocyte, the sperm, or the endometrium. With an extremely low penetrance level of such a trait, and the expected patient-to-patient variation, the relatively low incidence (1–3%) of MZ pregnancies observed after ART can be justified. With the same level of embryo–endometrium dyssynchronization, some patients may end up with a MZ pregnancy while others may not.

Compromised endometrial–embryo communication due to an advanced endometrium, the transfer of delayed embryos and/or an extended time period of separation between the embryo, and endometrium in genetically susceptible patients may contribute to the subsequent dyssynchrony between the uterus and embryo, being a more plausible explanation for the increased incidence of MC twinning seen after ART.

Discussion

For this model to be considered viable, it should be able to explain documented observations in literature related to MZ pregnancies after ART. Ovulation induction alone increases the incidence of MZ pregnancies, even before in vitro manipulation or culture [7]. When using clomiphene citrate only for ovulation induction, a significantly greater proportion (MZ twins:all twins) of MZ twins was observed when compared with cases where gonadotropins were used (12% versus 3.6%). The anti-estrogenic effect of clomiphene is known to have a direct negative effect on the endometrium. Based on the model, an inadvertent dyssynchronization or advancement of the endometrium secondary to ovarian stimulation may be enough to trigger a splitting event in susceptible patients.

MZ twinning rates are similarly increased after cleavage stage embryo transfer [17, 18] and frozen-thawed embryo transfers [25]; however, no more than with ovulation induction alone. This suggests that the increased rate of MZ pregnancies after cleavage stage transfers has little to do with in vitro culture or manipulation, but rather is a direct consequence of the unwanted endometrial effect resulting from the initial ovarian stimulation. When transferring frozen-thawed cleavage stage embryos or blastocysts, it is assumed that all thawed embryos are going to be at a perfectly matched morphological and physiological state, and the endometrium is prepared accordingly. In reality, when these embryos are thawed, they will represent a range of qualities, developmental stages, and levels of post-thaw survival and, for blastocysts, might even have been frozen on different days of development (day 5 or day 6). With this much developmental variation present in the post-thaw embryos, the increased rate of embryo splitting seen after non-stimulated transfers can be expected due to the embryos lagging behind a fixed-state endometrium.

When transferring blastocysts, however, the rate of MZ twinning is increased further over that of ovulation induction alone [26, 27], significantly more so than when transferring cleavage stage or frozen-thawed embryos. The same was observed in our program, where significantly more MZ pregnancies resulted from day-5 transfers than from cleavage stage transfers. According to the model this is to be expected, as under this circumstance, we expect an advanced endometrium due to ovarian stimulation as well as possibly delayed embryo development due to extended, and sometimes, suboptimum culture conditions. Furthermore, even if we do achieve optimum embryo development, the embryo and endometrium are now separated for up to 6 days, without the possibility to communicate and reestablish synchronized development. In contrast, continuous corrective communication is possible under natural conditions or, the lack thereof, at least attenuated after earlier cleavage stage embryo transfer. If substantiated, this will also explain why the impact of in vitro zona pellucida manipulation, such as ICSI or assisted hatching, is inconclusive at best [17, 18].

In our program, blastocysts are routinely thawed 12–15 hours before transfer. Furthermore, all frozen blastocysts are treated as day-5 blastocysts, regardless of the day of cryopreservation. These measures are an attempt to normalize possible blastocyst–endometrium dyssynchronization, resulting from slower in vitro embryos. Interestingly, when thawing in advance, MZ pregnancy rates for frozen-thawed blastocysts are not significantly different than those observed after ovulation induction alone or after fresh cleavage stage embryo transfer in our program or in others (Figure 7.2) [18, 25].

It is observed that the proportion of MC placentations is much higher (>90%) [8] for ART-generated MZ pregnancies than for naturally occurring MZ pregnancies (~69%) [28]. Based on the full spectrum of MZ placental variations observed in nature and after ART, we have to assume that the timing of the MZ twinning event and the mechanism leading to the splitting of the embryo varies [4, 29, 30]. However, MC, MZ pregnancies are still the most common placental type, regardless of whether they are naturally occurring or a consequence of ART. This suggests that the underlying causes of the most common type of MZ splitting in the human manifest themselves relatively late in embryogenesis, likely after embryo hatching. However, in our program, the proportion of MC, MZ pregnancies (75.3% of all MZ pregnancies; Table 7.1) was not higher than that reported in literature for naturally conceived pregnancies. It may be that the proportion of MC pregnancies is artificially inflated due to the underdiagnosis of DC, MZ pregnancies after ART [24]. During ART, the transfer of multiple embryos is the rule rather than the exception. Therefore, DC twins can easily be missed after the transfer of more than one embryo, followed by the ultrasonic confirmation of only two implantations.

According to the proposed model, it is accepted that the less frequently observed DC, MZ pregnancies (~25%) might be a different manifestation of the same underlying causes, or; more likely, that other mechanisms have their effect on the embryo during earlier developmental stages in vivo or in vitro. The occasional zona-induced, atypical hatching and mechanical splitting of a blastocyst [31] or the observance of a double ICM [21] will fit in this category. Atypical hatching or double ICMs will be non-routine causes of ART-related MZ pregnancies; and as expected, mostly result in DC, MZ pregnancies.

Armadillos always have a MC, quadro-amnionic placenta, with the timing of obligatory ICM splitting and subsequent MC placental formation linked to very specific circulating (progesterone) as well as paracrine signals from the uterus. Considering the similar MC-DA placenta type in the human, this sequence of events identified in the armadillo may not be unlike what is predicted in the human when the endometrium is advanced relatively to the embryo; or when the embryo and endometrium are separated and unable to communicate over an extended period of time (also progesterone related). Monochorionic placentations, being most-frequently observed among human MZ pregnancies, suggest that the most common cause of these MZ pregnancies after ART is a dyssynchrony between the embryo and endometrium, manifested only after embryo transfer [4, 24].

Ovulation induction is known to lead to an advanced endometrium [56] and an alteration in endometrial receptivity [57] as evidenced by elevated serum progesterone levels during stimulation and histopathology. For many years now, we have been faced with overcoming the suboptimum development of in vitro-produced embryos, being more difficult the longer we keep these embryos in culture. When encountering a MC, MZ pregnancy, one would expect to see evidence of slow embryos, an advanced endometrium, or both according to this model. In our study all 55 patients with MC, MZ pregnancies had one of two things in common: slightly elevated serum progesterone (1–2 ng/mL) during stimulation and/or poor quality blastocysts/morulae for transfer. The progesterone levels were not elevated and the embryos were not necessarily slow for patients with DC, MZ pregnancies. These observations fit with a hypothesis that the same mechanisms at work in the armadillo may be responsible for MC-DA pregnancies in the human after ART.

It is frequently noted that MZ twinning events occur in batches with long periods of no MZ twinning, followed by periods with several MZ twin pregnancies in a row [5]. Adverse events in the laboratory such as a period of poor air quality, a suboptimum batch of media/macromolecular supplement, or a drifting incubator may result in batches of compromised embryos, explaining the serial occurrence of ART-related MZ pregnancies in susceptible patients. This will also explain why there are significant variations in MZ rates between different ART programs [8]. Following improvements in laboratory and culture conditions, MZ pregnancy rates after blastocyst transfer may then be reduced over time to match those seen after cleavage stage embryo transfer [34, 58]. However, even with optimum blastocyst culture conditions in the best laboratories, the blastocyst-transfer MZ pregnancy rate could not be reduced to less than that seen with cleavage stage embryo transfer or with ovulation induction alone. This fits the model, as improved culture conditions do not completely address the advanced endometrium, delayed communication between the blastocyst and the endometrium, or the subsequent embryo–endometrial dyssynchrony.

It was reported that blastocysts transferred after co-culture were not as prone to result in MZ pregnancies as those blastocysts transferred after culturing in media alone [5, 35]. At the time of that study, improved quality blastocysts could routinely be produced using co-culture compared with blastocysts produced without co-culture in the blastocyst culture media of the time, likely attenuating the embryo–endometrium dyssynchrony when co-cultured. Similarly, it was shown that MZ twinning rates are different when embryos are cultured in different culture media or culture conditions, regardless of the day of transfer [36]. The lower MZ pregnancy rates were observed in the better culture conditions. Similarly, it is likely that better quality blastocysts reduce the asynchronous shock between embryo and endometrium.

DZ triplets (MZ twin and one DZ singleton) are more common than MZ twins [18, 26, 40] after ART. Similarly, in our program, it was more common for a MZ twin pregnancy to be associated with a third DZ singleton than for twin MZ pregnancies to be present by themselves. Frequently, when transferring poor quality day-5 blastocysts or morulae, two or three embryos are transferred. In contrast, an elective single blastocyst transfer typically is performed when confronted with an excellent quality blastocyst for transfer. Although rare, MC, MZ triplets are occasionally observed [16, 38, 39]. The most feasible explanation for MC, MZ triplets in the human is that they are formed by the same mechanism as the identical quadruplets in the armadillo. In the armadillo, the four identical quadruplets are achieved by two binary fissions along a dominant axis [48]. If one of these embryos dies in utero after the process of binary fusion in the human, MC, MZ triplets will be the result.

In our own program, the longer length of ovarian stimulation for patients with MZ pregnancies compared with the patients with non-MZ, IVF pregnancies strongly suggested an endometrial contribution. Similarly, the observed differences in MZ pregnancy rates between physicians directly correlated with the length of ovarian stimulation for each physician. The physician with the highest MZ pregnancy rate stimulated his patients, on average, almost one day longer than the other physicians. According to the model, it is feasible that the longer stimulations resulted in a more advanced endometrium and, therefore, an increased risk for MZ pregnancies. The concept of a more advanced endometrium with longer stimulations is supported by the consistent, albeit moderate, increase of serum progesterone during stimulation for all the MC pregnancies. As expected, this was not true for DC, MZ pregnancies.

If the notion of embryo–endometrial dyssynchronization as the most common under-lying cause for ART-related MZ pregnancies is true, we should find very little evidence of a contribution of in vitro zona micromanipulation such as assisted hatching or ICSI [59]. As expected, most larger studies and meta-analyses fail to observe any correlation between assisted hatching, ICSI, and MZ twinning, even though consistently documenting a signifi-cant increase in the MZ twinning rate after blastocyst transfer [17, 18]. Results from our study as well as the literature fail to support specific laboratory factors as a cause of MZ multiple gestation.

Even though very rare, we must keep in mind that hereditary MZ twinning can be transmitted by the father or the mother [43, 44]. Therefore, it can be assumed that some patients may be genetically prone to embryo splitting after ART if subjected to a certain threshold of embryo–endometrial dyssynchronization.

In summary, the two most convincing risk factors for MZ twinning supported by reputable studies still are: (1) ovulation induction and (2) extended embryo culture, which fit this model very well. Ovulation induction represents a sure way to advance the endometrium. Extended culture, especially under less-than-perfect culture conditions, is likely to result in delayed and suboptimum quality blastocysts, which do not have an opportunity to communicate with the advanced endometrium to reestablish synchrony for at least five to six days. When only one of these variables is affected such as observed with ovulation induction alone (advanced endometrium) or with frozen-thawed blastocyst transfers (delayed embryos), a threefold increase of MZ pregnancies can be expected. When both of these variables are affected (advanced endometrium and delayed embryos), for example when transferring fresh blastocysts, a further doubling of the already threefold increase in MZ pregnancies is predicted. Indeed, after blastocyst transfer, the incidence of MZ pregnancies is increased about seven times over what is commonly seen in the natural population.

How then to counter the epidemic of MZ pregnancies resulting from ART? It appears that a two-pronged approach is required as both the advanced endometrium and the tardy embryos should be addressed. Physicians should experiment with different stimulation protocols and consider milder stimulations (slower endometrium) to reduce or remove the impact of an advanced endometrium on an already compromised blastocyst. With the advent of successful blastocyst vitrification, banking all of the blastocysts for later transfer in an optimized, non-stimulated endometrium may now be feasible. Furthermore, these cryo-banked blastocysts may be warmed slightly in advance to ensure a bias towards more advanced embryos. Newer technologies, such as time-lapse photography, non-invasive culture medium screening, and the genetic screening of embryos, may allow for the earlier day-2 or day-3 transfer of embryos, with resulting similar or better implantation rates as blastocysts. The earlier transfers will allow for a timelier reestablishment of embryo–endometrial communication and synchronization. To ensure the best possible quality blastocysts available for transfer, all should be done to optimize the culture conditions. Optimized culture conditions should include the consideration of low-oxygen culture through all stages of embryo development, growth factor culture medium supplementation, the use of physiological culture media, optimized macromolecular culture medium supple-mentation, and incubation equipment capable of most reliably resembling the natural environment.

Realizing that the most probable etiology of MZ pregnancies after ART has to do with the dyssynchronization of the embryo and endometrium rather than zona pellucida hardening and zona manipulation, we may be able to identify the specific signals and pathways responsible for triggering the splitting event in blastocysts. With that knowledge, specific treatment protocols can be developed to block or alter these signals and to reduce or eliminate eventually the all too frequent and unwelcome occurrence of ART-related MZ pregnancies.

References

1. Imaizumi Y. A comparative study of zygotic twinning and triplet rates in eight countries, 1972–1999. *J Biosoc Sci* 2003;**35** (2):287–302.

2. Yovich JL, Stanger JD, Grauaug A, *et al.* Monozygotic twins from in vitro fertilization. *Fertil Steril* 1984;**41**(6):833–7.

3. Peramo B, Ricciarelli E, Cuadros-Fernandez JM, *et al.* Blastocyst transfer and monozygotic twinning. *Fertil Steril* 1999;**72** (6):1116–17.

4. Aston KI, Peterson CM, Carrell DT. Monozygotic twinning associated with assisted reproductive technologies: a review. *Reproduction* 2008;**136**:377–86.

5. Behr B, Fisch JD, Racowsky C, *et al.* Blastocyst-ET and monozygotic twinning. *J Assist Reprod Genet* 2000;**17**(6):349–51.

6. Kawachiya S, Bodri D, Shimada N, *et al.* Blastocyst culture is associated with an elevated incidence of monozygotic twinning after single embryo transfer. *Fertil Steril* 2011;**95**(6):2140–2.

7. Derom C, Vlietinck R, Derom R, *et al.*, Increased monozygotic twinning rate after ovulation induction. *Lancet* 1987;**8544**:1236–8.

8. Knopman J, Krey LC, Lee J, *et al.* Monozygotic twinning: an eight-year experience at a large IVF center. *Fertil Steril* 2010;**94**(2):502–10.

9. Minakami H, Honma Y, Matsubara S, *et al.* Effects of placental chorionicity on outcome in twin pregnancies. *J Reprod Med* 1999;**44**:595–9.

10. Cameron AH, Edwards JH, Derom R, *et al.* The value of twin surveys in the study of malformations. *Eur J Obstet Gynecol Reprod Biol* 1983;**14**:347–56.

11. Honma Y, Minakami H, Eguchi Y, *et al.* Relation between hemoglobin discordance and adverse outcome in monozygotic twins. *Acta Obstet Gynecol Scand* 1999;**78**:207–11.

12. Bulla M, Von Lilien T, Goecke H, *et al.* Renal and cerebral necrosis in survivor of in-utero fetal death of co-twin. *Arch Gynecol* 1987;**240**:119–24.

13. Sharara FI, Abdo G. Incidence of monozygotic twins in blastocyst and cleavage stage assisted reproductive technology cycles. *Fertil Steril* 2010;**93** (2):642–5.

14. Shieve LA, Meikle SF, Peterson HB, *et al.* Does assisted hatching pose a risk for monozygotic twinning in pregnancies conceived through in vitro fertilization? *Fertil Steril* 2000;**74**(2):288–94.

15. Sills ES, Tucker MJ, Palermo GD. Assisted reproductive technologies and monozygotic twins: implications for future study and clinical practice. *Twin Res* 2000;**3** (4):217–23.

16. Pantos K, Kokkali G, Petroutsou K, *et al.* Monochorionic triplet and monoamniotic twins gestation after intracytoplasmic sperm injection and laser-assisted hatching. *Fetal Diagn Ther* 2009;**25**(1):144–7.

17. Sills ES, Moomjy M, Zaninovic N, *et al.* Human zona pellucida micromanipulation and monozygotic twinning frequency after IVF. *Hum Reprod* 2000;**15**(4):890–5.

18. Schachter M, Raziel A, Friedler S, *et al.* Monozygotic twinning after assisted reproductive techniques: a phenomenon independent of micromanipulation. *Hum Reprod* 2001;**16**(6):1264–9.

19. Frankfurter D, Trimarchi J, Hackett R, *et al.* Monozygotic pregnancies from transfers of zona-free blastocysts. *Fertil Steril* 2004;**82**:483–5.

20. Chida S. Monozygous double inner cell masses in mouse blastocysts following fertilization in vitro and in vivo. *J In Vitro Fert Embryo Transf* 1990;**7**(3):177–9.

21. Meintjes M, Guerami AR, Rodriguez JA, *et al.* Prospective identification of an in vitro-assisted monozygotic pregnancy based on a double-inner-cell-mass blastocyst. *Fertil Steril* 2001;**76**(3) Suppl 1: S172–3.

22. Allegra A, Monni G, Zoppi MA, *et al.* Cojoined twins in a trichorionic quadruplet pregnancy after intracytoplasmic sperm injection and quarter laser-assisted zona thinning. *Fertil Steril* 2007;**87**(1):189.

23. Bulmer MG. *The Biology of Twinning in Man.* Oxford, Clarendon Press, 1970.

24. Derom C, Leroy F, Vlietinck R, *et al.* High frequency of iatrogenic monozygotic twins with administration of clomiphene citrate and a change in chorionicity. *Fertil Steril* 2006;**85**(3):755–7.

25. Domitrz J, Wolczynski S, Syrewicz M, *et al.* Monozygotic pregnancy after the treatment for infertility by transfer of frozen-thawed embryos. *Ginekol Pol* 1999;**70**(1):13–19.

26. Milki AA, Jun SH, Hinckley MD, *et al.* Incidence of monozygotic twinning with blastocyst transfer compared to cleavage-stage transfer. *Fertil Steril* 2003;**79**:503–6.

27. Chang HJ, Lee JR, Jee BC, *et al.* Impact of blastocyst transfer on offspring sex ratio and the monozygotic twinning rate: a systematic review and meta-analysis. *Fertil Steril* 2009;**91**(6):2381–90.

28. Paek B, Shields LE. Twin-to-twin transfusion syndrome: diagnosis and treatment. *Curr Woman Health Rev* 2005, **1**:43–7.

29. Scott L. The origin of monozygotic twinning. *Reprod Biomed Online* 2002;**5**:276–84.

30. Alikani M, Cekliniak NA, Walters E, *et al.* Monozygotic twinning following assisted conception: an analysis of 81 consecutive cases. *Hum Reprod* 2003;**18**(9):1937–43.

31. Van Lagendonckt A, Wyns C, Godin PA, *et al.* Atypical hatching of a human blastocyst leading to monozygotic twinning: a case report. *Fertil Steril* 2000;**74**(5):1047–50.

32. Jain JK, Boostanfar R, Slater CC, *et al.* Monozygotic twins and triplets in association with blastocyst transfer. *J Assist Reprod Genet* 2004;**21**:103–7.

33. Papanikalaou EG, Fatemi H, Venetis C, *et al.* Monozygotic twinning is not increased after single blastocyst transfer compared with single cleavage-stage embryo transfer. *Fertil Steril* 2010;**93**(2):592–7.

34. Moayeri SE, Behr B, Lathi RB, *et al.* Risk of monozygotic twinning with blastocyst transfer decreases over time. An 8-year experience. *Fertil Steril* 2007;**5**:1028–32.

35. Menezo YZ, Sakkas D. Monozygotic twinning is related to apoptosis in the embryo? *Hum Reprod* 2002;**17**:247–8.

36. Cassuto G, Chavrier M, Menezo YZ. Culture conditions and not prolonged culture time are responsible for monozygotic twinning in human in vitro fertilization. *Fertil Steril* 2003;**80**:462–3.

37. Yanaihara A, Yorimitsu T, Motoyama H, *et al.* Monozygotic multiple gestation following in vitro fertilization: analysis of seven cases from Japan. *J Exp Clin Assist Reprod* 2007;**4**:4.

38. Ferreira M, Bos-Mikich A, Höner M, *et al.* Dichorionic twins and monochorionic triplets after the transfer of two blastocysts. *J Assist Reprod Genet* 2010;**9–10**:545–8.

39. Dessolle L, Allaoua D, Freour T, *et al.* Monozygotic triplet pregnancies after single blastocyst transfer: two cases and literature review. *Reprod Biomed Online* 2010;**21**(3):283–9.

40. Elizur SE, Levron J, Shrim A, *et al.* Monozygotic twinning is not associated with zona pellucida micromanipulation procedures but increases with high-order pregnancies. *Fertil Steril* 2004;**82**(2):500–1.

41. MacGillivary I. Epidemiology of twin pregnancy. *Semin Perinatol* 1986;**10**:4–8.

42. Hall JG. Twinning. *Lancet* 2003;**362**:735–43.

43. Unger S, Hoopmann M, Bald R, *et al.* Monozygotic triplets and monozygotic twins after ICSI and transfer of two blastocysts: case report. *Hum Reprod* 2003;**19**(1):110–13.

44. Steinman G. Mechanisms of twinning. VI. Genetics and etiology of monozygotic

twinning in in vitro fertilization. *J Reprod Med* 2003;**48**(8):583–90.

45. Cyranoski D. Developmental biology: two by two. *Nature* 2009;**458**:826–9.

46. Loughry WJ, Prodöhl PA, McDonough CM, et al. Polyembryony in Armadillos. *Am Scientist* 1998;**86**:274–9.

47. Prodöhl PA, Loughry WJ, McDonough CM, Nelson WS, Avise JC. Molecular documentation of polyembryony and the micro-spatial dispersion of clonal sibships in the nine-banded armadillo, *Dasypus novemcinctus*. *Proc Biol Sci* 1996;**263** (1377):1643–9.

48. Blickstein I, Keith LG. On the possible cause of monozygotic twinning: lessons from the 9-banded armadillo and from assisted reproduction. *Twin Res Hum Genet* 2006;**10**(2):394–9.

49. Li Y, Yang D, Zhang Q. Dichorionic quadramnionic quadruple gestation with monochorionic triamnionic triplets after two embryos transferred and selective reduction of twin pregnancy: case report. *Fertil Steril* 2009;**92**(6):2038.

50. Peppler RD, Canale J. Quantitive investigation of the annual pattern of follicular development in the nine-banded armadillo (*Dasypus novemcinctus*). *J Reprod Fertil* 1980;**59**(1):193–7.

51. Lopez FL, Desmarais JA, Murphy BD. Embryonic diapause and its regulation. *Reproduction* 2004;**128**:669–78.

52. Bagatto B, Crossley DA, Burggren WW. Physiological variability in neonatal armadillo quadruplets: within- and between-litter differences. *J Exp Biol* 2000;**203**(11):1733–40.

53. Tarin JJ, Cano A. Do human concepti have the potential to enter into diapause? *Hum Reprod* 1999;**14**:2434–6.

54. Warnes GM, Quinn P, Kirby CA, et al. The effect of transferring pronuclear embryos on pregnancy outcome after in vitro fertilization. *Ann N Y Acad Sci* 1988;**541**:465–71.

55. Hamamy MB, Ajlouni HK, Ajlouni KM. Familial monozygotic twinning: report of an extended multi-generation family. *Twin Res* 2004;**7**:219–22.

56. Bazy P, Ghaffari M, Soleimanirad J, et al. Morphometrical effects of the effects of ovulation induction drugs in long protocol on ultrastructure of human endometrial epithelium during the implantation window. *J Reprod Infertil* 2004;**5**(2):105–14.

57. Valbuena D, Jasper M, Remohi J, et al. Ovarian stimulation and endometrial receptivity. *Hum Reprod* 1999;**14**(Suppl 2):107–11.

58. Papanikalaou EG, Camus M, Kolibianakis EM, et al. In vitro fertilization with single blastocyst-stage versus single cleavage-stage embryos. *N Engl J Med* 2006;**354**:1139–46.

59. Abusheika N, Salha O, Sharma V, et al. Monozygotic twinning and IVF/ICSI treatment: a report of 11 cases and review of literature. *Hum Reprod Update* 2000;**6**(4):396–403.

60. Machin GA, Keith LG. *An Atlas of Multiple Pregnancy. Biology and Pathology.* New York, Parthenon Publishing. 1999;99.

Chapter

8

Amino acids and ammonium

Deirdre Zander-Fox and Michelle Lane

Introduction

The introduction of amino acids to the culture media for the mammalian oocyte and embryo is arguably the most important advance made in regards to the successful culture of viable embryos. Currently all media for the culture of human embryos contain amino acids as a core component of their formulation. Amino acids are molecules containing an amine group (NH_2) as well as a carboxylic acid group (COOH) and a variable side chain. In mammals there are 20 proteinogenic amino acids that are naturally incorporated into polypeptides within the body, while some other organisms have 22 (Table 8.1). Traditionally amino acids have been shown to be important in cellular metabolism and in many organisms as energy substrates and osmolytes. However, there is growing evidence in other tissues that amino acids are able to control many cellular functions including regulation of cell signaling and gene expression. Interestingly, although it is clear that their addition to a culture medium formulation improves embryo development and viability, the cellular function of amino acids in regulating embryo development is largely unknown. This chapter will review the current knowledge and history of the use of amino acids in culture media for the mammalian embryo as well as the in vitro artifact of by-product accumulation of ammonium in the medium.

Amino acids in the reproductive tract

The first hint to the importance of amino acids for the development of the mammalian embryo came from early analyses of the reproductive tract which identified the presence of high levels of amino acids within oviduct and uterine fluid [1–6]. There was a large degree of homology in the composition of amino acids between all species [5]. Throughout the lumen of the tract, glycine is the most abundant amino acid comprising up to 50% of the total amino acid pool [5]. Alanine, asparagine, glutamate, glycine, taurine, and threonine are present at relatively high concentrations in the female tract whilst other amino acids are present at lower or trace levels (Table 8.2). It is also evident that the levels of amino acids in the reproductive tract alter both with the estrous cycle, the presence of an embryo, and also between the oviduct and uterus [5, 7]. Interestingly, the amino acids at high levels in the tracts, glycine, taurine, alanine, glutamate, serine, and aspartate, are also present in high concentrations in oocytes and embryos themselves [8] as well as in the blastocoelic fluid of the blastocyst [5, 9].

It is of interest that the amino acids found at highest concentrations in the lumen of the female reproductive tract show a large degree of homology with those defined by Eagle as

Culture Media, Solutions, and Systems in Human ART, ed. Patrick Quinn. Published by Cambridge University Press. © Cambridge University Press 2014.

Table 8.1. Proteinogenic amino acid reference list including name, abbreviation, molecular weight, and chemical properties

	Amino acid	Abbreviation		Molecular weight (kDa)	Eagle's tissue culture classification	Chemical properties
		Long	Short			
1	Alanine	Ala	A	89	Non	Non-polar, hydrophobic, aliphatic
2	Arginine	Arg	R	174	Ess	Polar, basic
3	Asparagine	Asn	N	132	Non	Polar neutral, uncharged
4	Aspartic acid	Asp	D	133	Non	Polar, acidic
5	Cytesine	Cys	C	121	Ess	Polar neutral, uncharged
6	Glutamic acid	Glu	E	147	Non	Polar, acidic
7	Glutamine	Gln	Q	146	Non	Polar neutral, uncharged
8	Glycine	Gly	G	75	Non	Polar, uncharged
9	Histidine	His	H	155	Ess	Polar, basic
10	Isoleucine	Ile	I	131	Ess	Non-polar, hydrophobic, aliphatic
11	Leucine	Leu	L	131	Ess	Non-polar, hydrophobic, aliphatic
12	Lysine	Lys	K	146	Ess	Polar, basic
13	Methionine	Met	M	149	Ess	Non-polar, hydrophobic
14	Phenylalanine	Phe	F	131	Ess	Non-polar, hydrophobic, aromatic
15	Proline	Pro	P	115	Non	Non-polar, hydrophobic
16	Serine	Ser	S	105	Non	Polar neutral, uncharged
17	Threonine	Thr	T	119	Ess	Polar neutral, uncharged
18	Tryptophan	Trp	W	204	Ess	Non-polar, hydrophobic, aromatic
19	Tyrosine	Tyr	Y	181	Ess	Polar, uncharged, aromatic
20	Valine	Val	V	117	Non	Non-polar, hydrophobic, Aliphatic
21	Selenocytosine*	Se-Cys	U	168		Polar, uncharged,
22	Pyrrolysine*	Pyl	O	255		
	Taurine**	Tau		125		Non-proteinogenic amino acid

 * Selenocytosine and pyrrolysine are currently not added to embryo culture media
** Taurine is a non-proteinogenic amino acid; however, due to its abundance in the reproductive tract it is added to culture media.

Table 8.2. Comparison of the amino acid composition of fluid from the female reproductive tract of several species

	Human serum (mM)	Bovine oviduct (mM)	Ovine oviduct (mM)	Murine oviduct (mM)	Ovine uterus (mM)	Rabbit uterus (mM)	Murine uterus (mM)
Non-essential amino acids							
Alanine	0.289	0.51	0.45	2.5	0.39	2.8	1.3
Asparagine	0.043	0.35	–	0.23	–	–	0.09
Aspartate	0.019	0.05	0.097	0.93	0.22	0.28	0.43
Glutamate	0.055	0.36	0.43	1.37	0.42	3.36	1.69
Glutamine	0.468	–	–	1.44	–	–	0.47
Glycine	0.215	0.78	1.42	3.22	0.69	4.15	1.38
Proline	0.169	–	–	–	–	–	–
Serine	0.118	0.04	0.017	0.59	0.04	1.09	0.26
Arginine	0.084	–	0.13	0.05	0.23	0.3	0.03
Essential amino acids							
Cysteine	0.087	0.01	Trace	–	Trace	–	–
Histidine	0.078	0.08	0.11	0.18	0.10	0.23	0.07
Isoleucine	0.065	0.11	0.11	0.20	0.12	0.21	0.12
Leucine	0.116	0.14	0.24	0.38	0.28	0.49	0.22
Lysine	0.187	0.31	0.29	0.26	0.28	0.26	0.24
Methionine	0.026	0.04	0.06	0.17	0.05	0.32	0.08
Phenylalanine	0.050	0.07	0.14	0.20	0.11	0.11	0.12
Threonine	0.137	–	Trace	0.80	Trace	1.85	0.33
Tryptophan	–	–	trace	0.05	trace	–	0.05
Tyrosine	0.052	0.05	0.01	0.25	0.01	0.12	0.14
Valine	0.197	0.18	0.27	0.35	0.41	0.33	0.21
Taurine	–	–	0.8	6.64	0.1	3.41	3.76

non-essential amino acids for the development of somatic cells in culture (Table 8.2) [10]. In contrast, those required for the normal growth and development of somatic cells in culture, defined by Eagle as essential amino acids [10], are present at either low or trace concentrations in fluid of the female reproductive tract (Table 8.2).

Amino acid transport in oocytes and embryos

Several studies have assessed the activity of amino acid transporters within the developing embryo to establish their role in regulating amino acid uptake. It is clear that the preimplantation embryo possesses several transport systems for amino acids including Na^+-dependent transporters for zwitterionic amino acids, BO+ as well as those used for the regulation of volume, β-amino acid transporters, Gly transporters, and SIT1 transporters [11–15]. Correlations between developmental changes in Na^+-dependent transport activities for taurine, glycine, and aspartate and changes in internal content of these amino acids within the embryo have previously been demonstrated [16]. Similarly, the amino acid content of the blastocyst increases when cultured in the presence of glycine, alanine, glutamine, taurine, and glutamate from the 2-cell stage, and systems for their transport are present during preimplantation development [17, 18]. Amino acid transport systems of the precompaction stage embryo differ substantially to the post-compaction embryo, suggesting differences in amino acid requirements at different stages of development.

Amino acids in embryo culture media for embryos

Initial attempts to culture the mammalian embryo in vitro routinely used a medium lacking amino acids, with compositions most commonly consisting of balanced salt solutions with the triad of carbohydrates pyruvate, lactate, and glucose. Mammalian embryos, including human embryos, can develop to the blastocyst stage in the absence of amino acids; however, development is delayed, blastocysts exhibit perturbed gene expression including an altered epigenome all culminating in substantially reduced viability. Additionally, amino acid-free media for culturing mouse embryos reduces fetal growth rates as well as affecting offspring health and cognitive function. Even a brief exposure to medium lacking amino acids (5 minutes) can deplete the intracellular amino acid stores, impairing blastocyst development and cell number [19].

One of the first studies on the effect of amino acids in culture media reported that the four amino acids glutamine, phenylalanine, methionine, and isoleucine were essential for hamster oocyte maturation in vitro [20]. Furthermore, glutamine was shown to stimulate rabbit oocyte maturation [21]. These same four amino acids were able to support the cleavage of hamster zygotes to the 2-cell stage [22] and also enabled hamster embryos to overcome the 8-cell block to development in vitro [23]. However, it was not until the 1990s that work on amino acids in the culture medium for mammalian embryos began in earnest. Studies of individual amino acids asparagine, aspartate, glycine, serine, and taurine demonstrated stimulation of blastocyst formation and cell number, whilst cysteine, isoleucine, leucine, phenylalanine, tyrosine, and valine all inhibited embryo development in culture [24, 25]. Subsequently, the importance of amino acid inclusion in embryo culture media has been demonstrated in a variety of species, including mice [26–31], hamster [32, 33], cattle [34], sheep [35], and human [36], with improvements in rates of development, molecular and metabolic health, and viability.

One approach to examining the role of amino acids on embryo development was to consider those amino acids found at the highest concentrations in the female reproductive tract (alanine, aspartate, glutamate, glutamine, glycine, and serine). These amino acids have considerable homology with those defined by Eagle as non-essential amino acids (Table 8.1). Supplementation of culture medium with non-essential amino acids and glutamine, for the development of mouse zygotes, stimulated both blastocyst formation and cell number in vitro and increased viability [26, 35]. In contrast, the amino acids which are present at low or trace concentrations in the reproductive tract (Eagle's essential amino acids) inhibited cleavage stage development; however, essential amino acids were shown to be important in the development of later stage embryos after compaction. In particular, their presence in culture media stimulates the development of the inner cell mass (ICM) and significantly improves viability after transfer [28, 37].

Similar results of improved embryo and blastocyst development and quality due to the addition of specific amino acids during different stages of embryo development have also been shown in the sheep and cow [35, 38–40]. Supplementation of culture medium with Eagle's non-essential amino acids stimulated sheep blastocyst formation [35], whilst culture with Eagle's 20 amino acids stimulated both blastocyst formation and cell number and resulted in pregnancy rates equivalent to in vivo developed controls [35]. In addition, the development of cattle zygotes derived from in vitro maturation and fertilization to the blastocyst stage is stimulated by the presence of 20 Eagle's amino acids [41, 42]. Further, a study on human embryos demonstrated that embryo development to the blastocyst stage was increased with provision of non-essential amino acids for cleavage development and all 20 amino acids for post-compaction development, significantly increasing blastocyst cell number and reducing apoptosis [36].

There have been several studies investigating the role of glutamine in preimplantation embryo development. Glutamine is an important amino acid in the culture of many somatic cells as it can be used both as an energy source and as a precursor for macromolecules [43]. The importance of glutamine in the culture media to stimulate embryo development has been demonstrated for many species [32, 33, 44–46], including the human [47, 48]. In addition, preimplantation embryos can take up [49, 50] and metabolize glutamine [51–53] from the culture medium and glutamine has been shown to be important in the regulation of reactive oxygen species in the pig [46].

The amino acid taurine is one of the most abundant amino acids in the female reproductive tract. Studies on the mouse embryo revealed that taurine when present as the sole amino acid stimulated oocyte maturation as well as blastocyst formation and cell number [54, 55]. Taurine as the sole amino acid has also been shown to stimulate the development of pig embryos in vitro [56] while hypotaurine, a derivative of taurine, has been shown to be particularly important for hamster in vitro embryo development [57]. Taurine has also been shown to stimulate human blastocyst development when present as the sole amino acid [48].

Currently commercially available media for the culture of the human embryo all contain amino acids as a core ingredient. Most culture systems use a sequential provision of amino acids beginning with non-essential amino acids and glutamine (stable derivative) for the first phase of culture, often with the addition of a more complex composition of amino acids (20 amino acids) for development to the blastocyst stage. This sequential provision of amino acids has enabled routine development to the blastocyst stage of human embryos, with high rates of viability.

Traditional functions of amino acids

It has been thought for many years that the improvement in embryo development that occurs when embryos are cultured in the presence of amino acids is likely a result of their roles as energy substrates, osmolytes, and chelators (usually those described as Eagle's non-essential amino acids) and as substrates for protein (non-essential and essential amino acids) (Figure 8.1).

Most organisms have a highly conserved mechanism for the protection of cells from osmotic stress utilizing organic solutes; either non-essential amino acids, methylamines, or

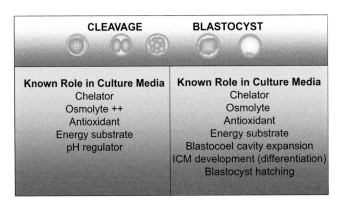

Figure 8.1 Schematic depicting the amino acid requirements of the embryo at the cleavage and blastocyst stage as well as their varying roles in maintaining homeostasis and promoting development.

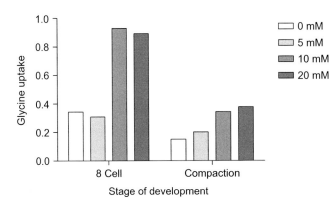

Figure 8.2 Glycine uptake by mouse embryos at both the 8-cell and compacting embryos in response to varying concentrations of extracellular Na^+ stress.

polyols [58, 59]. Intracellular accumulation of non-essential amino acids has been shown to be non-perturbing to cellular enzyme function and can stabilize proteins within a cell [60]. In the precompaction stage embryo it has been demonstrated that the amino acids glycine, β-alanine, L-alanine, glutamine, and proline can protect mammalian embryos from elevated organic solute concentrations in vitro [61, 62]. It appears, however, that the amino acids used by the post-compaction stage embryo for osmoregulation differ, with only alanine, glutamine, glycine, and β-alanine able to act as osmolytes [11]. It also appears that the reliance on amino acids for osmoprotection may also decline after compaction (Figure 8.2).

It has also been proposed that specific amino acids such as alanine and glycine may also act as regulators of intracellular pH (pH_i). Although amino acids exist primarily as zwitterions, a small percentage would be present as the disassociated acid form which could accept a proton and transport it out of the blastomere [63]. Given that the early embryo does not possess robust mechanisms for regulation of pH_i, with either poor or no function of Na^+/H^+ antiporter [64], it is probable that this role may be more important in the precompaction stage embryo.

Several non-essential amino acids can also be oxidized as energy sources via the tricarboxylic acid (TCA) cycle, which for the cleavage stage embryo is the primary energy-generating pathway. Glutamine in particular has been demonstrated to be taken up and metabolized by the cleavage stage and blastocyst stage embryo [50, 53].

Studies have also demonstrated that amino acids also play an essential role as chelators and antioxidants and can regulate metabolism and cell differentiation [28, 65–69]. Glycine is also a very effective chelator of inorganic and organic minerals, including heavy metals, which are detrimental to embryos.

Clearly, a role for amino acids in all cells is to act as substrates for proteins, with all 20 amino acids being proteinogenic. This on the surface seems to be contrary to the provision of only the non-essential amino acids during cleavage stage development. However, the early embryo prior to embryonic genome activation has low biosynthetic activity, while exhibiting high protein turnover and degradation. Therefore, it would seem likely that the availability of substrates from protein turnover is sufficient to meet the biosynthetic needs of the embryo.

Amino acids as regulators of cellular signaling: the new role

While such traditional cellular functions of amino acids such as metabolites, osmolytes, and chelators are well known, recent data from other tissues make it clear that levels of extracellular amino acids have a role in cell signaling. In other tissues there are several amino acid-sensing receptors that respond to changes in the extracellular concentrations of amino acids. L-amino acid sensors have been shown to be present in a wide variety of tissues such as kidney, liver, pancreas, muscle, brain, and pituitary. In these tissues there is evidence of both sensors of extracellular amino acids levels as well as intracellular sensors. It has been demonstrated that amino acid availability can control gene expression, where changes in amino acid provision in culture can result in >1500 differentially expressed genes, with the majority involved in pathways of cell growth and proliferation, cell cycle, gene expression, cell death, and development [70]. Several of these pathways also have been shown to involve mTor and GCN2 pathways, which are important cellular kinases having a major role in the regulation of protein synthesis, transcription, and mRNA turnover. Further, the depletion or lack of amino acids in other tissues has also been shown to result in significant alterations in gene expression and has been shown to induce a stress signaling response involving ATF/CREB transcription factors and the Jun/Fos pathways [71]. Interestingly, these pathways have been shown to be elevated in embryos cultured in vitro in Human Tubal Fluid (HTF) in the absence of amino acids, implying a similar stress response in the absence of amino acids [71].

There are an increasing number of molecules that are being identified that sense amino acid content in cells. Each of these transporters respond to different families of amino acids and some to specific amino acids, meaning that changes in the level of even one amino acid can alter cell signaling pathways. One well-documented amino acid sensor is the Ca^{2+}-sensing receptor (CaR), which senses the levels of aromatic, aliphatic, and polar amino acids (L-Phe, L-Trp, L-Tyr, L-His, L-Thr, L-Ser, L-Ala, L-Gln, L-Asn, and Gly) to enhance the sensitivity of the CaR to Ca^{2+}, acting to stimulate intracellular Ca^{2+} mobilization. As the CaR has been shown to have significant roles in both calcium homeostasis and signaling pathways associated with control of differentiation, the presence of this receptor indicates that changes in amino acid concentrations can regulate calcium metabolism (as reviewed by Conigrave and Hampson [72]). Other broad-spectrum extracellular amino acid sensors include the G-coupled protein receptor superfamily (GPRC6A) which has a preference for L-Arg and L-Lys and is similarly widely expressed in mammalian tissues [73]. In addition, there are several sensor receptors, such as mGlu, Casr, Tas1r1, and GABA B, that are highly selective for specific amino acids [72, 74].

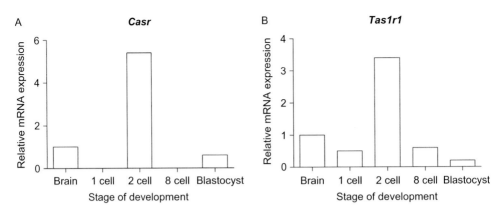

Figure 8.3 Relative mRNA expression of (A) *Casr* and (B) *Tas1r1* in the mouse zygote, 2-cell, 8-cell, and blastocyst. *18S* was used as the housekeeper and mouse brain mRNA expression was used as the calibrator.

The role of these amino acid-sensing receptors in controlling the gene expression and cell signaling of the preimplantation embryo has not been contemplated to date. However, we show here that mRNAs for the amino acid sensors *Casr* and *Tas1r1* are present in preimplantation mouse embryos, possibly indicating a role for these sensors in embryo cell signaling (Figure 8.3).

Further searches of the US National Institute of Child Health and Human Development (NIH) websites for uploaded arrays also confirm the presence of mRNA for all of these receptors (http://www.ncbi.nlm.nih.gov/geo/). Therefore, it is highly likely that these amino acid sensors may have a role in the regulation of development of the mammalian embryo and explain some of the observations of the improved development in the presence of amino acids and the alterations in gene expression in the absence of amino acids. The presence of these transporters and their specificity for different amino acids would suggest that even the mildest changes in the amino acid content of the culture media, either singly or by altering the concentrations of the aromatic > basic > acidic amino acids, for the mammalian embryo may have significant impacts on intracellular signaling, stress response, and consequently development and viability.

Amino acids and embryonic stem cell culture/pluripotency

An interesting new finding as to the role of amino acids comes from their roles in embryonic stem (ES) cell culture media. It has been demonstrated that two amino acids have an involvement in the pluripotency and metastability of human ES cells. Addition of threonine to the medium has been shown to have a positive effect by stimulating ES cell proliferation by up-regulation of the PI3K/Akt, MAPK, and mTOR signaling pathways [75]. Threonine was also shown to be able to regulate gene expression. In contrast, threonine depletion for the culture of ES cells resulted in a down-regulation of pluripotency markers Oct4 and Nanog, and increased trophectoderm markers Cdx2 and Fibroblast growth factor 4 (FGF4) [75].

In contrast, proline added to the culture medium at concentrations > 100 μM (usually present in embryo culture media at 100 μM) resulted in differentiation of ES cells into primitive ectoderm-like cells with concomitant changes in gene expression, while a concentration of 40 μM did not affect ES cell development and differentiation [76]. This effect was related to changes in the mTOR pathway although other amino acids that can also activate the mTOR signaling complex, glycine and leucine, did not alter differentiation.

Although this work is from ES cells, this is of interest for the mammalian preimplantation embryo in that the maintenance of the ICM, and in particular a pluripotent epiblast, is a prerequisite for a successful pregnancy. It is also of interest that specific amino acids in the culture medium have been shown to stimulate the ICM of the blastocyst and that embryos cultured in the absence of amino acids have very low number of cells in the ICM of which few are epiblast. It is likely that as more emerges from ES cells as to how amino acids regulate cellular signaling, we will begin to gain some insight into the roles of amino acids in regulating the blastocyst, and in particular the ICM.

Amino acids (methionine) and epigenetic regulation

The addition of methyl groups to nucleic acids, proteins, lipids, and secondary metabolites facilitates multiple biological processes; in particular, the addition of methyl groups to CpG islands (methylation) within chromatin results in changes to DNA transcription. During development, cells acquire different programmed gene expression, many of which are regulated by epigenetic modifications such as DNA methylation. Therefore, each cell type has its own epigenetic signature that reflects genotype, the environment which it is exposed to, and developmental history, all of which is then reflected in the phenotype of the cell [77–79].

For most cell types, these epigenetic marks become fixed after differentiation; however, in the early embryo both the paternal and maternal genomes undergo reprogramming to erase gamete epigenetic marks and reset the genome of the zygote for totipotency and later establishment of the embryo's own genetic marks; therefore, preimplantation embryo development is a crucial stage of epigenetic regulation [80, 81].

Methylation is influenced by the availability of methyl donors and the derivative of the amino acid methionine, S-adenosyl methionine (SAM), acts as a methyl donor thus linking amino acid concentration to epigenetic regulation (Figure 8.4).

Whole animal studies, utilizing the agouti mouse strain, which modulates its coat color based on epigenetic variation, have demonstrated that feeding pregnant dams methyl supplements (including methionine) can alter the coat color of resultant offspring, indicative of alterations to DNA methylation [82]. In addition, studies have demonstrated that maternal oral supplementation of methionine assists in the prevention of fetal congenital malformations, in particular neural tube defects (NTD), possibly due to methylation changes [83–86].

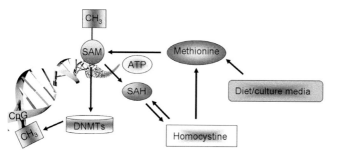

Figure 8.4 Schematic depicting the methionine pathway leading to DNA methylation. Figure adapted from Sergio and Lamprecht Nature Review 2003. SAM (S-adenosyl methionine), ATP (adenosine triphosphate) DNMT (DNA methyltransferase), SAH (S-adenosyl homocystine), CH_3 (methyl group), CpG (CpG island with the DNA strand). See plate section for color version.

As mentioned previously, amino acids have vital importance in maintaining the viability of the developing embryo, with embryos displaying a perturbed epigenetic profile when cultured in media without amino acids, resulting in loss of paternal imprinting and altered methylation of H19 when compared to embryos cultured in media containing amino acids [87]. It has been suggested that this could be due to a decline in the availability of methyl donors such as methionine and has resulted in renewed interest into the need of methionine in the culture media for the mammalian embryo.

Methionine is transported into the embryo via specific transporters and can play a role in polypeptide production, DNA synthesis and methylation, and reactive oxygen species control [82, 88–90]. The addition of methionine to culture media for development of in vitro maturation (IVM)/in vitro fertilization (IVF) zygotes increases blastocyst development in the cow, and rat embryos grown in media without methionine exhibit abnormal neural tube closure which can be prevented by the addition of methionine back into the culture media [88, 91].

Interestingly, there have also been studies that have demonstrated that excess methionine in culture can have a negative impact on fetal development. Mouse embryos cultured during the time of cranial neural tube closure in the presence of increasing concentration of methionine (> 5 mM) resulted in a dose-dependent increase in excencephaly [92]. This also corresponded to alterations to the SAM:SAH ratio which are expected to result in suppression of DNA methyltransferase activity, decreased methylation, and increased rates of NTD [92]. Interestingly, a study using bovine oocytes and blastocysts demonstrated undetectable levels of critical enzymes involved in the methionine cycle, demonstrating that the early embryo may not be equipped to metabolize high levels of methionine [93]. Therefore, the conclusion of these studies is that although methionine supplementation may be beneficial for the later stage blastocyst and beyond, due care must be taken when using high levels as this may result in suppression of the methylation cycle and altered programming.

Currently, methionine is present in embryo culture media, often at super-physiological levels [94]. The actual methionine requirements for human embryos and the impact of variable methionine levels on DNA methylation and programming are currently unknown. As altered DNA methylation can impact on the long-term health outcomes of offspring, this demonstrates a knowledge gap and should be the focus of future research.

By-products of amino acid metabolism: ammonium

The transport of ammonium ions or ammonia across cellular membranes is a homeostatic process for many eukaryote cells. At low concentrations, ammonium/ammonia can act as a nitrogen source; however, at high concentrations it becomes cytotoxic.

Ammonium is formed in culture media by the spontaneous breakdown of amino acids and by the transamination of amino acids by the embryo (although this is a relatively small contribution to the overall ammonium concentration), where the amino group is removed from the amino acid and converted to ammonia. Ammonia (NH_3) is normally encountered as a gas and is also a proton acceptor. In water (pH 7), a very small percentage of NH_3 is converted into the ammonium cation (NH_4^+). The ammonium ion level increases upon increasing the pH of the solution; at "physiological" pH (~7.4) about 99% of the ammonia molecules are protonated (converted to NH_4^+). Temperature and salinity also affect the proportion of NH_4^+; therefore, in embryo culture media (pH 7.2–7.4 at 5–7% CO_2) the ammonium concentration can increase quite substantially, as NH_3 is converted to NH_4^+ [26].

In culture media the majority of ammonia and ammonium production is believed to be due to the most volatile amino acid, glutamine. The toxicity of glutamine in tissue culture media is well known and is attributed to the accumulation of ammonium, which arises because of glutamine metabolism or breakdown [95–97]. In culture media containing amino acids, the concentration of ammonium can increase significantly over time; particularly in media containing the labile amino acid glutamine (170 µM after 24 hours and up to 545.2 µm after 120 hours) [98]. These media may result in reduced embryo viability and pregnancy outcomes in the human, as well as possibly confound experimental results in the laboratory [99].

However when substituted with alanyl-L-glutamine, N-acetyl-glutamine, or glycyl-L-glutamine, dipeptides of glutamine which have increased stability in culture, significantly lower levels of ammonium (10–20 µM) are produced [26, 98]. In the case of alanyl-L-glutamine and glycyl-L-glutamine, they have been shown to stimulate embryo development and increase viability in a manner either similar or superior to glutamine [100, 101].

Research in the mouse has shown that the presence of ammonium in the culture media during preimplantation development, from the zygote to the blastocyst stage, can have a detrimental effect on the embryo, as it can decrease embryo cleavage and blastocyst development, decrease blastocyst cell number, alter gene imprinting and metabolism, and increase apoptosis in a concentration-dependent manner [26, 98, 102]. Concentrations as low as 18.8 µM can decrease the number of ICM cells within the resultant blastocysts and increase apoptosis, and 37.5 µM and above decreases total blastocyst cell number [98].

Additionally, moderate levels of ammonium during the entire preimplantation stage also decrease implantation rates and fetal development rates as well as increasing fetal abnormalities and decreasing fetal maturity after transfer [98, 102, 103]. There is also evidence that the presence of ammonium in culture media at concentrations ≥ 300 µM can also increase the occurrence of birth defects such as exencephaly [98, 104].

The effects of ammonium have also been assessed in ruminant species, as high plasma levels have been linked to decreased fecundity in cattle. The level to which bovine embryos are susceptible to ammonia/ammonium in vitro is dependent on concentration, duration, and stage of exposure [105]. It was demonstrated that exposure to moderate concentrations of ammonium chloride (29–88 µM) during fertilization increased blastocyst development and hatching rates, while continuous exposure of embryos to moderate to high concentrations of ammonium chloride (29–356 µM) increased the number of degenerate ova and decreased blastocyst development and hatching rates. Interestingly, continuous exposure during IVM, IVF, and in vitro culture (IVC) to moderate levels (88 µM) increased development to the morula stage and did not affect blastocyst development at any concentration used, which is perhaps indicative of an adaptation process, although the longer-term consequences on pregnancy and offspring are unclear [105].

One study on human embryos found a statistically significant negative correlation between ammonium concentration in the media on day 4 and blastocyst development, with a reduction of 26%, regardless of whether the cycle was stimulated or natural [99]. Increased ammonium also significantly increased the number of arrested embryos by 16%. No correlation was observed between the number of embryos per drop and the ammonium concentration, indicating that the majority of ammonium buildup was due to spontaneous deamination of amino acids. However, the mean ammonium concentration in media incubated without embryos was 56 µmol/L, indicating that embryo amino acid metabolism does contribute to the overall ammonium concentration.

Despite its obvious effect on the embryo, the mechanism by which ammonium causes these perturbations is currently unknown. It has been suggested that one mechanism may be by reducing intracellular pH, but this remains to be elucidated.

As mentioned earlier, to alleviate the buildup of ammonium in culture media, culture systems have been developed that contain a dipeptide of glutamine, the most volatile amino acid, which keeps ammonium buildup to a minimum [106]. This is compared to a medium without the stable form of glutamine that had levels of ammonium of approximately 250 μM after the same incubation time [98]. Therefore, both the storage of media containing glutamine and the length of time that a medium is left in the incubator before embryo culture can have a significant effect on the levels of ammonium produced and therefore on the embryo development and viability outcomes [98]. Although ammonium production is reduced by the presence of a stable glutamine form, all amino acids are labile at 37 °C. Therefore, irrespective of the source of glutamine, it is essential for consistent high levels of development that care is taken to limit the amount of time that amino acid-containing medium is incubated at 37 °C. It is important that media are not placed into the incubator for extended periods.

Conclusions: the future of the amino acid

It is now standard practice to include amino acids in culture media formulations as their presence significantly increases embryo development and viability. As mentioned previously, this is not surprising, due to the fact that the female reproductive tract contains significant concentrations of amino acids and that the embryo expresses the transporters required to uptake and utilize amino acids. However, despite their importance, there has been little attention paid to optimizing further their concentrations in culture media or investigating their role as precursors for epigenetic regulation and stem cell development. Due to the fact that preimplantation embryo developmental period is a crucial time for erasing and resetting of the embryonic epigenetic profile, the concentration of certain amino acids may influence epigenetic programming and therefore the long-term developmental trajectory of the offspring. In addition, amino acid concentration may also impact stem cell development. Due to the fact that the developing cleavage embryo is totipotent and the blastocyst is pluripotent, the concentration of amino acids may have the ability to influence differentiation, resulting in changes to the developmental trajectory of these cells.

In conclusion, amino acids have long been added to culture media due to their importance as chelators, osmolytes, and metabolic precursors. However, these new emerging roles may result in a new era for amino acids in culture media, as their presence is further refined and their role in epigenetics and cell differentiation within the embryo is determined.

Acknowledgements

The authors would like to acknowledge gratefully Dr. Kathryn Gebhardt for her assistance with determining the level of gene expression of *Casr* and *Tas1r1* in embryos and Tod Fullston for his assistance with primer design.

References

1. Perkins JL, Goode L. Free amino acids in the oviduct fluid of the ewe. *J Reprod Fertil* 1967;**14**(2):309–11.

2. Fahning ML, Schultz RH, Graham EF. The free amino acid content of uterine fluids and blood serum in the cow. *J Reprod Fertil* 1967;**13**(2):229–36.

3. Menezo Y, Laviolette P. [Amino constituents of tubal secretions in the rabbit. Zymogram–proteins–free amino acids]. *Ann Biol Anim Biochim Biophys* 1972;**12**(3):383–96.

4. Stanke DF, Sikes JD, DeYoung DW, Tumbleson ME. Proteins and amino acids in bovine oviducal fluid. *J Reprod Fertil* 1974;**38**(2):493–6.

5. Miller JG, Schultz GA. Amino acid content of preimplantation rabbit embryos and fluids of the reproductive tract. *Biol Reprod* 1987;**36**(1):125–9.

6. Casslen BG. Free amino acids in human uterine fluid. Possible role of high taurine concentration. *J Reprod Med* 1987;**32**(3):181–4.

7. Elhassan YM, Wu G, Leanez AC, et al. Amino acid concentrations in fluids from the bovine oviduct and uterus and in KSOM-based culture media. *Theriogenology* 2001;**55**(9):1907–18.

8. Schultz GA, Kaye PL, McKay DJ, Johnson MH. Endogenous amino acid pool sizes in mouse eggs and preimplantation embryos. *J Reprod Fertil* 1981;**61**(2):387–93.

9. Jaszczak S, Hafez ES, Moghissi KS, Kurrie DA. Concentration gradients of amino acids between the uterine and blastocoelic fluid in the rabbit. *Fertil Steril* 1972;**23**(6):405–9.

10. Eagle H. Amino acid metabolism in mammalian cell cultures. *Science* 1959;**130**(3373):432–7.

11. Richards T, Wang F, Liu L, Baltz JM. Rescue of postcompaction-stage mouse embryo development from hypertonicity by amino acid transporter substrates that may function as organic osmolytes. *Biol Reprod* 82(4):769–77.

12. Steeves CL, Hammer MA, Walker GB, et al. The glycine neurotransmitter transporter GLYT1 is an organic osmolyte transporter regulating cell volume in cleavage-stage embryos. *Proc Natl Acad Sci U S A* 2003;**100**(24):13982–7.

13. Van Winkle LJ, Campione AL, Farrington BH. Development of system B0,+ and a broad-scope Na(+)-dependent transporter of zwitterionic amino acids in preimplantation mouse conceptuses. *Biochim Biophys Acta.* 1990;**1025**(2): 225–33.

14. Anas MK, Lee MB, Zhou C, et al. SIT1 is a betaine/proline transporter that is activated in mouse eggs after fertilization and functions until the 2-cell stage. *Development* 2008;**135**(24):4123–30.

15. Anas MK, Hammer MA, Lever M, Stanton JA, Baltz JM. The organic osmolytes betaine and proline are transported by a shared system in early preimplantation mouse embryos. *J Cell Physiol* 2007;**210**(1):266–77.

16. Van Winkle LJ. Amino acid transport regulation and early embryo development. *Biol Reprod* 2001;**64**(1):1–12.

17. Van Winkle LJ, Dickinson HR. Differences in amino acid content of preimplantation mouse embryos that develop in vitro versus in vivo: in vitro effects of five amino acids that are abundant in oviductal secretions. *Biol Reprod* 1995;**52**(1):96–104.

18. Van Winkle LJ, Mann DF, Weimer BD, Campione AL. Na(+)-dependent transport of anionic amino acids by preimplantation mouse blastocysts. *Biochim Biophys Acta* 1991;**1068**(2):231–6.

19. Gardner DK, Lane M. Alleviation of the '2-cell block' and development to the blastocyst of CF1 mouse embryos: role of amino acids, EDTA and physical parameters. *Hum Reprod* 1996;**11**(12):2703–12.

20. Gwatkin RB, Haidri AA. Requirements for the maturation of hamster oocytes in vitro. *Exp Cell Res* 1973;**76**(1):1–7.

21. Bae IH, Foote RH. Utilization of glutamine for energy and protein synthesis by

cultured rabbit follicular oocytes. *Exp Cell Res* 1975;**90**(2):432–6.

22. Juetten J, Bavister BD. The effects of amino acids, cumulus cells, and bovine serum albumin on in vitro fertilization and first cleavage of hamster eggs. *J Exp Zool* 1983;**227**(3):487–90.

23. Bavister BD, Leibfried ML, Lieberman G. Development of preimplantation embryos of the golden hamster in a defined culture medium. *Biol Reprod* 1983;**28**(1):235–47.

24. Bavister BD, Arlotto T. Influence of single amino acids on the development of hamster one-cell embryos in vitro. *Mol Reprod Dev* 1990;**25**(1):45–51.

25. McKiernan SH, Clayton MK, Bavister BD. Analysis of stimulatory and inhibitory amino acids for development of hamster one-cell embryos in vitro. *Mol Reprod Dev* 1995;**42**(2):188–99.

26. Gardner DK, Lane M. Amino acids and ammonium regulate mouse embryo development in culture. *Biol Reprod* 1993;**48**(2):377–85.

27. Ho Y, Wigglesworth K, Eppig JJ, Schultz RM. Preimplantation development of mouse embryos in KSOM: augmentation by amino acids and analysis of gene expression. *Mol Reprod Dev* 1995;**41**(2):232–8.

28. Lane M, Gardner DK. Differential regulation of mouse embryo development and viability by amino acids. *J Reprod Fertil* 1997;**109**(1):153–64.

29. Nakazawa T, Ohashi K, Yamada M, *et al.* Effect of different concentrations of amino acids in human serum and follicular fluid on the development of one-cell mouse embryos in vitro. *J Reprod Fertil* 1997;**111**(2):327–32.

30. Summers MC, McGinnis LK, Lawitts JA, Raffin M, Biggers JD. IVF of mouse ova in a simplex optimized medium supplemented with amino acids. *Hum Reprod* 2000;**15**(8):1791–801.

31. Biggers JD, McGinnis LK, Raffin M. Amino acids and preimplantation development of the mouse in protein-free potassium simplex optimized medium. *Biol Reprod* 2000;**63**(1):281–93.

32. Kane MT, Bavister BD. Protein-free culture medium containing polyvinylalcohol, vitamins, and amino acids supports development of eight-cell hamster embryos to hatching blastocysts. *J Exp Zool* 1988;**247**(2):183–7.

33. Kane MT, Carney EW, Bavister BD. Vitamins and amino acids stimulate hamster blastocysts to hatch in vitro. *J Exp Zool* 1986;**239**(3):429–32.

34. Lee ES, Fukui Y. Synergistic effect of alanine and glycine on bovine embryos cultured in a chemically defined medium and amino acid uptake by vitro-produced bovine morulae and blastocysts. *Biol Reprod* 1996;**55**(6):1383–9.

35. Gardner DK, Lane M, Spitzer A, Batt PA. Enhanced rates of cleavage and development for sheep zygotes cultured to the blastocyst stage in vitro in the absence of serum and somatic cells: amino acids, vitamins, and culturing embryos in groups stimulate development. *Biol Reprod* 1994;**50**(2):390–400.

36. Devreker F, Hardy K, Van den Bergh M, *et al.* Amino acids promote human blastocyst development in vitro. *Hum Reprod* 2001;**16**(4):749–56.

37. Lane M, Gardner DK. Nonessential amino acids and glutamine decrease the time of the first three cleavage divisions and increase compaction of mouse zygotes in vitro. *J Assist Reprod Genet* 1997;**14**(7):398–403.

38. Pinyopummintr T, Bavister BD. Effects of amino acids on development in vitro of cleavage-stage bovine embryos into blastocysts. *Reprod Fertil Dev* 1996;**8**(5):835–41.

39. Steeves TE, Gardner DK. Temporal and differential effects of amino acids on bovine embryo development in culture. *Biol Reprod* 1999;**61**(3):731–40.

40. Thompson JG, Gardner DK, Pugh PA, McMillan WH, Tervit HR. Lamb birth weight is affected by culture system utilized during in vitro pre-elongation development of ovine embryos. *Biol Reprod* 1995;**53**(6):1385–91.

41. Pinyopummintr T, Bavister BD. In vitro-matured/in vitro-fertilized bovine oocytes

can develop into morulae/blastocysts in chemically defined, protein-free culture media. *Biol Reprod* 1991;**45**(5):736–42.

42. Takahashi Y, First NL. In vitro development of bovine one-cell embryos: influence of glucose, lactate, pyruvate, amino acids and vitamins. *Theriogenology* 1992;**37**(5):963–78.

43. Zielke HR, Zielke CL, Ozand PT. Glutamine: a major energy source for cultured mammalian cells. *Fed Proc* 1984;**43**(1):121–5.

44. McKiernan SH, Bavister BD, Tasca RJ. Energy substrate requirements for in-vitro development of hamster 1- and 2-cell embryos to the blastocyst stage. *Hum Reprod* 1991;**6**(1):64–75.

45. Carney EW, Bavister BD. Stimulatory and inhibitory effects of amino acids on the development of hamster eight-cell embryos in vitro. *J In Vitro Fert Embryo Transf* 1987;**4**(3):162–7.

46. Suzuki C, Yoshioka K, Sakatani M, Takahashi M. Glutamine and hypotaurine improves intracellular oxidative status and in vitro development of porcine preimplantation embryos. *Zygote* 2007;**15**(4):317–24.

47. Devreker F, Winston RM, Hardy K. Glutamine improves human preimplantation development in vitro. *Fertil Steril* 1998;**69**(2):293–9.

48. Devreker F, Van den Bergh M, Biramane J, *et al.* Effects of taurine on human embryo development in vitro. *Hum Reprod* 1999;**14**(9):2350–6.

49. Lewis AM, Kaye PL. Characterization of glutamine uptake in mouse two-cell embryos and blastocysts. *J Reprod Fertil* 1992;**95**(1):221–9.

50. Gardner DK, Clarke RN, Lechene CP, Biggers JD. Development of a noninvasive ultramicrofluorometric method for measuring net uptake of glutamine by single preimplantation mouse embryos. *Gamete Res* 1989;**24**(4):427–38.

51. Chatot CL, Tasca RJ, Ziomek CA. Glutamine uptake and utilization by preimplantation mouse embryos in CZB medium. *J Reprod Fertil* 1990;**89**(1):335–46.

52. Rieger D, Loskutoff NM, Betteridge KJ. Developmentally related changes in the metabolism of glucose and glutamine by cattle embryos produced and co-cultured in vitro. *J Reprod Fertil* 1992;**95**(2):585–95.

53. Rieger D, Loskutoff NM, Betteridge KJ. Developmentally related changes in the uptake and metabolism of glucose, glutamine and pyruvate by cattle embryos produced in vitro. *Reprod Fertil Dev* 1992;**4**(5):547–57.

54. Dumoulin JC, Evers JL, Bakker JA, *et al.* Temporal effects of taurine on mouse preimplantation development in vitro. *Hum Reprod* 1992;**7**(3):403–7.

55. Dumoulin JC, Evers JL, Bras M, Pieters MH, Geraedts JP. Positive effect of taurine on preimplantation development of mouse embryos in vitro. *J Reprod Fertil* 1992;**94**(2):373–80.

56. Reed ML, Illera MJ, Petters RM. In vitro culture of pig embryos. *Theriogenology* 1992;**37**:95–109.

57. Barnett DK, Bavister BD. Hypotaurine requirement for in vitro development of golden hamster one-cell embryos into morulae and blastocysts, and production of term offspring from in vitro-fertilized ova. *Biol Reprod* 1992;**47**(2):297–304.

58. Yancey PH, Clark ME, Hand SC, Bowlus RD, Somero GN. Living with water stress: evolution of osmolyte systems. *Science* 1982;**217**(4566):1214–22.

59. Somero GN. Protons, osmolytes, and fitness of internal milieu for protein function. *Am J Physiol* 1986;**251**(2 Pt 2): R197–213.

60. Arakawa T, Timasheff SN. The stabilization of proteins by osmolytes. *Biophys J* 1985;**47**(3):411–14.

61. Dawson KM, Baltz JM. Organic osmolytes and embryos: substrates of the Gly and beta transport systems protect mouse zygotes against the effects of raised osmolarity. *Biol Reprod* 1997;**56**(6):1550–8.

62. Hammer MA, Baltz JM. Beta-alanine but not taurine can function as an organic osmolyte in preimplantation mouse embryos cultured from fertilized eggs. *Mol Reprod Dev* 2003;**66**(2):153–61.

63. Bavister BD, McKiernan SH. Regulation of hamster embryo development in vitro by amino acids. In: Bavister BD, ed. *Preimplantation Embryo Development.* New York, Plenum Press. 1993;57–72.

64. Baltz JM, Biggers JD, Lechene C. Two-cell stage mouse embryos appear to lack mechanisms for alleviating intracellular acid loads. *J Biol Chem* 1991;**266**(10):6052–7.

65. Lindenbaum A. A survey of naturally occurring chelating ligands. *Adv Exp Med Biol* 1973;**40**:67–77.

66. Gardner DK. Changes in requirements and utilization of nutrients during mammalian preimplantation embryo development and their significance in embryo culture. *Theriogenology* 1998;**49**(1):83–102.

67. Liu Z, Foote RH. Effects of amino acids on the development of in-vitro matured/in-vitro fertilization bovine embryos in a simple protein-free medium. *Hum Reprod* 1995;**10**(11):2985–91.

68. Lane M, Gardner DK. Mitochondrial malate-aspartate shuttle regulates mouse embryo nutrient consumption. *J Biol Chem* 2005;**280**(18):18361–7.

69. Martin PM, Sutherland AE. Exogenous amino acids regulate trophectoderm differentiation in the mouse blastocyst through an mTOR-dependent pathway. *Dev Biol* 2001;**240**(1):182–93.

70. Shan J, Lopez MC, Baker HV, Kilberg MS. Expression profiling after activation of the amino acid deprivation response in HepG2 human hepatoma cells. *Physiol Genomics* 2010 Mar 9 [Epub ahead of print].

71. Wang Y, Puscheck EE, Lewis JJ, et al. Increases in phosphorylation of SAPK/JNK and p38MAPK correlate negatively with mouse embryo development after culture in different media. *Fertil Steril* 2005;**83** (Suppl 1):1144–54.

72. Conigrave AD, Hampson DR. Broad-spectrum L-amino acid sensing by class 3 G-protein-coupled receptors. *Trends Endocrinol Metab* 2006;**17**(10):398–407.

73. Kuang D, Yao Y, Lam J, Tsushima RG, Hampson DR. Cloning and characterization of a family C orphan G-protein coupled receptor. *J Neurochem* 2005;**93**(2):383–91.

74. Nelson G, Chandrashekar J, Hoon MA, et al. An amino-acid taste receptor. *Nature* 2002;**416**(6877):199–202.

75. Ryu JM, Han HJ. L-threonine regulates G1/S phase transition of mouse embryonic stem cells via PI3K/Akt, MAPKs, and mTORC pathways. *J Biol Chem* **286** (27):23667–78.

76. Washington JM, Rathjen J, Felquer F, et al. L-Proline induces differentiation of ES cells: a novel role for an amino acid in the regulation of pluripotent cells in culture. *Am J Physiol Cell Physiol* **298**(5):C982–92.

77. Morgan HD, Santos F, Green K, Dean W, Reik W. Epigenetic reprogramming in mammals. *Hum Mol Genet* 2005;**14** Spec No 1:R47–58.

78. Bird A. DNA methylation patterns and epigenetic memory. *Genes Dev* 2002;**16** (1):6–21.

79. Li E. Chromatin modification and epigenetic reprogramming in mammalian development. *Nat Rev* 2002;**3**(9):662–73.

80. Reik W, Dean W, Walter J. Epigenetic reprogramming in mammalian development. *Science* 2001;**293** (5532):1089–93.

81. Rideout WM, 3rd, Eggan K, Jaenisch R. Nuclear cloning and epigenetic reprogramming of the genome. *Science* 2001;**293**(5532):1093–8.

82. Wolff GL, Kodell RL, Moore SR, Cooney CA. Maternal epigenetics and methyl supplements affect agouti gene expression in Avy/a mice. *FASEB J* 1998;**12**(11):949–57.

83. Essien FB, Wannberg SL. Methionine but not folinic acid or vitamin B-12 alters the frequency of neural tube defects in Axd mutant mice. *J Nutr* 1993;**123**(1):27–34.

84. Ehlers K, Elmazar MM, Nau H. Methionine reduces the valproic acid-induced spina bifida rate in mice without altering valproic acid kinetics. *J Nutr* 1996;**126**(1):67–75.

85. Shaw GM, Velie EM, Schaffer DM. Is dietary intake of methionine associated with a reduction in risk for neural tube defect-affected pregnancies? *Teratology* 1997;**56**(5):295–9.

86. Dunlevy LP, Burren KA, Mills K, et al. Integrity of the methylation cycle is

essential for mammalian neural tube closure. *Birth Defects Res A Clin Mol Teratol* 2006;**76**(7):544–52.

87. Doherty AS, Mann MR, Tremblay KD, Bartolomei MS, Schultz RM. Differential effects of culture on imprinted H19 expression in the preimplantation mouse embryo. *Biol Reprod* 2000;**62**(6):1526–35.

88. Bonilla L, Luchini D, Devillard E, Hansen PJ. Methionine requirements for the preimplantation bovine embryo. *J Reprod Dev* 2010;**56**(5):527–32.

89. Metayer S, Seiliez I, Collin A, *et al.* Mechanisms through which sulfur amino acids control protein metabolism and oxidative status. *J Nutr Biochem* 2008;**19**(4):207–15.

90. Menezo Y, Khatchadourian C, Gharib A, *et al.* Regulation of S-adenosyl methionine synthesis in the mouse embryo. *Life Sci* 1989;**44**(21):1601–9.

91. Coelho CN, Klein NW. Methionine and neural tube closure in cultured rat embryos: morphological and biochemical analyses. *Teratology* 1990;**42**(4):437–51.

92. Dunlevy LP, Burren KA, Chitty LS, Copp AJ, Greene ND. Excess methionine suppresses the methylation cycle and inhibits neural tube closure in mouse embryos. *FEBS Lett* 2006;**580**(11):2803–7.

93. Kwong WY, Adamiak SJ, Gwynn A, Singh R, Sinclair KD. Endogenous folates and single-carbon metabolism in the ovarian follicle, oocyte and pre-implantation embryo. *Reproduction* **139**(4):705–15.

94. Steele W, Allegrucci C, Singh R, *et al.* Human embryonic stem cell methyl cycle enzyme expression: modelling epigenetic programming in assisted reproduction? *Reprod Biomed Online* 2005;**10**(6):755–66.

95. Visek W, Kolodny G, Gross P. Ammonia effects in cultures of normal and transformed 3T3 cells. *J Cell Physiol* 1972;**80**:373–81.

96. McLimans W, Blumenson L, Repasky E, Ito M. Ammonia loading in cell culture systems. *Cell Biol Int Rep* 1981;**5**:653–60.

97. Heeneman S, Deutz N, Buurman W. The concentrations of glutamine and ammonia in commercially available cell culture media. *J Immunol Methods* 1993;**166**:85–91.

98. Lane M, Gardner DK. Ammonium induces aberrant blastocyst differentiation, metabolism, pH regulation, gene expression and subsequently alters fetal development in the mouse. *Biol Reprod* 2003;**69**(4):1109–17.

99. Virant-Klun I, Tomazevic T, Vrtacnik-Bokal E, *et al.* Increased ammonium in culture medium reduces the development of human embryos to the blastocyst stage. *Fertil Steril* 2006;**85**(2):526–8.

100. Biggers JD, McGinnis LK, Lawitts JA. Enhanced effect of glycyl-L-glutamine on mouse preimplantation embryos in vitro. *Reprod Biomed Online* 2004;**9**(1):59–69.

101. Summers MC, McGinnis LK, Lawitts JA, Biggers JD. Mouse embryo development following IVF in media containing either L-glutamine or glycyl-L-glutamine. *Hum Reprod* 2005;**20**(5):1364–71.

102. Zander DL, Thompson JG, Lane M. Perturbations in mouse embryo development and viability caused by ammonium are more severe after exposure at the cleavage stages. *Biol Reprod* 2006;**74**(2):288–94.

103. Lane M, Gardner DK. Increase in postimplantation development of cultured mouse embryos by amino acids and induction of fetal retardation and exencephaly by ammonium ions. *J Reprod Fertil* 1994;**102**(2):305–12.

104. Sinawat S, Hsaio WC, Flockhart JH, *et al.* Fetal abnormalities produced after preimplantation exposure of mouse embryos to ammonium chloride. *Hum Reprod* 2003;**18**(10):2157–65.

105. Hammon DS, Wang S, Holyoak GR. Effects of ammonia during different stages of culture on development of in vitro produced bovine embryos. *Anim Reprod Sci* 2000;**59**(1–2):23–30.

106. Gardner DK, Lane M. Towards a single embryo transfer. *Reprod Biomed Online* 2003;**6**(4):470–81.

Chapter

9

Growth factors and cytokines in embryo development

Sarah A. Robertson and Jeremy G. Thompson

Introduction

Embryos developing naturally in the mother's reproductive tract experience a substantially different environment to those developing in a culture dish after in vitro fertilization (IVF). A key distinction between the two is the presence of an array of growth factors and cytokines produced naturally by the maternal tissues in vivo. The majority of modern embryo culture media does not contain these agents. The biological function of growth factors and cytokines in vivo is to mediate communication between the maternal tissues and the embryo. Although embryos clearly can develop in simple culture media in vitro in the absence of exogenous growth factors, there is compelling evidence that in the physiological situation, these growth factors and cytokines have paracrine cell–cell signaling actions that contribute to yielding healthier embryos than those produced in a culture dish [1, 2]. Their actions in the embryo include modulation of cell gene expression and metabolic function that in turn influence cell survival and differentiation, ultimately impacting embryo implantation competence and post-implantation development [2, 3]. Despite growing information on how cytokines influence embryos, there is a lack of consensus opinion regarding whether any maternally derived factors are truly essential for "normal" development of human embryos in vitro, when high quality embryo culture medium is utilized. The benefits and possibility of any risks of their use in IVF is an important ongoing research question in reproductive medicine [4].

Given the lack of any major advance in IVF success rates in recent years, there is keen interest in exploring whether growth factors can be added to embryo culture media to improve embryo development in vitro and the value of their utility for achieving better rates of successful implantation and healthy pregnancy. Importantly, expanding the clinical utility of growth factors in IVF embryo development depends on first achieving (1) a robust understanding of their functions in the in vivo situation and (2) a complete and consensus view of what is "normal" development. While embryos can certainly develop in the absence of exogenous growth factors into blastocysts that are able to implant and develop after transfer, there is a growing appreciation amongst reproductive biologists that disruption of growth factor signaling in embryos may be a factor limiting their optimal growth and long-term developmental potential. Since the peri-conceptual environment influences the early embryo to impart long-term consequences for the fetus and neonate, it is important to ensure that the early environment provides the best possible experience for embryos at the outset of life. An absence of growth factors from most embryo culture

Culture Media, Solutions, and Systems in Human ART, ed. Patrick Quinn. Published by Cambridge University Press. © Cambridge University Press 2014.

media may in part explain why IVF success is limited especially for some subsets of patients, and may have consequences for all embryos, contributing to the subtle changes in birth-weight and health outcomes evident in children conceived by IVF [5–9]. This viewpoint is supported by animal studies showing there are subtle but important differences between the trajectory of embryo development after in vitro conception and culture, compared with development in the female reproductive tract in vivo, and that growth factor addition to embryo culture can protect embryos from cellular stress and in part alleviate these adverse effects.

This chapter reviews current knowledge on the synthesis of endometrial growth factors and cytokines and their different roles in promoting, or sometimes constraining, embryo development. We describe the physiological communication pathways by which cells of the preimplantation embryo are regulated by cytokines of female reproductive tract origin, and our views on how this fundamental biology might be applied to human reproductive medicine. Preceding this is a brief description of the biological nature of the cytokine family of molecules, with emphasis on those characteristics that are relevant to embryo development. The intention of this chapter is not to provide a comprehensive review of every cytokine targeting the embryo, but rather to highlight central and emerging concepts. Because of space constraints we are unable to reference many important primary papers and instead refer readers to excellent reviews. The discussion will focus where possible on studies in women, but also includes information from animal models since experiments in rodents and livestock species generally precede and inform human research. In the human, the precise roles of cytokines in early pregnancy are more difficult to define than in animals, and are constrained by limited availability of human embryos and tissue for research. Notwithstanding this, there is now compelling evidence that at least one cytokine, granulocyte–macrophage colony-stimulating factor (GM-CSF; also known as CSF2), is a beneficial addition to human embryo culture media that improves the likelihood of successful pregnancy, particularly in women who are prone to miscarriage.

Growth factors, cytokines, and cell communication

"Growth factors" are polypeptide glycoproteins (usually 6–30 kDa in size) that bind to receptors on the cell surface, with the primary result of activating cellular proliferation and/or differentiation in the target cell. The term "cytokines" refers to a broader class of signaling proteins used extensively in cellular communication to exert autocrine, paracrine, and endocrine effects, which may include stimulatory as well as inhibitory functions, ranging from maintenance of cell survival to induction of cell death. In the context of regulation of embryo development, a wide range of both positive and negative cytokine regulators are involved, so "cytokine" will be employed as the more correct terminology for the purpose of this chapter.

Cytokines were originally described on the basis of their actions in the immune and hematopoietic systems, but have since been shown to have a wide range of activities with many different cell types producing and responding to these molecules. Cytokines are usually named after the biological function for which they were first discovered, and so their nomenclature can be misleading and even anomalous. On the basis of structural similarities, gene organization, chromosomal location, and receptor usage they can be classified into six families; the hematopoietins (including the colony-stimulating factors [CSFs], interferons [IFNs], and most of the interleukins [ILs]), epidermal growth factors, β-trefoils (fibroblast growth factors and IL1), the tumor necrosis factors (TNFs), the cysteine knot cytokines (including the transforming growth factor [TGF]-β family), and the chemokines [10].

Generally, cytokines are produced in relatively small quantities and exert their actions at nanomolar or picomolar concentrations. Most cytokines are secreted into the extracellular fluid, but some can be sequestered into the extracellular matrix or anchored to the cell membrane. Together with their short half-life, this usually restricts their sphere of influence to autocrine, paracrine, or juxtacrine actions within the immediate neighborhood of production. However, some cytokines such as IL6 and TNFα can be produced in large amounts to have systemic actions through the entire body, for example in times of infection or inflammatory stress.

Cytokines bind to specific, high affinity receptors in the cytoplasmic membrane on the surface of the target cell, which triggers a cascade of intracellular events that ultimately cause changes in the pattern of gene expression and protein synthesis. In this way, cytokine signals act to promote or inhibit multiple aspects of target cell behavior, including survival, proliferation, and reversible and irreversible transitions in cell differentiation and phenotype. Cytokines are remarkably promiscuous and pleiotropic in their actions. A single factor can elicit extraordinarily diverse and sometimes apparently opposite responses in a range of different target cells that are generally dose-dependent. The response of a cell to a given cytokine depends not only on its lineage and differentiation state, but also on the local microenvironment, particularly the concentration of other cytokines and growth factors, and the extracellular matrix [11].

For many cytokines, individual factors bind only to a single cognate receptor, but other factors share receptor components or whole receptors. This underpins the considerable degree of overlap in activity between different cytokine family members. The capacity for duplication of function between individual cytokines is clearly borne out by the surprising lack of severe consequences of null mutation of many cytokine genes in mice. An individual cytokine is usually found to be absolutely essential in only a small number of cellular events, presumably because most biological responses can be achieved by more than one cytokine. Rather than suggesting that many cytokines are therefore essentially dispensable, cytokine "knockout" experiments indicate that critical cellular functions are usually backed up by "fail-safe" mechanisms where the loss of one cytokine can be compensated by another factor with similar activities. This principle is particularly evident in the reproductive system, where null mutations in only a few cytokines lead to complete infertility. However, while deletion of individual cytokines may be consistent with viable pregnancy, the resulting perturbation in maternal tract cytokine balance can compromise the quality of placental and fetal development, leading to fetal growth retardation and reduced health of offspring in neonatal and adult life.

Cytokines are generally not expressed constitutively and are usually produced only in response to specific excitants such as hormones, other cytokines, and bacterial or viral products. A variety of elaborate extracellular and intracellular control mechanisms exist to limit the duration and spread of a cytokine response. These ensure that the potent effects of cytokines are confined to the immediate vicinity of the producing cell, and limit the lifespan of the response in the target cell. Down-regulation of cytokine receptors on responding cells is achieved through a reduction in the rate of receptor synthesis, or by internalization and subsequent degradation of receptor–ligand complexes. Cytokine activities are further counterbalanced and modulated by other cytokines that oppose their effects, as well as by naturally occurring cytokine antagonists.

Cytokine and chemokine synthesis in the endometrium

In the endometrium and oviduct, the most prominent cellular source of cytokines able to influence the embryo is the epithelial cells lining the surface of the tract, together with the leukocyte populations residing immediately beneath the epithelial surface. Literally thousands of studies are now published detailing the expression patterns of a wide range of cytokines and their receptors in the endometrium and oviduct in many mammalian species, and these have been reviewed comprehensively [12–17]. Together these studies show that cytokines are expressed in distinct spatial and temporal patterns during the menstrual cycle, particularly in the secretory phase endometrium, and are detectable in uterine lavage fluid recovered at this time [18]. Their synthesis is regulated primarily by ovarian steroid hormones, but also by local factors secreted by adjacent endometrial cells as well as introduced factors emanating from the male partner's seminal fluid, the conceptus itself, or various microorganisms present as sexually transmitted infections, or the normal microbial flora. Further influences on endometrial cytokine expression occur in the form of systemic factors such as nutritional status and micronutrient availability, stress and neuroendocrine signals, and genetic polymorphisms in cytokine and cytokine receptor genes (Figure 9.1).

Cytokine production by endometrial and oviductal epithelial cells

Epithelial cells forming the luminal surface of the endometrium and the oviduct, and lining the surface of the endometrial glands, secrete an extensive repertoire of cytokines which are secreted into the luminal cavity where the embryo develops. The first factors identified include CSF1, GM-CSF, leukemia inhibitory factor (LIF), TNFα, IL6, and TGFβ and later IL11, IL13, IL15, and IL18 were added to the repertoire [12–17, 19–22]. Epithelial cells also produce an array of chemokines [23] which primarily act to regulate recruitment of leukocytes into the female reproductive tract, but may also target developing embryos [23].

Epithelial cytokine synthesis is not constitutive, but is regulated over the course of the reproductive cycle by ovarian sex steroids acting at the transcriptional (mRNA) level. Individual cytokine genes show different temporal patterns, suggesting their independent regulation or sequential activation, by mechanisms that are not fully defined but likely to involve crosstalk between cytokine transcription factors and steroid hormone receptors. Cytokine production in epithelial cells is most dynamic during the luteal phase, when these cells orchestrate local changes necessary to support embryo development and prepare for blastocyst implantation.

Factors other than steroid hormones – such as cytokines, growth factors, and prostaglandins (PGs) derived from leukocytes, seminal fluid, and the conceptus – can further modulate epithelial cell cytokine expression. This was originally described in mice, where a surge in expression of pro-inflammatory cytokines including GM-CSF, IL6, and an array of chemokines is induced in estrogen-primed uterine and oviductal epithelial cells after the introduction of seminal fluid at mating [24]. The secretion pattern alters again around the time of implantation, when increasing concentrations of circulating progesterone begin to suppress GM-CSF and chemokine synthesis [20], and drive a switch to CSF1 and LIF expression [21, 22].

There is considerable similarity between steroid hormone-regulated cytokine secretion patterns in the rodent and human female reproductive tract. Estrogen-regulated cytokines including CSF1, GM-CSF, and TNFα increase in abundance over the course of the

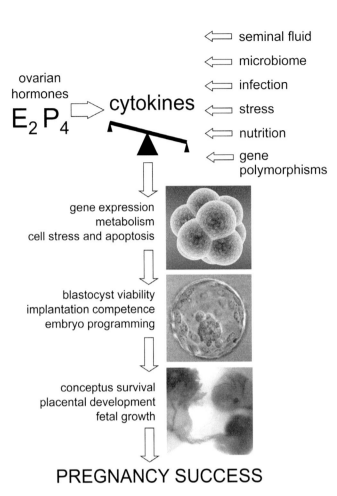

Figure 9.1 Cytokine expression in the female reproductive tract is regulated by ovarian steroid hormones and a variety of intrinsic and extrinsic factors. The cytokine environment influences gene expression, metabolism, cell stress, and apoptosis pathways in the preimplantation embryo to initiate downstream events impacting implantation, placental development, and fetal growth, and ultimately healthy pregnancy outcome. E_2 = estradiol; P_4 = progesterone.

proliferative phase and into the early luteal phase in women. A late secretory phase decline in GM-CSF and further increase in CSF1, TNFα, and LIF match patterns occurring early in the mouse [19, 21, 25, 26]. Seminal factors including TGFβ and PGE$_2$ are capable of inducing expression of IL8, GM-CSF, IL6, and other cytokines and chemokines in human cervical epithelial cells [27] and may influence cytokine expression in the endometrium as well [28]. In the event of implantation of an embryo, CSF1, LIF, and other progesterone-induced epithelial cytokines are up-regulated and then predominate for the duration of the pregnancy [21, 22]. In the absence of pregnancy, a switch back to expression of pro-inflammatory cytokines including several chemokines occurs in response to premenstrual progesterone withdrawal [29, 30].

Factors associated with microorganisms bind to Toll-like receptors (TLRs) expressed by epithelial cells in the cervix and uterus and can induce production of pro-inflammatory cytokines in uterine and endocervical epithelial cells. Cervical epithelial cells respond to chlamydia infection with increased mRNA expression and secretion of IL1, IL8, growth-related oncogene (GRO)-α, GM-CSF, and IL6 [31], and lipo-oligosaccharides from

Escherichia coli or *Neisseria gonorrheae* similarly induce inflammatory cytokine expression [32]. It is likely that cytokine networks induced after infection act in an amplifying cascade, with factors such as IFNγ and TNFα elicited in endometrial leukocytes implicated as potent stimulators of cytokine and chemokine expression in epithelial cells [33]. The TLR-mediated response to bacterial and viral entities plays a central role in recognizing presence of infection and eliciting the cytokine response necessary to activate protective immunity and limit tissue damage. However, excessive stimulation of the TLR-induced pro-inflammatory pathway can override the normal hormone-regulated expression of endometrial cytokines and may be an underappreciated pathway through which sexually transmitted infection interferes with fertility.

Cytokine production by endometrial and oviductal leukocytes

The endometrium and oviduct are richly populated with leukocyte populations, particularly macrophages, dendritic cells, granulocytes, lymphocytes, and mast cells, all of which are potent sources of a variety of cytokines that could reasonably access the luminal cavity and the developing embryo within. The secretory profile of leukocytes is highly variable depending on their activation state. Endometrial macrophages can secrete an array of cytokines in patterns that are flexible and responsive to the ovarian steroid environment, signals derived from the conceptus and semen, and infection [34]. Uterine and decidual macrophages can secrete cytokines with immune-activating or immunosuppressive properties. In healthy pregnancies decidual macrophages synthesize anti-inflammatory and tolerance-inducing cytokines TGFβ and IL10 [35, 36] and IL1 receptor antagonist [37] consistent with an anti-inflammatory M2 phenotype. Human leukocyte antigen-G (HLA-G) expressed by the embryo may contribute to sustaining this decidual macrophage phenotype, resulting in increased TGFβ synthesis [38]. However, in the event of infection, TLR ligands profoundly alter the secretory profile of decidual macrophages, activating expression of pro-inflammatory cytokines IFNγ and IL12 which are linked with fetal loss [39].

Lymphocytes are very important contributors to the uterine cytokine environment because their cytokine products, particularly IFNγ, are extremely potent and act in low picomolar concentrations. A large proportion of the lymphocytes found in the uterus and decidua are termed uterine natural killer (uNK) cells, and these cells are distributed throughout the decidual tissue in the cycle and during pregnancy. Several cytokines are synthesized by uNK cells (IL4, IL5, IL10, IL13, GM-CSF, G-CSF [CSF3], CSF1, TNFα, IFNγ, and LIF) [40]. Heterogeneity in the patterns of expression of these cytokines indicates that a variety of subsets of uNK cells exist in the decidua and while uNK cells expressing immunosuppressive cytokines normally predominate, their cytokine production can change in response to infection or other environmental triggers [40, 41].

T-lymphocytes are more sparsely distributed in endometrial tissues and these cells also exhibit complex phenotypes with different patterns of cytokine production. Helper (CD4+) and suppressor/cytotoxic (CD8+) T-lymphocytes aggregating in the human endometrium and decidua can secrete an array of cytokines including all of those listed for uNK cells, plus IL2 and IL4 [42, 43]. A pivotal T-lymphocyte population conferring maternal immune tolerance in pregnancy is the CD4+CD25+ T regulatory (Treg) cells. The suppressive function of this population is linked to synthesis of copious TGFβ and IL10 [44].

Eosinophils, neutrophils, and mast cells exist in varying abundance in the cycling and pregnant endometrium and these cells also have the potential to synthesize a variety of different cytokines and chemokines in a regulated manner. Neutrophils are a potent source of IFNγ in the human endometrium, with expression regulated by bacterial components, IL12, and TNFα [45]. Uterine mast cells may contribute significantly to local GM-CSF and TNFα content, with release during early pregnancy being induced by the neuropeptide substance P and embryo-derived factors [46].

Cytokine regulation of embryo development
Maternal tract cytokine–embryo communication

Cytokines originating from the oviductal and endometrial epithelium bathe the developing embryo as it traverses the reproductive tract prior to implantation. Comprehensive studies in mainly mouse embryos show that embryos express cytokine receptors from conception until implantation and beyond, and several cytokines exert different effects on embryo cell number and viability, gene expression, and developmental competence. Through promoting and in some cases inhibiting the timing and extent of blastomere survival, proliferation, and differentiation, these factors appear to have important roles in synchronizing embryo growth with the maternal changes that lead to uterine receptivity. The identity and biological effects of growth factors and cytokines targeting the preimplantation embryo have been reviewed previously [2, 47–51]. Strategies including supplementation of exogenous cytokines to the embryo culture, neutralization of ligand or receptors, or studying mice with null mutations in ligand or receptor genes show that factors including GM-CSF, CSF1, LIF, heparin-binding epidermal growth factor (HB-EGF), insulin-like growth factor (IGF)-I, and IGF-II all promote blastocyst development. Others including TNFα and IFNγ exert potent inhibitory effects, with TNFα acting to reduce the viability of cells in the inner cell mass of murine embryos [52] while IFNγ has embryotoxic effects over a wide concentration range and limits trophectoderm proliferation [53].

The embryo itself synthesizes several cytokines, including IL1, LIF, EGF, TGFβ, and IL6, which have autocrine roles in neighboring cells within the embryo [54], as well as providing signals to maternal tissues. Embryo-derived IL1 may function in signaling events that increase endometrial receptivity to implantation. In sheep and cattle, IFNτ produced by the preimplantation embryo acts to mediate maternal recognition of pregnancy through preventing regression of the corpus luteum [55].

Cytokine regulation of human embryo development

In human embryos, rates of embryo development to the blastocyst stage are characteristically less than 50% and human IVF embryo development is characterized by arrested, delayed, and abnormal cell division [2]. Human embryos express cognate receptors for several cytokines and at least four cytokines have been shown, in well-conducted studies with sufficient embryos, to exert substantial biological effects to improve blastocyst development in vitro. Using embryos surplus to patient requirements, GM-CSF, LIF, HB-EGF, and IGF-I have each been shown to improve the rate of proliferation and viability of blastomeres, and/or the proportion of embryos that develop to the blastocyst stage and beyond.

We have reported profound embryotrophic effects of GM-CSF in human embryos [56], where addition to culture medium increased the proportion of embryos that developed to the blastocyst stage from 30% to 76%. The developmental competence of these blastocysts, as assessed by hatching and attachment to extracellular matrix-coated culture dishes, was also improved by GM-CSF. The period in culture required to yield 50% blastocyst development was reduced by 14 hours, and blastocysts grown in GM-CSF were found to contain approximately 35% more cells, due primarily to an increase in the size of the inner cell mass [56].

In another study, addition of LIF to a complex serum-free human embryo culture media increased the blastulation rate from 18% to 44% [57], although this was not reflected in any advance in attachment and trophectoderm outgrowth. Addition of HB-EGF also improved the proportion of embryos developing to the blastocyst stage, as well as their developmental competence as assessed by hatching, adherence to extracellular matrix proteins, and trophectoderm outgrowth [58]. Blastulation rates increased from 41% in the control group to 71% in the presence of HB-EGF. In contrast to GM-CSF, however, HB-EGF did not accelerate the speed of development or increase cell number and its effect was limited to good quality embryos. Addition of IGF-I to culture media increased the blastulation rate from 35% in the controls to 60% in the treatment group and caused an increase in blastocyst cell number due to an increase in cells in the inner cell mass [59].

Cytokines and embryo developmental competence

The peri-conceptional period, when the embryo is formed and implantation occurs, is critical not just for establishing pregnancy but also for programming the course of fetal and placental development that results in a healthy neonate at birth. Indeed the life potential of the offspring is set in train from this early time, since disturbance to preimplantation embryo development or endometrial receptivity both impact later morphogenesis of the placenta and its capacity to support fetal growth [60]. Experimental perturbations at various stages of pregnancy implicate the first days of life as the most susceptible period for influencing later fetal health [61–64]. Altered embryo development, or insufficient maternal support of the conceptus at implantation can lead to miscarriage, or "shallow" placental development, resulting in preeclampsia, fetal growth restriction, and/or preterm delivery [60, 65]. In turn these conditions affect health after birth and can result in metabolic disorder and onset of chronic disease [66]. Several maternal stressors can act in the peri-conceptional period, including immunological, infectious, nutritional, metabolic, physiochemical, or even psychosocial perturbations – all of these have been shown to exert similar subtle but permanent alterations in fetal development and the life-course trajectory of offspring.

There is compelling epidemiological evidence from many human studies in a range of settings that is consistent with animal data, showing that variation in environment before birth alters the risk of disease in later life, and that early pregnancy is the most vulnerable period [67]. Constrained fetal growth in utero impacts perinatal events and growth after birth and can predispose an individual to obesity, heart disease, diabetes, and stroke in adulthood, to an extent comparable in magnitude to genetic predisposition and lifestyle factors such as obesity and smoking.

Cytokines and embryo programming

The impact of preimplantation development on later pregnancy progression, fetal growth, and postnatal health is known as embryo "programming." Indeed the biological process of early programming of later development is the key to defining the difference between a "viable" embryo and a "healthy" embryo – that is, not every embryo that appears morphologically normal in the culture dish has equivalent competence to generate a healthy baby and adult. The cytokine environment is implicated as a major factor in programming future development in embryos.

The means by which "memory" of environment in early life may be perpetuated into later fetal and postnatal growth remain ill-defined. Several parameters contribute to embryo programming; two critical factors are cell number in the blastocyst, and genetic imprinting. Even small perturbations in blastomere number and inner cell mass/trophectoderm allocation in the blastocyst influence the growth trajectory of the fetus and after birth [66]. Aberrant genetic imprinting, with defects evident in imprinted genes *Igf2*, *H19*, *Grb10*, and *Grb7*, occurs when mouse embryos are cultured in the presence of serum [68] or in suboptimal culture media [69] and is linked with later growth changes. Fetal over-growth in cattle and sheep after embryo culture (the "large offspring syndrome") has been attributed to imprinting errors in *Igf2r* as a direct consequence of metabolic stress in culture [70]. Through influencing blastomere division rate and viability, as well as gene expression and possibly methylation of genes, cytokines present in the reproductive tract during the periconceptional period likely contribute to embryo programming. Because expression of methyltransferases and other methylation machinery are cell cycle-regulated, disruption in their function may occur after the timing of embryo development is slowed in culture [71], whereas embryotrophic growth factors that accelerate blastomere cell division would oppose this effect.

The full range of effects of early cytokine exposure on later fetal and postnatal growth is not yet understood, as virtually all studies on cytokine-mediated effects during embryo culture are limited to the developmental endpoint of the blastocyst stage embryo. Only a few studies report the effects of cytokines on implantation success after embryo transfer in rodents. When embryos were transferred to recipients after culture in medium supplemented with EGF, a key autocrine growth factor in preimplantation embryos [54], implantation rates were increased [72]. Insulin stimulates cell proliferation in the inner cell mass in vitro in the rat [73] and after transfer, rates of implantation, fetal survival, and weight at birth were all increased both in rats [74] and in mice [75]. Addition of LIF to embryo culture increases cell number in blastocysts which after transfer generate fetuses with higher birthweights, although this is partially attributable to prolonged gestation [76]. Conversely, embryo transfer experiments show that exposure of embryos to TNFα during the preimplantation period does not alter implantation rate, but predisposes to later miscarriage and fetal growth retardation [77].

A major criticism we have of research in this field is that, rather inexplicably, the consequences of cytokine treatments following embryo transfer have been poorly reported. Investigation of long-term effects in rodent models is relatively easy to perform and allows examination in detail of placentation and fetal development, as well as subsequent neo-natal growth. However, effects on fetal development and subsequent intergenerational effects have only been evaluated for one cytokine, GM-CSF (discussed in the following section). Perhaps more understandably, data from ruminant species are also restricted to a few studies recording subsequent pregnancy rate following embryo transfer, and are largely limited to LIF [78], GM-CSF (CSF2) [79], IGF-I [80], and EGF plus IGF-I [81]. In each of these studies, substantially improved implantation rates were observed and for GM-CSF, this was linked with reduced pregnancy loss in later gestation. In each study normal calves were born and no adverse effects on offspring were reported.

Cytokine regulation of embryo sensing and adaptation

These observations on developmental programming raise the question of why the mammalian embryo has evolved such exquisite responsiveness to the external environment when it might be argued that a fully autonomous developmental program would be less risky for long-term viability and health. It seems likely that developmental plasticity in the preimplantation embryo is desirable so that the embryo can respond to the demands and opportunities of the outside world by adaptation, rather than by adhering to a standard fixed phenotype that may be inappropriate to the changing external environment and could place the mother at health risk [82]. Plasticity can be exerted at the cellular level by adjustment of cell numbers and lineage fate, and at the molecular level by changes in gene expression pathways or the more permanent effects of epigenetics [83, 84]. Together these processes exert modifications through which the environment can modulate the phenotype to "suit best" the prevailing or predicted after-birth environment.

Changes in cell numbers and lineage allocation or in gene expression in blastocysts due to perturbation in the local physiochemical or cytokine environment cause differences in placental structure and nutrient transport function, which is the key limiting factor in fetal growth [62, 63, 85]. With plasticity comes the risk of poor outcomes – when embryo sensing of the external environment fails to indicate and match the reality correctly, or where compromises made to favor immediate survival are suboptimal for later metabolic, neurodevelopmental, or immune health after birth. In broad terms it seems that extreme adaptation causes loss of functional capacity and resistance to future stressors, while maintenance of capacity in early intrauterine life improves the likelihood of subsequent health and resilience in adulthood [86].

The molecular mechanisms underlying communication between the female tract and the embryo, through which information about environment is transmitted, are not fully defined. There is evidence from our group and others that in the peri-conceptional period, inflammatory insults lead to altered oviductal cytokine patterns which correlate with changes in embryo development and long-term outcomes [64, 87]. Thus, we argue that maternal tract cytokines are a key pathway through which inflammatory, infectious, and chemical insults can converge and integrate, since all of these factors alter cytokine expression in the reproductive tract [87]. We predict that cytokines operate together with availability of nutrients (amino acids, hexose sugars, and lipids) and physiochemical parameters including oxygen, ionic composition, and ammonia [61] to provide the signals through which embryos sense the prevailing environment and adjust their developmental program accordingly.

Cytokines and maternal tract quality control

A related action of the local cytokine network present during the pre- and peri-implantation period may be to ensure that pregnancy does not occur when the mother is not adequately prepared or the environment is not suitable [88]. Stringent maternal quality control processes appear to operate as pregnancy is established – in humans, the majority of early embryos perish before implantation and only ~60% of embryos that implant survive beyond the second week. In the event that infection, nutritional deprivation, stress, or injury is overwhelming, the cytokine network is a pathway through which these environmental cues and intrinsic factors can converge to prevent an embryo from implanting. Key candidate cytokines that in sufficiently high concentrations can terminate embryo development are TNFα and IFNγ, which are produced by maternal tract tissues, particularly immune cells, when these insults are present.

GM-CSF and embryo development

One cytokine that has received considerable attention for its utility in human IVF embryo culture is GM-CSF, and since this is the first cytokine now incorporated into commercial culture medium, we shall discuss the biology of GM-CSF regulation of embryo development in greater detail. GM-CSF was originally identified as a regulator of the proliferation, differentiation, and activation of myeloid hematopoietic cells. A considerable body of literature now demonstrates the key role of this cytokine in the events of early pregnancy and particularly its actions as an important cytokine for supporting preimplantation embryo development.

GM-CSF is secreted into the oviduct and uterus during the period following conception under regulation by estrogen and is further induced by factors present in male seminal fluid. In women, GM-CSF is secreted by epithelial cells lining the Fallopian tube and the uterus where its expression fluctuates over the course of the menstrual cycle, being maximal in the mid-luteal phase [26, 89].

In vitro studies indicate that GM-CSF is a potent embryotrophic factor with survival- and development-promoting effects in mouse, cattle, and human preimplantation embryos [56, 90, 91]. Embryos express GM-CSF receptors (GM-Rα), indicating that in vivo, GM-CSF secreted from maternal uterine epithelial cells acts on embryos in a paracrine manner. Both mouse and human embryos synthesize GM-Rα from the time of fertilization through blastocyst stages of development [91, 92]. Expression occurs in both the outer trophecto-derm layer and the inner cell mass cells, with receptor protein detectable on the cell membrane of trophectoderm cells [91, 92].

The most obvious effect of supplementing culture medium with GM-CSF in human and mouse blastocysts in vitro is an increased number of blastomeres after the same period in culture [56, 91]. When mouse embryos are flushed from the reproductive tract early after fertilization and cultured ex vivo to the blastocyst stage, embryos develop faster, attain higher number of viable blastomeres, and hatch and attach to the culture dish more frequently if GM-CSF is added to the culture medium [91]. GM-CSF appears to exert a stronger beneficial effect when embryos are exposed to stressors such as protein deprivation [93]. Blastocysts recovered from mice with a null mutation in the *Csf2* gene have fewer cells than wild-type control mice, showing GM-CSF is essential for normal blastocyst develop-ment even in the in vivo situation where other cytokines might be expected to compensate for any deficiency [91].

The embryotrophic effects of GM-CSF are more profound in human embryos [56]. In studies involving several hundred frozen human embryos, addition of the cytokine to culture medium from the 2- to 4-cell stage onwards was found to exert a twofold increase in the proportion of IVF embryos that develop to the blastocyst stage [56, 92]. The developmental competence of these blastocysts, as assessed by zona pellucida dissolution and attachment to extracellular matrix-coated culture dishes, was substantially improved with GM-CSF. Embryos cultured in the presence of GM-CSF reached blastocyst stage on average 14 hours quicker, and contain approximately 35% more cells [56]. This is due primarily to an increase in the size of the inner cell mass compartment, associated with a 50% reduction in apoptotic nuclei [92]. Even in the presence of other cytokines, GM-CSF seems to have a paramount role, since when human IVF embryos were co-cultured with autologous endometrial cells, the amount of GM-CSF secreted into culture medium correlated with likelihood of successful pregnancy after embryo transfer [94].

Effects of GM-CSF on promoting blastocyst development in vitro are now also reported for bovine [90] and porcine [95] embryos. In sheep embryos [96] and cattle embryonic tropectoderm cells [97], GM-CSF acts to promote blastocyst secretion of IFNτ, the pregnancy recognition molecule important for activating maternal support of embryo development.

GM-CSF and fetal programming

GM-CSF signaling in early embryos impacts not only short-term survival, but also long-term developmental competence. In a large embryo transfer study in mice comparing the effects of presence and absence of GM-CSF in in vitro embryo culture medium, fetal and postnatal growth, and the likelihood of obesity in adult progeny were influenced by early growth factor exposure [63]. In mice, embryo culture is known to have adverse effects on the fetus that manifest as growth restriction in utero, rapid compensatory growth after birth, and larger body mass with increased fat deposits in adults. Addition of GM-CSF to embryos prior to transfer was found to improve embryo implantation rate, correct deficiencies in placental structure and fetal growth trajectory, and partly alleviate the long-term adverse effects of embryo culture on postnatal growth [63]. This result shows GM-CSF exposure in the preimplantation period is essential for programming optimal fetal development after implantation. It also suggests that reproductive deficiency seen in GM-CSF null mutant mice, which show fetal growth restriction and high rates of fetal loss and abnormality in late gestation [98], is at least in part the consequence of GM-CSF deprivation in the preimplantation embryo.

GM-CSF and protection of embryos from cell stress and apoptosis

The means by which GM-CSF exerts its embryotrophic and programming influence in embryos is not fully defined, but several factors point to a mechanism involving protection of embryos from cell stress and the programmed cell death (apoptosis) that ultimately results from severe cell stress. The rates of cell division, differentiation, and/or cell death that accompany progression from zygote to blastocyst are highly sensitive to disruption by environmental stressors [99]. Embryo culture, particularly in suboptimal culture media, exerts cell stress in developing embryos, which results in fewer blastomeres due equally to retarded progression through the cell cycle and elevated incidence of apoptosis [100]. Growth factor and cytokine deprivation in vitro has been proposed to be a potential stressor in vitro [3], along with metabolic and substrate deficiency [101] and oxidative stress [102].

While it seems clear that a small percentage of cells in the preimplantation embryo usually die by apoptosis even under optimal conditions in vivo, a greater than normal activation of the apoptosis pathway is part of the adaptive response to culture stress in embryos, where it is presumed to ensure removal of irreversibly damaged cells [103, 104]. Culture-induced stress is demonstrated by the elevated expression of Bcl-2 family genes and the TRP53 stress response pathways in cultured mouse [105] and human embryos [106]. A response to stress in embryos that precedes apoptosis is activation of the heat shock protein (HSP) or stress response pathway, which acts to limit cell damage and facilitate recovery to help cells survive stress. HSPs interact with and modulate the apoptosis pathway, and influence commitment to either cell death or survival, depending on the severity of cell damage. Mild thermal, oxidative, and osmotic stresses or culture in vitro induces HSPs in embryos from as early as the blastocyst stage [107].

Several studies show that GM-CSF inhibits the cellular stress response and apoptosis pathways, implicating this as a key mechanism underpinning improved embryo growth and survival. TUNEL staining in in vitro cultured human embryos shows GM-CSF protects blastomeres from apoptosis, particularly in the inner cell mass [92], and mouse embryos cultured with GM-CSF also show evidence of reduced apoptosis [108]. Microarray and RT-PCR analyses of gene transcription profile in mouse embryos show that GM-CSF suppresses the stress response that activates the apoptosis pathway [108, 109]. In in vivo developed blastocysts, *Csf2* null mutation caused elevated expression of some stress response genes but the effect was less severe than in vitro [109], indicating the protective effect of GM-CSF is particularly important in in vitro culture media, compared with in vivo where other cytokines can partly compensate for absence of GM-CSF.

GM-CSF utilty in IVF embryo culture media

On the basis of the large number of animal studies and in vitro human data, plus three small pilot studies in Australia, Korea, and the USA, a clinical trial to evaluate the potential benefit of GM-CSF in human clinical IVF has recently been completed by the Danish company ORIGIO A/S. Initially, a preclinical safety study was completed using human oocytes from 73 women, and it was confirmed that there is no increase in chromosomal abnormality in embryos cultured with GM-CSF [110]. The embryo transfer study comprised a multicenter, randomized, placebo-controlled, double-blinded prospective study involving 1332 Danish and Swedish patients recruited from 14 fertility clinics. Fertilization, embryo culture until day 3, and embryo transfer were performed in either control medium, or medium supplemented with GM-CSF. GM-CSF was associated with a significant increase in implantation rate at gestational week 12, with ongoing implantation rate (number of fetal heart beats as a fraction of embryos transferred) of 23.0% for the GM-CSF group, compared with 18.7% for the control group (P = 0.02). The most profound effect of GM-CSF was evident in a subgroup of 327 women who had previously experienced miscarriage after conception by IVF or naturally, where ongoing implantation rate at gestational week 12 was increased by 40%, from 16.5% in control medium to 23.2% with GM-CSF (P = 0.001). Follow-up on children born in the completed study shows that embryo culture in GM-CSF increased the number of women achieving a live birth in the miscarriage subgroup by 28%, while perinatal parameters including birthweight, gestational age at birth, and rate of birth defects were similar in both treatment groups. On the basis of this outcome, ORIGIO has now released EmbryoGen®, the world's first embryo culture medium containing a cytokine or growth factor.

Together these data from the largest IVF clinical trial conducted to date provide solid evidence that there are benefits of addition of cytokine to embryo culture media in terms of establishing successful pregnancy and increasing the chance of a healthy infant at term. These benefits are most apparent in women who are prone to miscarriage, where for various reasons the maternal tract may be less than optimal for supporting healthy embryo growth or the embryos might be more vulnerable to culture-induced stress. Importantly, the absence of any evidence of adverse outcome in the children born after embryo culture in cytokine is reassuring for the safety of using GM-CSF, although it will be important to follow the development of these children over the longer term.

Conclusions

In vitro conditions for culture of human embryos are generally suboptimal and are believed to compromise embryo quality and contribute to the high rates of implantation failure and impaired fetal outcomes seen in human IVF and related reproductive technologies [5–9]. Thus, there is scope for improving the quality of IVF embryo culture media, to increase both the number of embryos suitable for transfer and the likelihood of establishing healthy pregnancy after transfer. An attractive avenue worthy of exploration is the naturally produced cytokines that, when added to culture medium, provide a culture environment that more closely mimics the physiological situation. In vivo, cytokines can be viewed as important agents for mediating maternal tract–embryo communication, with fluctuations in the relative abundance of positive agents, including GM-CSF, LIF, HB-EGF, and IGF-II, against negative agents such as TNFα and IFNγ, implicated in mediating the biological effects of embryo programming, embryo plasticity and adaptation, and maternal tract quality control. While cytokines have sometimes been viewed as simply "fine-tuning agents" in the reproductive tract that are dispensable in vitro, the weight of evidence from animal studies is that deprivation of growth factors from culture medium is a major cause of the culture-induced stress that leads to altered growth trajectories and compromises health in offspring after embryo culture. Consistent with this, the results of a large human clinical trial demonstrate that at least one cytokine, GM-CSF, is efficacious in maximizing developmental competence in human embryos and can be utilized as a new therapeutic strategy to protect against fetal loss after IVF in women who are prone to miscarriage.

The utility of combining additional cytokines together with GM-CSF to improve further human embryo development in vitro, perhaps utilizing LIF, HB-EGF, and/or IGF-II, remains to be explored. Research to evaluate the additive interactions of cytokines would improve the likelihood of eventually defining an embryo growth medium that truly replicates the in vivo milieu. However, given our knowledge of cytokine intracellular signaling and redundancy amongst ligands activating these pathways, it seems likely that the full benefit will be achieved with at most two or three factors and will not require all of the cytokines known to be present in vivo. Additionally, as emphasized by Harper and colleagues [4], it is critical that new innovations in IVF practice, particularly including use of cytokines, are founded in a solid understanding of the underlying biology and carefully evaluated for safety and efficacy in well-designed, sufficiently powered clinical trials.

Conflict of interest statement

Sarah Robertson is an inventor on patents concerning utility of GM-CSF in IVF culture medium and receives royalty income from ORIGIO A/S. Jeremy Thompson is a consultant to Cook Medical Pty. Ltd. and has patents on methods for in vitro oocyte maturation.

References

1. Kaye PL. Preimplantation growth factor physiology. *Rev Reprod* 1997;**2**: 121–7.

2. Hardy K, Spanos S. Growth factor expression and function in the human and mouse preimplantation embryo. *J Endocrinol* 2002;**172**:221–36.

3. O'Neill C. The potential roles for embryotrophic ligands in preimplantation embryo development. *Hum Reprod Update* 2008;**14**:275–88.

4. Harper J, Magli MC, Lundin K, *et al.* When and how should new technology be introduced into the IVF laboratory? *Hum Reprod* 2012;**27**:303–13.

5. Schieve LA, Meikle SF, Ferre C, *et al.* Low and very low birth weight in infants conceived with use of assisted reproductive technology. *N Engl J Med* 2002;**346**:731–7.

6. Jackson RA, Gibson KA, Wu YW, *et al.* Perinatal outcomes in singletons following in vitro fertilization: a meta-analysis. *Obstet Gynecol* 2004;**103**:551–63.

7. Hansen M, Kurinczuk JJ, Bower C, *et al.* The risk of major birth defects after intracytoplasmic sperm injection and in vitro fertilization. *N Engl J Med* 2002;**346**:725–30.

8. Maher ER, Afnan M, Barratt CL. Epigenetic risks related to assisted reproductive technologies: epigenetics, imprinting, ART and icebergs? *Hum Reprod* 2003;**18**:2508–11.

9. Gosden R, Trasler J, Lucifero D, *et al.* Rare congenital disorders, imprinted genes, and assisted reproductive technology. *Lancet* 2003;**361**:1975–7.

10. Callard RE, Gearing AJH. *The Cytokine Facts Book.* Academic Press, London, UK, 1994.

11. Nathan C, Sporn M. Cytokines in context. *J Cell Biol* 1991;**113**:981–6.

12. Robertson SA, Seamark RF, Guilbert LJ, *et al.* The role of cytokines in gestation. *Crit Rev Immunol* 1994;**14**:239–92.

13. Tabibzadeh S. Role of cytokines in endometrium and at the fetomaternal interface. *Reprod Med Rev* 1994;**3**:11–28.

14. Pollard, JW. Role of cytokines in the pregnant uterus of interstitial implanting species. In: Bazer FW, ed. *The Endocrinology of Pregnancy.* Totowa, NJ, Humana Press Inc. 1998;59–82.

15. Salamonsen LA, Dimitriadis E, Robb L. Cytokines in implantation. *Semin Reprod Med* 2000;**18**:299–310.

16. Dimitriadis E, White CA, Jones RL, *et al.* Cytokines, chemokines and growth factors in endometrium related to implantation. *Hum Reprod Update* 2005;**11**:613–30.

17. Kelly RW, King AE, Critchley HO. Cytokine control in human endometrium. *Reproduction* 2001;**121**:3–19.

18. Hannan NJ, Paiva P, Meehan KL, *et al.* Analysis of fertility-related soluble mediators in human uterine fluid identifies VEGF as a key regulator of embryo implantation. *Endocrinology* 2011;**152**:4948–56.

19. Hunt JS. Expression and regulation of the tumour necrosis factor-alpha gene in the female reproductive tract. *Reprod Fertil Dev* 1993;**5**:141–53.

20. Robertson SA, Mayrhofer G, Seamark RF. Ovarian steroid hormones regulate granulocyte-macrophage colony-stimulating factor synthesis by uterine epithelial cells in the mouse. *Biol Reprod* 1996;**54**:183–96.

21. Daiter E, Pollard JW. Colony stimulating factor-1 (CSF-1) in pregnancy. *Reprod Med Rev* 1992;**1**:83–97.

22. Kimber SJ. Leukaemia inhibitory factor in implantation and uterine biology. *Reproduction* 2005;**130**:131–45.

23. Hannan NJ, Salamonsen LA. Role of chemokines in the endometrium and in embryo implantation. *Curr Opin Obstet Gynecol* 2007;**19**:266–72.

24. Robertson SA. Seminal plasma and male factor signalling in the female reproductive tract. *Cell Tissue Res* 2005;**322**:43–52.

25. Charnock-Jones DS, Sharkey AM, Fenwick P, *et al.* Leukaemia inhibitory factor mRNA concentration peaks in human endometrium at the time of implantation and the blastocyst contains mRNA for the receptor at this time. *J Reprod Fertil* 1994;**101**:421–6.

26. Giacomini G, Tabibzadeh SS, Satyaswaroop PG, *et al.* Epithelial cells are the major source of biologically active granulocyte macrophage colony-stimulating factor in human endometrium. *Hum Reprod* 1995;**10**:3259–63.

27. Sharkey DJ, Tremellen KP, Jasper MJ, Gemzell-Danielsson K, Robertson SA. Seminal fluid induces leukocyte recruitment and cytokine and chemokine mRNA expression in the human cervix after coitus. *J Immunol* 2012;**188**:2445–54.

28. Gutsche S, von Wolff M, Strowitzki T, *et al.* Seminal plasma induces mRNA expression

of IL-1beta, IL-6 and LIF in endometrial epithelial cells in vitro. *Mol Hum Reprod* 2003;**9**:785–91.

29. Zhang J, Lathbury LJ, Salamonsen LA. Expression of the chemokine eotaxin and its receptor, CCR3, in human endometrium. *Biol Reprod* 2000;**62**:404–11.

30. Jones RL, Hannan NJ, Kaitu'u TJ, *et al.* Identification of chemokines important for leukocyte recruitment to the human endometrium at the times of embryo implantation and menstruation. *J Clin Endocrinol Metab* 2004;**89**:6155–67.

31. Rasmussen SJ, Eckmann L, Quayle AJ, *et al.* Secretion of proinflammatory cytokines by epithelial cells in response to *Chlamydia* infection suggests a central role for epithelial cells in chlamydial pathogenesis. *J Clin Invest* 1997;**99**:77–87.

32. Fichorova RN, Cronin AO, Lien E, *et al.* Response to *Neisseria gonorrhoeae* by cervicovaginal epithelial cells occurs in the absence of toll-like receptor 4-mediated signaling. *J Immunol* 2002;**168**:2424–32.

33. Fichorova RN, Anderson DJ. Differential expression of immunobiological mediators by immortalized human cervical and vaginal epithelial cells. *Biol Reprod* 1999;**60**:508–14.

34. Hunt JS, Robertson SA. Uterine macrophages and environmental programming for pregnancy success. *J Reprod Immunol* 1996;**32**:1–25.

35. Chen HL, Yelavarthi KK, Hunt JS. Identification of transforming growth factor-beta 1 mRNA in virgin and pregnant rat uteri by in situ hybridization. *J Reprod Immunol* 1993;**25**:221–33.

36. Heikkinen J, Mottonen M, Komi J, *et al.* Phenotypic characterization of human decidual macrophages. *Clin Exp Immunol* 2003;**131**:498–505.

37. Tabibzadeh S, Sun XZ. Cytokine expression in human endometrium throughout the menstrual cycle. *Hum Reprod* 1992;**7**: 1214–21.

38. Petroff MG, Sedlmayr P, Azzola D, *et al.* Decidual macrophages are potentially susceptible to inhibition by class Ia and class Ib HLA molecules. *J Reprod Immunol* 2002;**56**:3–17.

39. Haddad EK, Duclos AJ, Antecka E, *et al.* Role of interferon-gamma in the priming of decidual macrophages for nitric oxide production and early pregnancy loss. *Cell Immunol* 1997;**181**:68–75.

40. Croy BA, van den Heuvel MJ, Borzychowski AM, *et al.* Uterine natural killer cells: a specialized differentiation regulated by ovarian hormones. *Immunol Rev* 2006;**214**:161–85.

41. Higuma-Myojo S, Sasaki Y, Miyazaki S, *et al.* Cytokine profile of natural killer cells in early human pregnancy. *Am J Reprod Immunol* 2005;**54**:21–9.

42. Piccinni MP, Romagnani S. Regulation of fetal allograft survival by a hormone-controlled Th1- and Th2-type cytokines. *Immunol Res* 1996;**15**:141–50.

43. Jokhi PP, King A, Sharkey AM, *et al.* Screening for cytokine messenger ribonucleic acids in purified human decidual lymphocyte populations by the reverse-transcriptase polymerase chain reaction. *J Immunol* 1994;**153**:4427–35.

44. Guerin LR, Prins JR, Robertson SA. Regulatory T-cells and immune tolerance in pregnancy: a new target for infertility treatment? *Hum Reprod Update* 2009;**15**:517–35.

45. Yeaman GR, Collins JE, Currie JK, *et al.* IFN-gamma is produced by polymorphonuclear neutrophils in human uterine endometrium and by cultured peripheral blood polymorphonuclear neutrophils. *J Immunol* 1998;**160**:5145–53.

46. Cocchiara R, Albeggiani G, Azzolina A, *et al.* Effect of substance P on uterine mast cell cytokine release during the reproductive cycle. *J Neuroimmunol* 1995;**60**:107–15.

47. Pampfer S, Arceci RJ, Pollard JW. Role of colony stimulating factor-1 (CSF-1) and other lympho-hematopoietic growth factors in mouse pre-implantation development. *Bioessays* 1991;**13**:535–40.

48. Kaye PL, Harvey MB. The role of growth factors in preimplantation development. *Prog Growth Factor Res* 1995;**6**:1–24.

49. Stewart CL, Cullinan EB. Preimplantation development of the mammalian embryo and its regulation by growth factors. *Dev Genet* 1997;**21**:91–101.

50. Kane MT, Morgan PM, Coonan C. Peptide growth factors and preimplantation development. *Hum Reprod Update* 1997;**3**:137–57.

51. Diaz-Cueto L, Gerton GL. The influence of growth factors on the development of preimplantation mammalian embryos. *Arch Med Res* 2001;**32**:619–26.

52. Pampfer S, Moulaert B, Vanderheyden I, *et al*. Effect of tumour necrosis factor alpha on rat blastocyst growth and glucose metabolism. *J Reprod Fertil* 1994;**101**:199–206.

53. Hill JA, Haimovici F, Anderson DJ. Products of activated lymphocytes and macrophages inhibit mouse embryo development in vitro. *J Immunol* 1987;**139**:2250–4.

54. Paria BC, Dey SK. Preimplantation embryo development in vitro: cooperative interactions among embryos and role of growth factors. *Proc Natl Acad Sci U S A* 1990;**87**:4756–60.

55. Bazer FW, Spencer TE, Ott TL. Interferon tau: a novel pregnancy recognition signal. *Am J Reprod Immunol* 1997;**37**:412–20.

56. Sjoblom C, Wikland M, Robertson SA. Granulocyte-macrophage colony-stimulating factor promotes human blastocyst development in vitro. *Hum Reprod* 1999;**14**:3069–76.

57. Dunglison GF, Barlow DH, Sargent IL. Leukaemia inhibitory factor significantly enhances the blastocyst formation rates of human embryos cultured in serum-free medium. *Hum Reprod* 1996;**11**:191–6.

58. Martin KL, Barlow DH, Sargent IL. Heparin-binding epidermal growth factor significantly improves human blastocyst development and hatching in serum-free medium. *Hum Reprod* 1998;**13**:1645–52.

59. Lighten AD, Moore GE, Winston RM, *et al*. Routine addition of human insulin-like growth factor-I ligand could benefit clinical in-vitro fertilization culture. *Hum Reprod* 1998;**13**:3144–50.

60. Fowden AL, Forhead AJ, Coan PM, *et al*. The placenta and intrauterine programming. *J Neuroendocrinol* 2008;**20**:439–50.

61. Thompson JG, Lane M, Robertson SA. Adaptive responses of embryos to their microenvironment and consequences for post-implantation development. In: Owens JS, Wintour M, eds. *Early Life Origins of Health and Disease*. Austin, TX, Landes Bioscience. 2005;58–69.

62. Kwong WY, Wild AE, Roberts P, *et al*. Maternal undernutrition during the preimplantation period of rat development causes blastocyst abnormalities and programming of postnatal hypertension. *Development* 2000;**127**:4195–202.

63. Sjoblom C, Roberts CT, Wikland M, *et al*. Granulocyte-macrophage colony-stimulating factor alleviates adverse consequences of embryo culture on fetal growth trajectory and placental morphogenesis. *Endocrinology* 2005;**146**:2142–53.

64. Williams CL, Teeling JL, Perry VH, *et al*. Mouse maternal systemic inflammation at the zygote stage causes blunted cytokine responsiveness in lipopolysaccharide-challenged adult offspring. *BMC Biol* 2011;**9**:49.

65. Maltepe E, Bakardjiev AI, Fisher SJ. The placenta: transcriptional, epigenetic, and physiological integration during development. *J Clin Invest* 2010;**120**:1016–25.

66. Thompson JG, Kind KL, Roberts CT, *et al*. Epigenetic risks related to assisted reproductive technologies: short- and long-term consequences for the health of children conceived through assisted reproduction technology: more reason for caution? *Hum Reprod* 2002;**17**:2783–6.

67. Barker DJ, Clark PM. Fetal undernutrition and disease in later life. *Rev Reprod* 1997;**2**:105–12.

68. Khosla S, Dean W, Brown D, *et al*. Culture of preimplantation mouse embryos affects fetal development and the expression of imprinted genes. *Biol Reprod* 2001;**64**:918–26.

69. Doherty AS, Mann MR, Tremblay KD, et al. Differential effects of culture on imprinted H19 expression in the preimplantation mouse embryo. *Biol Reprod* 2000;**62**:1526–35.

70. Young LE, Fernandes K, McEvoy TG, et al. Epigenetic change in IGF2R is associated with fetal overgrowth after sheep embryo culture. *Nat Genet* 2001;**27**:153–4.

71. De Rycke M, Liebaers I, Van Steirteghem A. Epigenetic risks related to assisted reproductive technologies: risk analysis and epigenetic inheritance. *Hum Reprod* 2002;**17**:2487–94.

72. Morita Y, Tsutsumi O, Taketani Y. In vitro treatment of embryos with epidermal growth factor improves viability and increases the implantation rate of blastocysts transferred to recipient mice. *Am J Obstet Gynecol* 1994;**171**: 406–9.

73. De Hertogh R, Vanderheyden I, Pampfer S, et al. Stimulatory and inhibitory effects of glucose and insulin on rat blastocyst development in vitro. *Diabetes* 1991;**40**:641–7.

74. Zhang X, Armstrong DT. Presence of amino acids and insulin in a chemically defined medium improves development of 8-cell rat embryos in vitro and subsequent implantation in vivo. *Biol Reprod* 1990;**42**:662–8.

75. Kaye PL, Gardner HG. Preimplantation access to maternal insulin and albumin increases fetal growth rate in mice. *Hum Reprod* 1999;**14**:3052–9.

76. Cheung LP, Leung HY, Bongso A. Effect of supplementation of leukemia inhibitory factor and epidermal growth factor on murine embryonic development in vitro, implantation, and outcome of offspring. *Fertil Steril* 2003;**80**(Suppl 2):727–35.

77. Wuu YD, Pampfer S, Becquet P, et al. Tumor necrosis factor alpha decreases the viability of mouse blastocysts in vitro and in vivo. *Biol Reprod* 1999;**60**:479–83.

78. Fry RC, Batt PA, Fairclough RJ, et al. Human leukaemia inhibitory factor improves the viability of cultured ovine embryos. *Biol Reprod* 1992;**46**:470–4.

79. Loureiro B, Bonilla L, Block J, et al. Colony-stimulating factor 2 (CSF-2) improves development and posttransfer survival of bovine embryos produced in vitro. *Endocrinology* 2009;**150**:5046–54.

80. Block J, Hansen PJ, Loureiro B, et al. Improving post-transfer survival of bovine embryos produced in vitro: actions of insulin-like growth factor-1, colony stimulating factor-2 and hyaluronan. *Theriogenology* 2011;**76**:1602–9.

81. Sakagami N, Umeki H, Nishino O, et al. Normal calves produced after transfer of embryos cultured in a chemically defined medium supplemented with epidermal growth factor and insulin-like growth factor I following ovum pick up and in vitro fertilization in Japanese black cows. *J Reprod Dev* 2012;**58**:140–6.

82. Hochberg Z, Feil R, Constancia M, et al. Child health, developmental plasticity, and epigenetic programming. *Endocr Rev* 2011;**32**:159–224.

83. Young LE. Imprinting of genes and the Barker hypothesis. *Twin Res* 2001;**4**: 307–17.

84. Morgan HD, Santos F, Green K, et al. Epigenetic reprogramming in mammals. *Hum Mol Genet* 2005;**14** Spec No 1: R47–58.

85. Lane M, Gardner DK. Differential regulation of mouse embryo development and viability by amino acids. *J Reprod Fertil* 1997;**109**:153–64.

86. Watkins AJ, Papenbrock T, Fleming TP. The preimplantation embryo: handle with care. *Semin Reprod Med* 2008;**26**:175–85.

87. Robertson SA, Chin PY, Glynn DJ, et al. Peri-conceptual cytokines–setting the trajectory for embryo implantation, pregnancy and beyond. *Am J Reprod Immunol* 2011;**66**(Suppl 1):2–10.

88. Robertson SA. Immune regulation of conception and embryo implantation – all about quality control? *J Reprod Immunol* 2010;**85**:51–7.

89. Zhao Y, Chegini N, Flanders KC. Human fallopian tube expresses transforming growth factor (TGF beta) isoforms, TGF beta type I-III receptor messenger

ribonucleic acid and protein, and contains [125I]TGF beta-binding sites. *J Clin Endocrinol Metab* 1994;**79**:1177–84.

90. de Moraes AA, Hansen PJ. Granulocyte-macrophage colony-stimulating factor promotes development of in vitro produced bovine embryos. *Biol Reprod* 1997;**57**:1060–5.

91. Robertson SA, Sjoblom C, Jasper MJ, *et al.* Granulocyte-macrophage colony-stimulating factor promotes glucose transport and blastomere viability in murine preimplantation embryos. *Biol Reprod* 2001;**64**:1206–15.

92. Sjoblom C, Wikland M, Robertson SA. Granulocyte-macrophage colony-stimulating factor (GM-CSF) acts independently of the beta common subunit of the GM-CSF receptor to prevent inner cell mass apoptosis in human embryos. *Biol Reprod* 2002;**67**:1817–23.

93. Karagenc L, Lane M, Gardner DK. Granulocyte-macrophage colony-stimulating factor stimulates mouse blastocyst inner cell mass development only when media lack human serum albumin. *Reprod Biomed Online* 2005;**10**:511–18.

94. Spandorfer SD, Barmat LI, Liu HC, *et al.* Granulocyte macrophage-colony stimulating factor production by autologous endometrial co-culture is associated with outcome for in vitro fertilization patients with a history of multiple implantation failures. *Am J Reprod Immunol* 1998;**40**:377–81.

95. Cui XS, Lee JY, Choi SH, *et al.* Mouse granulocyte-macrophage colony-stimulating factor enhances viability of porcine embryos in defined culture conditions. *Anim Reprod Sci* 2004;**84**:169–77.

96. Imakawa K, Helmer SD, Nephew KP, *et al.* A novel role for GM-CSF: enhancement of pregnancy specific interferon production, ovine trophoblast protein-1. *Endocrinology* 1993;**132**:1869–71.

97. Michael DD, Wagner SK, Ocon OM, *et al.* Granulocyte-macrophage colony-stimulating-factor increases interferon-tau protein secretion in bovine trophectoderm cells. *Am J Reprod Immunol* 2006;**56**:63–7.

98. Robertson SA, Roberts CT, Farr KL, *et al.* Fertility impairment in granulocyte-macrophage colony-stimulating factor-deficient mice. *Biol Reprod* 1999;**60**:251–61.

99. Xie Y, Liu J, Proteasa S, *et al.* Transient stress and stress enzyme responses have practical impacts on parameters of embryo development, from IVF to directed differentiation of stem cells. *Mol Reprod Dev* 2008;**75**:689–97.

100. Xie Y, Puscheck EE, Rappolee DA. Effects of SAPK/JNK inhibitors on preimplantation mouse embryo development are influenced greatly by the amount of stress induced by the media. *Mol Hum Reprod* 2006;**12**:217–24.

101. Leese HJ. Quiet please, do not disturb: a hypothesis of embryo metabolism and viability. *Bioessays* 2002;**24**:845–9.

102. Nasr-Esfahani MM, Johnson MH. The origin of reactive oxygen species in mouse embryos cultured in vitro. *Development* 1991;**113**:551–60.

103. Brison DR, Schultz RM. Apoptosis during mouse blastocyst formation: evidence for a role for survival factors including transforming growth factor alpha. *Biol Reprod* 1997;**56**:1088–96.

104. Hardy K. Cell death in the mammalian blastocyst. *Mol Hum Reprod* 1997;**3**:919–25.

105. Jurisicova A, Latham KE, Casper RF, *et al.* Expression and regulation of genes associated with cell death during murine preimplantation embryo development. *Mol Reprod Dev* 1998;**51**:243–53.

106. Wells D, Bermudez MG, Steuerwald N, *et al.* Expression of genes regulating chromosome segregation, the cell cycle and apoptosis during human preimplantation development. *Hum Reprod* 2005;**20**:1339–48.

107. Luft JC, Dix DJ. Hsp70 expression and function during embryogenesis. *Cell Stress Chaperones* 1999;**4**:162–70.

108. Behr B, Mooney S, Wen Y, *et al.* Preliminary experience with low concentration of granulocyte-macrophage colony-stimulating factor: a potential regulator in preimplantation mouse embryo development and apoptosis. *J Assist Reprod Genet* 2005;**22**:25–32.

109. Chin PY, Macpherson AM, Thompson JG, *et al.* Stress response genes are suppressed in mouse preimplantation embryos by granulocyte-macrophage colony-stimulating factor (GM-CSF). *Hum Reprod* 2009;**24**:2997–3009.

110. Agerholm I, Loft A, Hald F, *et al.* Culture of human oocytes with granulocyte-macrophage colony-stimulating factor has no effect on embryonic chromosomal constitution. *Reprod Biomed Online* 2010;**20**:477–84.

Chapter

10

Osmolality

Jay M. Baltz

Introduction

The success of an embryo culture medium depends on its chemical composition. Salts, metabolites, chelators, vitamins, trace elements, buffers, dissolved gases, and other constituents contribute to healthy embryo development in the variety of media currently used for human embryo culture in clinical embryology laboratories. Beyond the chemical composition, however, other characteristics of media are also important to the health of cultured embryos. Physical properties such as pH and temperature must also be carefully controlled to provide the optimal environment for the developing embryo in vitro. Another fundamental physical property of solutions is their osmolality. Although the role of osmolality in the success of embryo culture is generally not as well appreciated as that of the other parameters already mentioned, it is nonetheless of critical importance for healthy embryo development.

What is osmolality?

Osmolality is a measure of the osmotic pressure of a solution, which can be thought of as analogous to air pressure. In air, pressure is exerted on any surface that is impermeable to gases because a huge number of air molecules are constantly colliding with the surface, each imparting a tiny force. Any time there are more air molecules per unit volume on one side of the surface than the other, there will be a net force pushing on the surface from the direction of higher air density. For example, when a balloon is blown up, there are more air molecules in a given volume inside the balloon than outside, which means more total collisions with the inside surface than the outside. The greater number of collisions on the inside results in a net force pushing outward, so that the balloon is expanded even against the elastic force of its having to be stretched. Osmotic pressure behaves similarly, except the colliding molecules are solutes dissolved in water and the surface corresponds to a "semi-permeable" membrane, permeable to water but not the solute molecules.

Cells, including eggs and the cells of embryos, are surrounded by plasma membranes that are relatively permeable to water, but impermeable to most of the solutes dissolved in their cytoplasm or in the external fluid. Thus, cells have semipermeable membranes, and if there is a net difference in the total concentrations of osmotically active solutes (osmolytes) between the intracellular and extracellular fluids, there will be a net force on the membrane. Cells thus behave like tiny osmotic balloons. Because cell membranes are pliable, cells will

Culture Media, Solutions, and Systems in Human ART, ed. Patrick Quinn. Published by Cambridge University Press. © Cambridge University Press 2014.

swell or shrink until the osmotic pressure is equalized across the membrane. When this occurs, water crosses the membrane and either concentrates or dilutes the intracellular osmolytes until their concentration is equalized with that outside the cell, eliminating the osmotic gradient and reaching a new equilibrium.

What is described above is the effect osmolality has on cells. Osmolality itself is just a measure of the concentration of the osmolytes in a solution that exert osmotic pressure [1]. Osmolality is given in units of the total effective molar concentration of osmolytes (osmoles) per unit mass of solution, or osmoles/kg (analogous to moles/kg for expressing molality). As an example, an ideal 1.0 M solution of a single perfect osmolyte completely dissolved in water would have an osmolality of 1 osmole/kg. Alternatively, the osmotic contribution in a solution can be expressed as osmolarity, given in osmoles/L (osmolar or OsM). If the total concentration of osmolytes in a solution is high, osmolality and osmolarity diverge, since the density of the solution becomes significantly higher than 1 kg/L. However, for the dilute solutions used in embryo culture or present in the embryo's in vivo environment, osmolality and osmolarity are approximately interchangeable, with osmolarity often used because of the convenience of the units (usually expressed as mOsM, milliosmolar) and their correspondence with the commonly used expression of solute concentration as molarity. It should be borne in mind, though, that osmometers report osmolality, and this is the technically correct designation, usually expressed as mosmoles/kg (milliosmoles per kg) [2].

Osmolality of culture media

Preimplantation embryo culture has been practiced for about a century, starting with Brachet's work with rabbit embryos [3]. Early embryo culture was done in complex biological fluids, mainly blood plasma and serum [4]. The first major advances in developing defined media for embryo culture occurred in the 1950s, starting with Whitten's successful culture of mouse embryos through several preimplantation stages [5, 6]. Work during the next two decades produced the classic mouse embryo culture media such as M16 [7], which was the most widely used mouse embryo culture medium for many years [8, 9], and similar defined media for human embryo culture, such as Human Tubal Fluid (HTF) medium [10].

However, although these mouse media supported development of 1-cell mouse embryos to the 2-cell stage, and 2-cell embryos to blastocysts, they did not permit development of the embryos of most mouse strains from the 1-cell stage to blastocysts. Instead, embryos became arrested at the late 2-cell stage (a phenomenon known as the "2-cell block") [11]. Similar developmental blocks afflicted other species cultured in the media that were available, including a developmental block at the 4- to 8-cell stages in human [12].

During the 1980s, there was a concerted effort to overcome these in vitro blocks by improving embryo culture media. A key driver of this was a program funded by the US National Institute of Child Health and Human Development, NIH (National Cooperative Program on Non-Human In Vitro Fertilization and Preimplantation Development, informally known as the "Culture Club"). Successful media for mouse embryo culture were thus developed, the first of which were CZB [13] and SOM [14, 15]. SOM was modified soon after its initial formulation to produce the KSOM mouse embryo culture medium that is now widely used [16]. These media not only finally permitted complete preimplantation culture from fertilized eggs to blastocysts of most mouse embryos, but served as the basis for culture media that support similar successful development of embryos from fertilized eggs in humans.

Both CZB and KSOM had essentially the same components as earlier media such as M16 (and HTF), differing only by the addition of glutamine and ethylenediaminetetraacetic acid (EDTA) (and the omission of glucose specifically during the cleavage stages in CZB). A major difference, however, was that both CZB and KSOM had substantially lower osmolalities than previous media. While M16 had an osmolality of around 290 mosmoles/kg, KSOM's was approximately 250 mosmoles/kg and CZB's 275 mosmoles/kg. Lower osmolarity itself was a key factor that led to media which eliminated in vitro blocks to embryo development [17, 18]. Similarly, many current human embryo culture media have lower osmolalities, with a large proportion having average reported osmolality values in the range of 250–280 mosmoles/kg (Table 10.1).

Why was lowered osmolality beneficial for embryo development? One possibility was that embryos normally develop in an environment with low osmolality, so that the successful culture media simply replicate this. This, however, does not seem to be the case, since the available measurements of oviductal fluid osmolality indicate osmolalities in the range of 300–310 mosmoles/kg in the mouse [19, 20], 320 mosmoles/kg in the pig [21], and 290 mosmoles/kg in the rat [22]. In each case, these values are essentially the same as the osmolality of blood in the same species [1, 23, 24]. Assuming a similar correspondence between blood and Fallopian tube osmolalities applies in humans, Fallopian tube fluid should be approximately 290 mosmoles/kg to match that of human blood [25], which is

Table 10.1. Human embryo culture media osmolalities

Manufacturer	Culture medium	Developmental stages1	Osmolality range (average) mosmoles/kg
Cook®IVF²	Sydney IVF Cleavage	Cleavage	285–295 (290)
	Sydney IVF Blastocyst	Postcomp	285–295 (290)
CooperSurgical³ (SAGE®)	Quinn's Advantage® Cleavage	Cleavage	257–273 (265)
	Quinn's Advantage® Blastocyst	Postcomp	257–273 (265)
Fertipro⁴	Ferticult™ IVF	Cleavage	275–285 (280)
	Ferticult™ G3	Postcomp	270–290 (280)
GyneMed⁵	GM501	All	270–290 (280)
InVitroCare⁶	IVC-ONE™, IVC-TWO™	Cleavage	270–290 (280)
	IVC-THREE™	Postcomp	270–290 (280)
Irvine Scientific⁷	SSM™ (plain, SSS, DSS)	All	260–270 (265)
	P1® (plain, SSS, DSS)	Cleavage	282–298 (290)
	ECM® (plain, SSS, DSS)	Cleavage	282–295 (288)
	Multiblast® (plain, SSS, DSS)	Postcomp	281–291 (286)
	HTF (plain, SSS)	Cleavage	272–288 (280)

Table 10.1. (*cont.*)

Manufacturer	Culture medium	Developmental stages1	Osmolality range (average) mosmoles/kg
LifeGlobal® (IVFonline)[8]	Global®	All	260–270 (265)
	HTF	Cleavage	280–292 (286)
Origio (MediCult)[9]	Universal IVF	Cleavage	277–293 (285)
	ISM1™	Cleavage	272–288 (280)
	ISM2™	Postcomp	272–288 (280)
	EmbryoAssist™	Cleavage	272–288 (280)
	BlastAssist®	Postcomp	272–288 (280)
VitroLife[10]	G1™ (G5 series™)	Cleavage	256–266 (261)
	G1™ with HSA (G5 series™)[11]	Cleavage	249–259 (254)
	G2™ (G5 series™)	Postcomp	255–265 (260)
	G2™ with HSA (G5 series™)[11]	Postcomp	248–258 (253)

[1] "Cleavage" indicates precompaction embryos starting from fertilized eggs. "Postcomp" denotes post-compaction embryos, generally from about the 8-cell stage to blastocysts. "All" indicates single-stage media for culture from fertilized egg to blastocyst.

[2] The osmolarity ranges were obtained from the Cook Medical website: http://www.cookmedical.com/wh/familyListingAction.do?family=Assisted+Reproduction&subFamily=Embryo+Culture in the following documents for each medium: Sydney IVF Cleavage: http://www.cookmedical.com/wh/content/mmedia/WH-BWE-EMC-EN-200812–13.pdf and Sydney IVF Blastocyst: http://www.cookmedical.com/wh/content/mmedia/WH-BWE-EMC-EN-200812–17.pdf (all accessed September 14, 2011).

[3] Patrick Quinn, PhD, HCLD, CooperSurgical, Inc., personal communication, January 13, 2011.

[4] The osmolarity ranges were obtained from the Fertipro website: http://www.fertipro.com/index.php?page=home&sub=general in the following documents for each medium: Ferticult™ IVF: http://www.fertipro.com/index.php?page=media&sub=fecu, Ferticult™ G3: http://www.fertipro.com/index.php?page=media&sub=g3 (all accessed September 14, 2011).

[5] The osmolarity ranges were obtained from the GyneMed website: http://www.gynemed.de/Home.14+M52087573ab0.0.html from the following document for GM501 Basic: http://www.gynemed.de/GM501-Basic.98+M52087573ab0.0.html (both accessed September 14, 2011).

[6] Values for osmolalities of the InVitroCare IVC™ series of media were not found on the company website (http://www.invitrocare.com) and could not be obtained directly from the company. A brochure for InVitroCare products, however, was located online at http://www.genycell.com/images/productos/protocolos/__94.pdf reporting IVC™ media osmolalities as 270–290 mosmoles/kg, used here (both accessed September 8, 2011).

[7] Laura Mena, Associate Product Manager, and Wayne Caswell, Field Scientist, Irvine Scientific, personal communication, January 26, 2011.

[8] The osmolarity ranges were obtained from the LifeGlobal® (IVFonline) website: http://www.lifeglobal.com/default2.asp in the following documents for each medium: Global®: http://www.lifeglobal.com/asp/Products/ProductDetail.asp?ID=LGGG and HTF: http://www.lifeglobal.com/asp/Products/ProductDetail.asp?ID=GMHT (all accessed September 14, 2011).

[9] Rasmus Kiil-Nielsen, International Product Manager, ORIGIO A/S, personal communication, January 15, 2011.

[10] Susie Oliver, T.S., VitroLife, Inc., personal communication, January 13, 2011.

[11] The lower osmolalities for media with HSA added likely are due to the dilution of the media with 5% v/v HSA solution™ added to the media as directed: http://www.vitrolife.com/Global/Fertility/Products/Product%20insert%20pdfs/Product%20insert_HSA%20solution.pdf (accessed September 8, 2011).

near the upper range of most of the more recently developed human embryo culture media and well above many. Thus, the evidence does not support the idea that successful embryo culture media must mimic the osmolality of the in vivo environment, for animals or humans.

Instead, it appears that the lower osmolality of many culture media is an artifact of the original lack of an environmental component, present in vivo, that is required to permit embryo development at normal osmolality [9]. The lowered osmolality of culture media that were developed to overcome the in vitro developmental blocks, in this scenario, is the result of compensating for the lack of normal constituents of the in vivo environment. This compromise arose during the development of mouse embryo culture media that overcame the 2-cell block in that species, when the unbiased optimization methods used to produce SOM and KSOM media led to a marked decrease in the total solute content, particularly NaCl, in these media relative to the original M16 medium [14, 15, 26]. Subsequent media that were based on this work, and other contemporary efforts at media development, have maintained the lowered osmolality in many cases.

What was missing from older culture media that necessitated lowering osmolality below the normal in vivo environment? The answer to this is amino acids, not present in earlier culture media, and the underlying mechanism is their role in cell volume regulation in early preimplantation embryos.

Cell volume regulation in preimplantation embryos

Osmolality is inextricably linked to cell volume. Animal cells regulate their volumes osmotically, by importing or exporting osmolytes to control intracellular osmotic pressure and thus adjust their volumes against any perturbations [27]. Increasing external osmolarity would cause a cell to shrink (Figure 10.1A,B). The initial response of the cell to such a volume decrease is to accumulate inorganic ions by activating one or more of several osmotically regulated inorganic ion transporters, thus increasing intracellular osmotic pressure and restoring cell volume (Figure 10.1C,D) [28]. This homeostatic response alone appears to suffice for most mammalian somatic cells. However, in a number of cell types, particularly where external osmolality is high or variable (for example, in the kidney), maintaining enough intracellular inorganic ions to completely balance external osmotic pressure is detrimental over the long term. To avoid this, these cells replace a portion of the intracellular inorganic ions with "organic osmolytes" (Figure 10.1E) [29].

Organic osmolytes are small, neutral organic compounds that do not perturb cellular biochemistry or physiological functions even at very high concentrations. Many diverse compounds are used as organic osmolytes in different types of organisms and different cell types within an organism [29]. In contrast to when organic osmolytes are employed, the increase in ionic strength that can occur when inorganic ions alone are used to provide intracellular osmotic support can severely disrupt macromolecular function and biochemical reactions. Thus, by substituting organic osmolytes for a portion of inorganic ions, cells can maintain their volumes without risking deleterious effects from accumulating high levels of the latter. Most organic osmolytes used by mammalian somatic cells are transported by specialized transporters that are activated by increased external osmolarity and decreased cell volume, with four organic osmolyte transporters, which transport specific amino acids, some amino acid derivatives, or saccharides, identified in mammalian somatic cells [30, 31].

The observation that the newer, successful culture media had lowered total osmolality but otherwise similar composition to older media led to the hypothesis that dysregulation of cell volume homeostasis in early preimplantation embryos could be a major factor in the

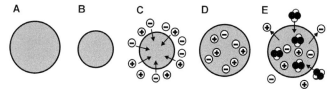

Figure 10.1 Model of mammalian cell volume regulation. When the normal physiological volume of a cell (A) decreases (B), the initial response is to activate transporters of inorganic ions such as Na⁺, K⁺, and Cl⁻ (C; ions represented by circles with positive and negative charges) and to import these ions until the amount of ions accumulated to a level where they can balance the external osmotic pressure and restore normal volume (D). In some cells, the increased ionic strength in the cytoplasm would be detrimental in the long term, as discussed in the text. Thus, these cells utilize organic osmolytes (represented by molecules composed of black and gray circles) that can be transported into the cells via specific transporters to replace a portion of the intracellular inorganic ions while still maintaining intracellular osmolality and normal cell volume (E).

developmental blocks that had previously occurred in culture. This in turn led Biggers and Van Winkle to propose independently that preimplantation embryos might normally require organic osmolytes [26, 32], which were missing from traditional culture media. Thus, organic osmolytes were obvious candidates for the "missing factor" that permits embryo development in vitro at the same osmolalities as in vivo. Organic compounds were then identified that were able to rescue mouse embryo development at higher osmolalities, including the amino acids glycine and glutamine [26, 32, 33].

As noted above, four organic osmolyte transporters have been identified in mammalian somatic cells. However, none of these could account for the ability of these amino acids to protect early mouse preimplantation embryos against increased osmolality, because either they did not accept these as substrates or the transporter was not present in embryos [17, 34]. Instead, the earliest stages of preimplantation embryos possess a unique mechanism of cell volume homeostasis that uses glycine as the principal organic osmolyte [35]. This mechanism relies on the glycine transporter GLYT1, a member of the neurotransmitter transporter family, which is normally found in the central nervous system [36]. GLYT1 also can accept glutamine as a substrate, but with much less affinity than glycine, so that glycine is highly preferred. The success of glutamine as an addition to the first culture media that successfully supported complete preimplantation development was at least partly due to its ability to substitute for glycine.

Sufficient glycine is available in vivo, since the half-maximally effective concentration of glycine for protecting 1-cell embryo development in hypertonic medium is about 0.05 mM, while there is 0.5–3.0 mM glycine in oviductal fluid [37, 38]. Early mouse embryos also accumulate very large amounts of glycine in vivo relative to any of the other common amino acids, with cytoplasmic glycine concentrations of over 20 mM found in 1- and 2-cell stage mouse embryos, reinforcing the idea that glycine is the normally preferred organic osmolyte in early embryos [39]. GLYT1 is also present and active, and appears to have a similar function, in human cleavage stage embryos [40].

Thus, early preimplantation embryos, from eggs up to about the 4-cell stage, use glycine accumulated as an organic osmolyte via GLYT1 as their major mechanism of cell volume control [17, 39]. This mechanism appears to be unique to early embryos, since a role for GLYT1 in cell volume control has not been found in somatic cells. The relatively low osmolalities of many culture media arose because the early media did not contain amino acids or any compounds that could be used by embryos as organic osmolytes. In vivo, or in culture media containing glycine (or glutamine in its absence), embryos accumulate a large amount of glycine that displaces inorganic ions from their cytoplasm. This permits them to develop at osmolalities that are similar to those in the oviduct or Fallopian tube. In contrast, in the absence of amino acids, embryos will not develop at higher osmolalities. However, by artificially lowering osmolality, embryo development becomes possible, since a lower total number of intracellular inorganic ions are then necessary to balance external osmotic pressure. Thus, cell volume control and osmolality have emerged as key parameters in determining whether healthy embryos will develop in vitro.

What is the optimal osmolality?

Like other properties of culture media, osmolality can be experimentally varied [33], allowing the question of what is the "best" osmolality for embryo culture to have been addressed by various researchers [41]. Brinster [42] appears to have been the first to alter systematically the osmolality of embryo culture media, finding that 2-cell mouse embryos would tolerate a relatively broad range of osmolalities in a simple culture medium, with development falling off above about 300 mosmoles/kg. In different culture media that also did not contain amino acids or other potential organic osmolytes, other researchers have similarly found that development of 2-cell embryos decreases sharply when osmolality is increased above thresholds that range from 300 to about 330 mosmoles/kg [18, 32, 41, 43, 44].

Culture from fertilized eggs is considerably more sensitive to increased osmolality than when the first cell cycle is completed in vivo and culture instead begins with 2-cell embryos. The corresponding thresholds above which development from 1-cell pronuclear embryos falls off range from about 240 to 310 mosmoles/kg [18, 26, 33, 44, 45]. When development was directly compared in the same media, 2-cell embryos developed in osmolalities up to 50 mosmoles/kg higher than when culture was instead started with fertilized eggs [18]. Since embryo culture in the clinic starts with fertilization, human embryos are therefore cultured through the stage at which they are most susceptible to the deleterious effects of increased osmolality.

The composition of the culture medium has a profound effect on the ability of embryos to tolerate increased osmolality. Mainly, this arises from the presence or absence of compounds that can be utilized as organic osmolytes. Thus, the upper range of osmolalities at which embryos can be cultured from fertilized eggs can be substantially extended if any effective organic osmolytes are present in the medium. As discussed above, glycine is the predominant organic osmolyte used by cleavage stage mouse embryos. Adding glycine to the medium allows mouse embryos to develop at osmolalities that are up to 70 mosmoles/kg higher than in its absence [18]. Similarly, glutamine in the medium increases the upper limit of permissible osmolalities by about 20 mosmoles/kg in the absence of glycine [26, 33].

Similar systematic determinations of development as a function of osmolality apparently have not been done for human embryos. The tolerance limits specified by the manufacturers of current commercial human embryo culture media include osmolalities that range from below 250 to almost 300 mosmoles/kg (Table 10.1). Likely, detrimental effects on human embryo culture would become evident if osmolality were to be increased substantially beyond this upper range. However, there is unlikely to be a single optimal osmolality for all human embryo culture media, which instead is almost certainly dependent on the composition of each medium. The main effect should arise from which, if any, compounds are present that can function as organic osmolytes in embryos. Thus, for example, media that contain glycine are likely to have a higher optimal osmolality range than those that do not.

Taking this all into account, there is not one answer to the question of what is the "best" osmolality for human embryo culture. Each culture system will instead have its own optimum, which, by analogy to the mouse embryo, may span a relatively broad range rather than represent a narrow peak. There will, however, be a threshold osmolality for each medium above which there is a negative impact on development and viability. To avoid being near this threshold, a medium with lower osmolality and that includes one or more compounds (particularly glycine) that function as organic osmolytes in embryos would be preferable, especially for the initial stages of development after fertilization. Evaporation should also be avoided, as this increases osmolality due to loss of water and consequent concentration of solutes, although detrimental effects of minor evaporation are clearly less likely to arise in media with lower osmolalities and organic osmolytes as constituents.

Conclusion

The osmolality of a culture medium is an important determinant of embryo viability and health. If osmolality is increased above a threshold, whose value varies depending on the composition of the medium, embryo development will be negatively affected. This is due to the perturbation of embryo cell volume. Negative effects can, however, be minimized if the normal physiological mechanisms of cell volume regulation in embryos are supported in vitro by the provision of compounds such as glycine that function as organic osmolytes in embryos. Recent work has revealed that early preimplantation embryos use a unique mechanism of cell volume regulation that involves the accumulation of glycine via the GLYT1 transporter. Thus, the presence of glycine, or another compound (such as glutamine) that can substitute in its absence, will help maintain normal cell volume homeostasis and promote healthy embryo development.

References

1. Waymouth C. Osmolality of mammalian blood and of media for culture of mammalian cells. *In Vitro* 1970;**6**:109–27.

2. Burton RF. Appendix A: Osmolality and Osmotic Coefficients. *Ringer Solutions and Physiological Salines.* Bristol, Wright Scientechnica. 1975;145–7.

3. Brachet A. Développement in vitro de blastodermes et de jeunes embryons de Mammifères. *C R Acad Sci, Paris* 1912;**155**:1191–3.

4. Alexandre H. A history of mammalian embryological research. *Int J Dev Biol* 2001;**45**:457–67.

5. Whitten WK. Culture of tubal mouse ova. *Nature* 1956;**177**:96.

6. Whitten WK. Culture of tubal ova. *Nature* 1957;**179**:1081–2.

7. Whittingham DG. Culture of mouse ova. *J Reprod Fertil Suppl* 1971;**14**:7–21.

8. Hogan B, Beddington R, Constantini F, Lacy E. *Manipulating the Mouse Embryo: A Laboratory Manual*, 2nd edn. Plainview, NY, Cold Spring Harbor Press, 1994.

9. Biggers JD. Reflections on the culture of the preimplantation embryo. *Int J Dev Biol* 1998;**42**:879–84.

10. Quinn P, Kerin JF, Warnes GM. Improved pregnancy rate in human in vitro fertilization with the use of a medium based on the composition of human tubal fluid. *Fertil Steril* 1985;**44**:493–8.

11. Goddard MJ, Pratt HPM. Control of events during early cleavage of the mouse embryo:

an analysis of the '2-cell block'. *Development* 1983;**73**:111–33.

12. Bolton VN, Hawes SM, Taylor CT, Parsons JH. Development of spare human preimplantation embryos in vitro: an analysis of the correlations among gross morphology, cleavage rates, and development to the blastocyst. *J In Vitro Fert Embryo Transf* 1989;**6**:30–5.

13. Chatot CL, Ziomek CA, Bavister BD, Lewis JL, Torres I. An improved culture medium supports development of random-bred 1-cell mouse embryos in vitro. *J Reprod Fertil* 1989;**86**:679–88.

14. Lawitts JA, Biggers JD. Optimization of mouse embryo culture media using simplex methods. *J Reprod Fertil* 1991;**91**:543–56.

15. Lawitts JA, Biggers JD. Overcoming the 2-cell block by modifying standard components in a mouse embryo culture medium. *Biol Reprod* 1991;**45**:245–51.

16. Lawitts JA, Biggers JD. Culture of preimplantation embryos. *Methods Enzymol* 1993;**225**:153–64.

17. Baltz JM, Tartia AP. Cell volume regulation in oocytes and early embryos: connecting physiology to successful culture media. *Hum Reprod Update* 2010;**16**:166–76.

18. Hadi T, Hammer MA, Algire C, Richards T, Baltz JM. Similar effects of osmolarity, glucose, and phosphate on cleavage past the 2-cell stage in mouse embryos from outbred and F1 hybrid females. *Biol Reprod* 2005;**72**:179–87.

19. Collins JL, Baltz JM. Estimates of mouse oviductal fluid tonicity based on osmotic responses of embryos. *Biol Reprod* 1999;**60**:1188–93.

20. Fiorenza MT, Bevilacqua A, Canterini S, *et al.* Early transcriptional activation of the hsp70.1 gene by osmotic stress in one-cell embryos of the mouse. *Biol Reprod* 2004;**70**:1606–13.

21. Li R, Whitworth K, Lai L, *et al.* Concentration and composition of free amino acids and osmolalities of porcine oviductal and uterine fluid and their effects on development of porcine IVF embryos. *Mol Reprod Dev* 2007;**74**:1228–35.

22. Waring DW. Rate of formation and osmolality of oviductal fluid in the cycling rat. *Biol Reprod* 1976;**15**:297–302.

23. Williams N, Kraft N, Shortman K. The separation of different cell classes from lymphoid organs. VI. The effect of osmolarity of gradient media on the density distribution of cells. *Immunology* 1972;**22**:885–99.

24. Knudsen JF, Litkowski LJ, Wilson TL, Guthrie HD, Batta SK. Follicular fluid electrolytes and osmolality in cyclic pigs. *J Reprod Fertil* 1979;**57**:419–22.

25. Case records of the Massachusetts General Hospital. Normal reference laboratory values. *N Engl J Med* 1980;**302**:37–48.

26. Lawitts JA, Biggers JD. Joint effects of sodium chloride, glutamine, and glucose in mouse preimplantation embryo culture media. *Mol Reprod Dev* 1992;**31**:189–94.

27. Hallows KR, Knauf PA. Principles of cell volume regulation. In: Strange K, ed. *Cellular and Molecular Physiology of Cell Volume Regulation.* Boca Raton, CRC Press. 1994;3–29.

28. Hoffmann EK, Lambert IH, Pedersen SF. Physiology of cell volume regulation in vertebrates. *Physiol Rev* 2009;**89**:193–277.

29. Yancey PH, Clark ME, Hand SC, Bowlus RD, Somero GN. Living with water stress: evolution of osmolyte systems. *Science* 1982;**217**:1214–22.

30. Kwon HM, Handler JS. Cell volume regulated transporters of compatible osmolytes. *Curr Opin Cell Biol* 1995;**7**:465–71.

31. Pastor-Anglada M, Felipe A, Casado FJ, Ferrer-Martinez A, Gomez-Angelats M. Long-term osmotic regulation of amino acid transport systems in mammalian cells. *Amino Acids* 1996;**11**:135–51.

32. Van Winkle LJ, Haghighat N, Campione AL. Glycine protects preimplantation mouse conceptuses from a detrimental effect on development of the inorganic ions in oviductal fluid. *J Exp Zool* 1990;**253**:215–19.

33. Dawson KM, Baltz JM. Organic osmolytes and embryos: substrates of the Gly and beta transport systems protect mouse zygotes

against the effects of raised osmolarity. *Biol Reprod* 1997;**56**:1550–8.

34. Jamshidi MB, Kaye PL. Glutamine transport by mouse inner cell masses. *J Reprod Fertil* 1995;**104**:91–7.

35. Dawson KM, Collins JL, Baltz JM. Osmolarity-dependent glycine accumulation indicates a role for glycine as an organic osmolyte in early preimplantation mouse embryos. *Biol Reprod* 1998;**59**:225–32.

36. Steeves CL, Hammer MA, Walker GB, *et al.* The glycine neurotransmitter transporter GLYT1 is an organic osmolyte transporter regulating cell volume in cleavage-stage embryos. *Proc Natl Acad Sci U S A* 2003;**100**:13982–7.

37. Guerin JF, Gallois E, Croteau S, *et al.* Techniques de récolte et aminogrammes des liquides tubaire et folliculaire chez les femelles domestiques. *Revue Med Vet* 1995;**146**:805–14.

38. Harris SE, Gopichandran N, Picton HM, Leese HJ, Orsi NM. Nutrient concentrations in murine follicular fluid and the female reproductive tract. *Theriogenology* 2005;**64**: 992–1006.

39. Tartia AP, Rudraraju N, Richards T, *et al.* Cell volume regulation is initiated in mouse oocytes after ovulation. *Development* 2009;**136**:2247–54.

40. Hammer MA, Kolajova M, Leveille M, Claman P, Baltz JM. Glycine transport by single human and mouse embryos. *Hum Reprod* 2000;**15**:419–26.

41. Baltz JM. Osmoregulation and cell volume regulation in the preimplantation embryo. In: Schatten GP, ed. *Current Topics in Developmental Biology*. San Diego, Academic Press. 2001;55–106.

42. Brinster RL. Studies on the development of mouse embryos in vitro. I. The effect of osmolarity and hydrogen ion concentration. *J Exp Zool* 1965;**158**:49–58.

43. Hay-Schmidt A. The influence of osmolality on mouse two-cell development. *J Assist Reprod Genet* 1993;**10**:95–8.

44. Davidson A, Vermesh M, Lobo RA, Paulson RJ. Mouse embryo culture as quality control for human in vitro fertilization: the one-cell versus the two-cell model. *Fertil Steril* 1988;**49**:516–21.

45. Whitten WK. Nutrient requirements for the culture of preimplantation embryos in vitro. *Adv Biosci* 1971;**6**:129–41.

Chapter

11

pH control in the embryo culture environment

Joe Conaghan

Introduction

The choice of culture medium [1, 2] with correct and optimized usage of incubators [3, 4] are essential components of the embryo culture environment. When embryos are developing poorly, or overall blastocyst formation rates appear low, it is tempting to want to change culture medium in an attempt to improve outcomes. However, since the quality of manufactured culture media is high, and the market offers stiff competition for these products, truly inferior media would likely not survive in the marketplace. Further, since these products are highly regulated and used worldwide under the watchful eye of many authorities and users, a medium that performs poorly in independent laboratories would be quickly identified, and it would become unpopular, leading to eventual discontinuation. Additionally, many solid choices of incubator are available, which have been used dependently by many users over long periods of time, and these have proved reliable [5]. It is probable therefore that long-term poor rates of embryo development are generally not attributed to a consistently substandard medium or poorly performing incubators, and are more likely to be the result of poor or improper use of the medium or incubators, with or without adequate quality control and monitoring of performance [6].

The factors that contribute to a superior culture environment, therefore, are less likely to be media or incubator choice, and more likely to be diligent monitoring and correct use of any medium and incubator. Parameters such as incubation temperature, gas quality and phase inside the incubator, overuse of the incubator, and incorrect use or handling of media are among the many causes of poor embryo development which are not related to the quality of the gametes used to make the embryos. Fortunately, procedures for careful monitoring and use of media and incubators are readily available [7–10], and widely used. Among these, the measurement and control of the pH in the culture environment can be established and used as a quality indicator (QI) of performance [11].

Just as clinical endocrinologists measure progesterone on cycle day 21 as a determination of a functioning menstrual cycle [12], the embryologist can use pH as a determinant of a functioning culture system. If the pH in the medium is at the target level, and it is stable, it is likely that the functioning of the incubator, the gas phase, and the stability of the culture dish are correct. Certainly, pH is not the only indicator of quality in the culture system [13] (see Wiemer *et al.* [14] for a review), but establishing that the pH is in line with the manufacturer's instructions and the lab's own in-house protocols and that it is stable over time and across all incubators should be an important part of daily quality assurance.

Culture Media, Solutions, and Systems in Human ART, ed. Patrick Quinn. Published by Cambridge University Press. © Cambridge University Press 2014.

The optimal range for pH for most culture media, as given by the manufacturer, is generally from 7.20 to 7.35. There is no definitive evidence that a pH of say 7.22 is any better or worse for human embryos than a pH of 7.32 in any particular medium [15]. The target pH for most products appears to be close to, but slightly lower than, that of blood plasma, which is generally given as 7.35–7.45 [16]. Early culture media design targeted a pH of 7.35 [17, 18), but over the years this value seems to have become established as the upper limit of acceptability for human embryo culture. The finding that the pH inside the embryo (pH_i) was about 6.98 to 7.12 [19] likely contributed to a downward trend in the pH of manufactured media, since most users would not want to create a stressful culture environment by having media pH that was significantly different from the expected pH_i.

The pH of embryo culture media is maintained by buffers that are optimized to work in the carbon dioxide (CO_2)-enriched culture environment at 37 °C [20]. When a sample of culture medium is first placed in the gas phase of the incubator, mild acidification occurs as CO_2 dissolves into the medium. After a period of exposure, the pH will stabilize and the medium is considered ready for use. The carbonic acid that is produced as CO_2 enters the medium is a weak acid that creates a strong buffer with its conjugate base, bicarbonate, in embryo culture medium. This combination maintains a stable pH in the embryo culture environment for as long as conditions are maintained. If embryos are to be moved outside the cell culture incubator and worked on for a period of time, it may be necessary to remove them to a solution that is buffered to maintain the target pH under ambient conditions [21]. In addition, since the pH of the medium largely depends on the interaction of carbonic acid (from CO_2 in the incubator) and bicarbonate, different media can be used at different target pHs in the same incubator by altering the bicarbonate concentration at manufacture [22].

What is pH?

For an excellent overview of the chemistry and biology of pH, including its regulation in the human embryo culture environment, see Pool [23]. This superb article is available online (http://embryologists.com/jce-archives/complete-issues/2004-issues/the-journal-of-clinical-embryology-volume-7-issue-3-fall-2004/) and should be a fundamental part of the library for any student of embryo culture.

pH is the measure of the molar concentration of hydrogen ions ($[H^+]$) in a solution; it is a negative logarithmic scale due to the possible ranges of hydrogen ion concentration, and is given in the formula :

$$pH = -\log[H^+]$$

A solution with an actual $[H^+]$ of 0.0001 M would therefore have a pH of 4, the later number being less unwieldy than the former. The addition of hydrogen ions to a solution will cause the solution to become more acidic (lower pH), and their removal turns a solution more alkaline or basic.

In the cell culture incubator, the CO_2 added to the gas phase readily dissolves into and equilibrates with culture medium (water) as is shown in the following formulae, first generating carbonic acid (a weak acid), and then liberating one or two protons in successive reactions, generating bicarbonate and then carbonate, resulting in an overall decrease in media pH. The equilibrium of these reactions is maintained only for as long as conditions remain constant, and a new equilibration will be quickly established if conditions change.

$$CO_2 + H_2O \rightleftharpoons H_2CO_3$$

$$H_2CO_3 \rightleftharpoons H^+ + HCO_3^-$$

$$HCO_3^- \rightleftharpoons H^+ + CO_3^{2-}$$

For example, a drop in the pressure of CO_2, such as occurs when moving from an area of high CO_2 pressure to an area of low pressure, will immediately affect the pH of the solution. An increase in temperature will have a similar effect as the solubility of CO_2 decreases at higher temperatures. This effect can sometimes be seen if cold equilibrated medium is placed directly from the refrigerator into an incubator at $37\,°C$, when small gas bubbles form in the medium.

Measuring pH

The measurement of the pH of a solution is easily and accurately accomplished with a readily available and compact pH meter. It is generally recommended that a pH meter purchased for the purpose of monitoring pH in a cell or embryo culture environment should be capable of being calibrated by the user with purchased pH standards prior to any working measurements being undertaken. Calibration is easily and quickly established using two to three standards that cover the range being measured (e.g., for culture media that have a working pH between 7.2 and 7.4, standards of pH 4, 7, and 10 could be used). Once the calibration is complete, it is also helpful to actually measure the pH of at least the closest standard (say pH 7) to the culture media to verify that the calibration is correct and has been saved. It is also important to consider that pH is influenced by other factors, as described below, so that the calibration and measurements should be made under the same circumstances. For example, using the calibration standards at room temperature but then measuring media pH at the working temperature of $37\,°C$ could introduce small but significant errors in the measurements. Similarly, measurements or calibrations made on one day may not be directly comparable to those on another day if significant changes in atmospheric pressure have occurred.

A standard inexpensive benchtop pH meter should be employed to check the pH of culture media in the IVF lab. Although the certificate of analysis for a purchased culture medium will usually state the pH, it is a good practice to verify this before placing the medium in use. Samples of medium should be prepared as they are intended to be used before attempting any measurements. For example, if albumin is to be added to the medium for embryo culture, it should be added to the medium for pH testing also. In this way, the pH measurements will most closely reflect the working pH of the medium. Also, since most benchtop pH meters have relatively large probes, the volume of medium needed for pH testing will necessarily be larger than that used for embryo culture. This should not be a problem, however, as a larger volume will be more stable during measurement. One approach is to place a 2 mL sample of working culture medium into the gas controlled incubator in a 15 mL polystyrene conical tube (BD Falcon, NJ, USA) and allow it to equilibrate overnight (see Figure 11.1). The following day, the pH meter can be calibrated and checked as mentioned above, before the media pH is measured. A running quality control log of media pH by batch, by incubator, and/or by day can be maintained depending on the preference of the user, and as a means of maintaining a stable and consistent culture environment.

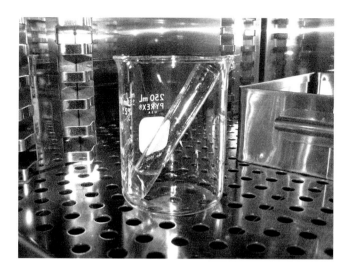

Figure 11.1 A 15 mL tube filled with 2 mL of working medium can be equilibrated overnight in the embryo culture incubator to allow measurement of pH.

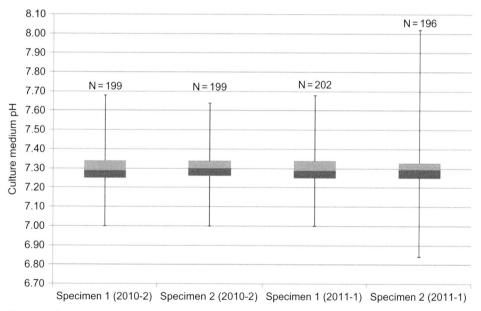

Figure 11.2 pH measurements of culture medium samples sent by the ABB proficiency testing service to laboratories performing human embryo culture. Proficiency testing samples from two dates are shown, with two medium samples on each date. Data courtesy of Ken Schill, ABB-PTS.

The measurement of pH may seem like a reasonably easy task for most embryologists, and their ability to check samples of embryo culture medium is tested during proficiency testing (PT) (see Figure 11.2). In general, most laboratories perform well at this task, with the mean (7.29) and median (7.30) readings remaining consistent across separate PT events, each supplying two media samples. However, about 25% of labs reporting PT results consistently report a pH that is outside the 7.20 to 7.35 range given for most commercial media and 20% of facilities participating in PT do not report pH at all. There are also occasional wild outliers that report pH values way outside the expected range. For example, for the data used in Figure 11.2, outliers reporting pHs of 3.69, 9.2, and 9.3 were omitted (all data courtesy of Ken Schill, American Association of Bioanalysis Proficiency Testing Service [AAB-PTS]).

Measuring pH in the petri dish where embryos are to be cultured is possible but likely requires dedicated equipment and may be more expensive. Since the volume of medium typically used for embryo culture is small, a miniature pH probe is needed that can be placed inside the culture incubator during use. A dish of medium which is identical to the users preferred embryo culture dish can then be used to check pH readings. One such system is the pH meter available from MTG (Bruckberg, Germany) which uses a proprietary disc in one well of a 4-well Nunc dish (Thermo Scientific, Waltham, MA, USA) that is pH sensitive and can relay pH readings continuously to a computer via optic fiber. Changes in pH in the medium covering the disc are detected and recorded in real time.

Factors that affect pH readings
Temperature
Increasing the temperature of a solution will favor the dissociation of hydrogen ions and therefore drive the pH down. But the differences are small, and may be considered negligible by many users. For example, the pH 7 standard solution from BDH Chemicals (Visalia, CA, USA) should have a pH of 7.12 at 0 °C, a pH of 7.02 at 20 °C, and a pH of 6.98 at 35 °C. These differences are probably not distinguishable with a standard pH meter, which likely has a margin of error of 0.02 to 0.1 depending on the model. However, temperature compensation is available for all but the most basic meters, and users that want maximum accuracy will opt for a meter that comes with a temperature probe.

pH at altitude
Atmospheric pressure is a measure of the weight of air above us. At sea level, the weight or pressure of air measured in Pascals (Pa) is about 101 kPa, which is defined as 1 standard atmosphere (atm) and is the equivalent of 760 mm of mercury if using a barometer to take measurements. The actual value fluctuates with weather, humidity, and temperature, and of course changes dramatically with altitude. Since the weight of air above us decreases as we climb, the actual measured pressure decreases by about 1.2 kPa per 100 m above sea level [24]. The pressure is also affected by local weather at any given altitude, with high or low pressure weather systems increasing or decreasing the weight of air above us. Similarly, an increase in temperature will cause expansion in the gases above us and cause a pressure decrease.

The pH of embryo culture media is largely determined by the amount of CO_2 in the gas phase of the incubator. If an optimal pH is achieved with an atmosphere containing 5% v/v CO_2, this pH can be largely maintained by keeping the gas phase constant, as well as maintaining temperature and humidity. Small fluctuations in atmospheric pressure will affect pH such that measurements of pH over time will not remain constant even if all other parameters remain constant. It is unrealistic therefore to expect to maintain an exact pH from day to day in a given incubator, and small changes should be expected. If a low pressure weather system moves in, the percentage CO_2 in the gas phase will be unaffected, but due to the less dense air, the number of CO_2 molecules in a given space will be reduced.

The pressure of CO_2 above the embryo culture dish will be lower and the actual number of CO_2 molecules contacting the surface of the medium will be fewer.

These differences are exacerbated by changes in altitude as the weight of air decreases steadily with increasing height above sea level. An incubator that is set to a gas phase of 6% CO_2 in air will maintain that concentration of gas at any altitude, but the effective amount of CO_2 in the incubator chamber will decrease steadily as the air pressure drops. A good analogy is a climber at the top of Mount Everest who is still breathing air that contains about 21% oxygen, but the air is so disperse (thin) that normal breathing cannot get enough oxygen molecules into the space in the lungs to sustain consciousness for most climbers. Similarly, an incubator at altitude that is set to 6% CO_2 in air still provides 6% CO_2 by volume, but there are simply not enough CO_2 molecules in the incubator chamber to maintain the same pH as the same incubator at sea level. At a 6% set point, the effective concentration of CO_2 will decrease steadily for every meter above sea level (see Figure 11.3). The net result is that an incubator moved from sea level to about 1500 m (the height of Guatemala City, and Kagali in Rwanda) will provide a CO_2 pressure that is significantly lower and about equivalent to 5% at sea level. At 3000 m (Quito, Ecuador is at about 2850 m), it is equivalent to about 4%.

These differences in the pressure of CO_2 inside the incubator chamber underscore the importance of measuring pH on a periodic basis in the laboratory to ensure that the desired pH is being maintained. The incubator display should continue to show the set level of CO_2 in the chamber for as long as the incubator, the CO_2 sensor, and the gas supply are maintained. However, normal changes in atmospheric pressure, humidity (humid air is denser), and temperature should be seen to have minimal effects on the pH of culture media. It should be possible with minimal effort to maintain pH within a narrow working

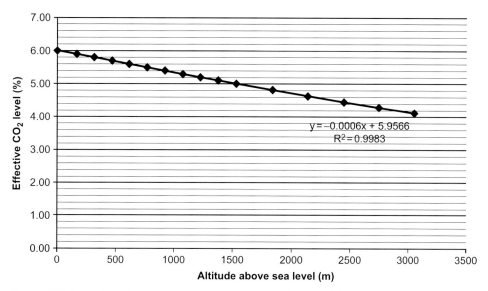

Figure 11.3 An incubator that is set to create a gas phase of 6% CO_2 in air will deliver effectively lower levels of gas at higher altitude due to decreasing atmospheric pressure. Note that the incubator display (and independent measurements) will correctly read 6% at all times.

range, and to take actual measurements according to a schedule to check periodically that significant changes have not occurred.

Choosing incubators for human embryo culture

Modern cell culture incubators have a feature that allows users to control the amount of CO_2 in the chamber. Pure CO_2 gas is supplied from a compressed cylinder or from liquid evaporation, and the incubator monitors the amount of gas in the internal environment, allowing it to reach a level preset by the user. Modern cell culture media are usually buffered to allow them to reach their optimum pH when the amount of CO_2 reaches approximately 5% by volume. Since ambient air has about 0.04% CO_2 by volume, the incubator has to monitor continuously the internal CO_2 level, and add CO_2 as necessary after a door opening or any other event that causes disruption in the gas phase.

The standard incubator monitors CO_2 using thermal conductivity, a method that works extremely well, but is affected by the humidification and temperature of the chamber. The resistance between two sensors in the incubator is altered by the presence of CO_2, so the incubator can be calibrated to tell accurately how much CO_2 is in the chamber. However, if the internal conditions that affect resistance change from those used at calibration, the incubator will not accurately be able to display the CO_2 level in the chamber. If for any reason the chamber loses humidity or the temperature drops, the incubator can no longer make a precise determination of the CO_2 percentage. After a door opening, which always causes a temperature drop and a loss of water vapor from the incubator, normal temperature and humidity levels have to be reestablished before the CO_2 can be returned to the set level. This can take 10 to 15 minutes (see Figure 11.4) depending on the size of the chamber, the operating temperature, the amount of water in the incubator, and other factors. If for any reason the water pan dries out, there is an immediate loss of function and the volume of CO_2 can no longer be controlled or measured. Adding water and restoring the humidified environment immediately corrects this problem and no lasting damage results to the

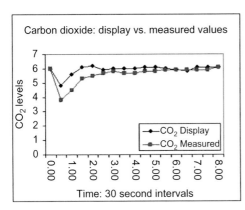
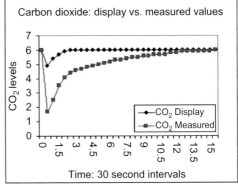

Figure 11.4 CO_2 measurements taken every 30 seconds after a 10-second incubator door opening. The incubator had a 150 liter chamber, was set at 6% CO_2 v/v, and was operating at 37 °C. The CO_2 level shown on the display was consistently higher than the actual CO_2 level as measured using an independent sensor. The left panel shows the CO_2 recovery when the incubator was equipped with six optional small inner doors to minimize gas loss. The right panel shows the results for the same incubator with the small inner doors removed. The small doors did reduce the overall loss of CO_2 and the incubator fully recovered in about 7 minutes. Without these doors, the drop in CO_2 after opening was much more drastic, and full recovery took almost twice as long.

incubator. However, the effect on the culture environment could be very damaging if the problem is not corrected quickly, as the change in CO_2 will directly cause a significant change in the pH of the medium.

This problem can be avoided by obtaining incubators that do not rely on chamber humidification for CO_2 determination. Infrared (IR) CO_2 sensors are an option that add to the cost of the incubator but may provide a higher level of assurance and safety for users. This type of sensor emits IR light, and has a sensor that determines the amount of IR present. Since CO_2 absorbs IR light, a linear reduction in IR reflects a linear increase in CO_2 levels and the incubator display is accurate at all times when the sensor is functioning. However, the IR sensor has a limited lifespan, and this should be determined at the time of purchase so that service and replacement can be scheduled before there is any risk of decline in the sensor's functionality. Periodic independent verification of CO_2 levels in the chamber should be performed to monitor for sensor failure. The benefits of the IR sensor, however, are likely to justify the cost to most users, as water is not required in the chamber and recovery of CO_2 is more rapid after a door opening.

Equilibrating embryo culture media in the CO_2 incubator

Embryos are traditionally cultured in plastic petri dishes or test tubes of a medium designed for that purpose and in a configuration that has changed little in decades [17]. Due to the small size of oocytes and embryos, the culture environment is designed to use small volumes of media so that they can be easily located and handled. These small volumes are typically covered with oil to prevent evaporation and to help maintain the temperature and pH of the media during short excursions from the gas phase inside the incubator. The equilibration times for these dishes of oil and medium depend on several factors, but most importantly on the surface area to volume ratios of the solutions in the dishes being used. For example, a Nunc 4-well dish (Thermo Scientific, Waltham, MA, USA) has a well surface area of 1.9 cm^2 and can hold a volume of medium of about 1 mL. Using this configuration, the medium in the well will equilibrate to a stable pH in about 2 hours under a gas phase of 5% CO_2 in air (see Table 11.1). However, if the volume of medium is reduced to 0.5 mL, the surface area to volume ratio changes dramatically, since the surface area remains the same but the volume is halved. The dish will now equilibrate in less than half the time and can be quickly available for use (Table 11.1).

If after equilibration, the dish is removed from the incubator, but kept at 37 °C, the pH begins to rise immediately, and reaches a maximum pH of 7.77 (0.5 mL of medium in the well) or 7.52 (1.0 mL of medium in the well) after 5 minutes in room air. With a surface area of 1.9 cm^2, the larger volume well has a surface area to volume ratio of 1.9 compared to 3.8 in the

Table 11.1. Time taken for G1 medium (Vitrolife, Denver, USA) with 10% SSS (Irvine Scientific, Santa Ana, USA) v/v to equilibrate to a pH of 7.30 after being placed in an embryo culture incubator with a gas phase of 5% CO_2 in air and running at 37°C. Dishes were removed from the incubator to room air but were maintained at 37°C

Volume of medium per well	0.5 mL	1 mL
Time taken to equilibrate	45	112
Maximum pH reached after 5 minutes outside the incubator	7.77	7.52
Time taken to re-equilibrate when returned to incubator	33	32

well with only 0.5 mL of medium. This higher ratio in the later well allows CO_2 in the incubator to equilibrate quickly with the medium in just 45 minutes, but then come out of solution rapidly, causing a dramatic rise in pH, when the dish is removed from the incubator. The effects are dampened significantly by lowering the surface area to volume ratio and the pH does not rise as much during the same 5-minute excursion from the incubator.

Equilibration and re-equilibration of embryo culture medium

Dishes of embryo culture media that are prepared and used without an oil overlay are extremely sensitive to changes in pH when traveling back and forth between room air and the gas controlled incubator (Figure 11.5). In this experiment, Nunc 4-well dishes (Thermo Scientific, Waltham, MA, USA) were prepared with 0.5 mL of medium per well, and placed in an incubator set to 37 °C and with a gas phase of 5% CO_2 in air. pH readings were taken every minute using an in-incubator pH meter (MTG, Germany). Initial equilibration took 45 minutes, by which time the medium had reached a stable pH of 7.32. The dish was then removed from the incubator for just 1 minute, and the pH was immediately seen to rise, reaching 7.53, a level that would be expected to be non-physiological and likely to be a source of stress for any embryos experiencing this pH. Since most media manufacturers recommend an upper pH of 7.35 to 7.4, cultures using 0.5 mL of medium in a Nunc 4-well

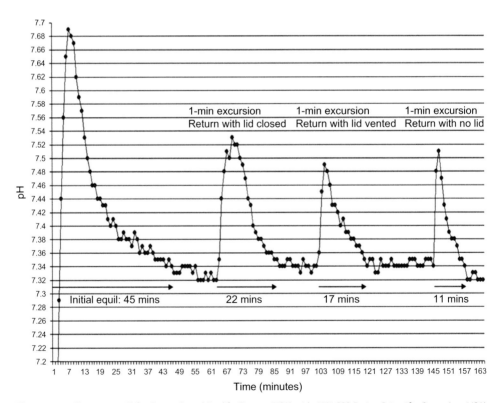

Figure 11.5 Changes in pH for G1 medium (Vitrolife, Denver, USA) with 10% SSS (Irvine Scientific, Santa Ana, USA) v/v during equilibration to a pH of 7.32 in an embryo culture incubator with a gas phase of 5% CO_2 in air and running at 37 °C. Dishes were removed from the incubator to room air for 1 minute but were maintained at 37 °C. Upon return to the incubator, re-equilibration time depended on how the lid was placed over the dish.

dish without an oil overlay would fail to stay under this ceiling. After just 1 minute outside the CO_2 environment of the incubator, the medium took 22 minutes to re-equilibrate. The media re-equilibration could be accelerated by returning the dish to the incubator with the lid tilted to one side (vented) or with the lid removed completely (Figure 11.5).

The data illustrate the difficulties for embryologists in working with dishes of medium without an oil overlay. Sometimes an oil overlay is avoided for convenience, or because oil might interfere with a particular procedure being performed, but without oil, the embryologist is dealing with a culture system that is prone to wild and dramatic shifts in pH that cannot be controlled. Further, in an alarmingly short time outside the incubator, a non-physiological pH is quickly reached and the media are being used outside the specifications set by the manufacturer. It is unknown what the effects on embryos are from such shifts in pH, but they are a likely source of stress and can be avoided.

Equilibration with an oil overlay

The rapid changes in pH that occur when moving a dish of culture medium between an incubator and room air can be controlled and dampened with the use of an oil overlay. However, the addition of oil dramatically increases the time taken for medium to first equilibrate when placed in the high CO_2 environment of the incubator (Figure 11.6). For a Nunc 4-well dish with 0.5 mL of medium and 0.5 mL of oil, the initial equilibration takes almost 12 hours, suggesting that the traditional practice of preparing embryo culture dishes

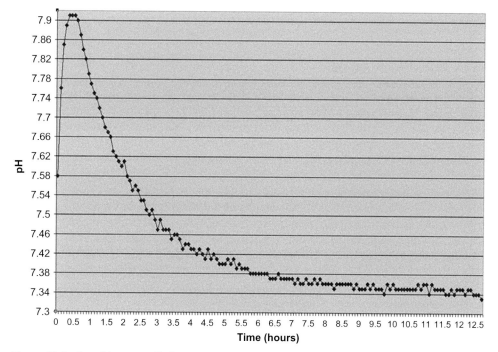

Figure 11.6 pH equilibration profile for 0.5 mL for G1 medium (Vitrolife, Denver, USA) with 10% SSS (Irvine Scientific, Santa Ana, USA) v/v under 0.5 mL mineral oil (also Irvine Scientific) during equilibration to a pH of 7.34 in an embryo culture incubator with a gas phase of 5% CO_2 in air and running at 37 °C.

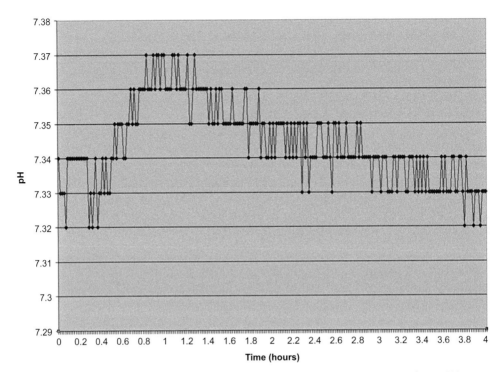

Figure 11.7 A change in pH was difficult to measure in G1 medium (Vitrolife, Denver, USA) with 10% SSS (Irvine Scientific, Santa Ana, USA) v/v equilibrated under oil (also Irvine Scientific) and removed from the gas phase of the incubator to room air. A dish removed from the incubator to room air for 10 minutes and maintained at 37 °C did register a small pH shift. Upon return to the incubator, re-equilibration took over 2 hours.

1 day in advance is justified. It also suggests that diffusion of CO_2 through the oil layer is extremely slow, and that it is unlikely that a dish could be prepared for use the same day when using an oil overlay. A dish made up with just 50 µL of medium under 0.5 mL of oil did equilibrate in just over 8 hours (data not shown), but this too is likely too long to allow same day making and use of culture dishes.

Once a dish with an oil overlay had been equilibrated, the pH of the media in the dish was extremely stable when removed from the incubator to room air at 37 °C. No measurable changes in pH were seen when removing the dish from the incubator for 1, 2, or 5 minutes (data not shown). It was not until the dish had been removed from the incubator for 10 minutes that a shift in the pH was observed, but even after a 10-minute exposure to room air, the pH only rose to 7.37 (from a baseline of 7.34). And the changes in pH were extremely slow with the rise to 7.37 taking almost half an hour, and re-equilibration taking over 2 hours (Figure 11.7). These data suggest that it is possible to keep pH stable in the embryo culture environment for up to 10 minutes, provided that the culture medium has been fully equilibrated in the gas phase of the incubator before use.

Summary and conclusions

Although an optimum pH has not been defined for human embryos, culture media are largely designed to work within a narrow pH range of approximately 7.20 to 7.35.

The working pH is only achieved after equilibration in a 37 °C incubator with a gas phase enriched with CO_2 to a concentration of 5% v/v or higher. Buffering of the medium is achieved through the use of bicarbonate in the medium and carbonic acid derived from CO_2 dissolving into solution. The exact pH of the medium can be determined using a standard laboratory pH meter, and these readings can form the backbone of a solid quality assurance program for the culture system. However, evidence suggests that many embryologists do not routinely measure media pH in their culture system, and some may be incapable of using a pH meter. This is worrying, as achieving and maintaining a target pH, as well as actually knowing the pH of the culture medium are good practices for the embryologist. If the pH of the medium is not known or controlled, embryo development and gene expression profiles can be negatively altered [25].

Once a working pH has been established, the incubation environment and the handling of the culture medium impact the ability to maintain a stable pH. The use of small volumes of medium without an oil overlay causes drastic swings in pH when dishes are moved from the incubator to room air and back again, and these changes cannot be controlled or dampened by the embryologist. Culturing and maintaining the medium under oil on the other hand allows pH to remain remarkably stable under most working conditions. A working knowledge of how pH is determined, the factors that affect pH, and the ability to measure and use pH as part of a quality management system are fundamental duties of the embryologist.

References

1. Biggers JD, Summers MC. Choosing a culture medium: making informed choices. *Fertil Steril* 2008;**90**(3):473–83.

2. Mantikou E, Youssef MA, van Wely M, *et al.* Embryo culture media and IVF/ICSI success rates: a systematic review. *Hum Reprod Update* 2013;**19**(3):210–20.

3. Cohen J, Rieger D. Historical background of gamete and embryo culture. *Methods Mol Biol* 2012;**912**:1–18.

4. Meintjes M, Chantilis SJ, Douglas JD, *et al.* A controlled randomized trial evaluating the effect of lowered incubator oxygen tension on live births in a predominantly blastocyst transfer program. *Hum Reprod* 2009;**24**(2):300–7.

5. Higdon HL, Blackhurst DW, Boone WR. Incubator management in an assisted reproductive technology laboratory. *Fertil Steril* 2008;**89**(3):703–10.

6. Magli MC, Van den Abbeel E, Lundin K, *et al.*; Committee of the Special Interest Group on Embryology. Revised guidelines for good practice in IVF laboratories. *Hum Reprod* 2008;**23**(6):1253–62.

7. Smith GD, Swain JE, Pool TB. (eds.) *Embryo Culture, Methods in Molecular Biology*, Vol. 912. New York, NY, Humana Press, 2012.

8. Mercader A, Valbuena D, Simón C. Human embryo culture. *Methods Enzymol* 2006;**420**:3–18.

9. Machtinger R, Racowsky C. Culture systems: single step. *Methods Mol Biol* 2012;**912**:199–209.

10. Quinn P. Culture systems: sequential. *Methods Mol Biol* 2012;**912**:211–30.

11. Swain JE. Optimizing the culture environment in the IVF laboratory: impact of pH and buffer capacity on gamete and embryo quality. *Reprod Biomed Online* 2010;**21**(1):6–16.

12. Pauerstein CJ, Eddy CA, Croxatto HD, *et al.* Temporal relationships of estrogen, progesterone, and luteinizing hormone levels to ovulation in women and infrahuman primates. *Am J Obstet Gynecol* 1978;**130**(8):876–86.

13. Quinn P, Warnes GM, Kerin JF, Kirby C. Culture factors affecting the success rate of in vitro fertilization and embryo transfer. *Ann N Y Acad Sci* 1985;**442**:195–204.

14. Wiemer KE, Anderson A, Weikert L. Quality control in the IVF laboratory. In: Gardner DK, Weissman A, Howles CM, Shoham Z, eds. *Textbook of Assisted Reproductive Techniques: Laboratory and Clinical Perspectives*. London, Martin Dunitz Ltd. 2001;27–33.

15. Swain JE. Is there an optimal pH for culture media used in clinical IVF? *Hum Reprod Update* 2012;18(3):333–9.

16. Waugh A, Grant A. *Ross and Wilson Anatomy and Physiology in Health and Illness*, 10th edn. Edinburgh, Churchill Livingstone Elsevier. 2007;22.

17. Brinster RL. A method for in vitro cultivation of mouse ova from 2-cell to blastocyst. *Exp Cell Res* 1963;32:205–8.

18. Quinn P, Kerin JF, Warnes GM. Improved pregnancy rate in human in vitro fertilization with the use of a medium based on the composition of human tubal fluid. *Fertil Steril* 1985;44(4);493–8.

19. Phillips KP, Léveillé MC, Claman P, Baltz JM. Intracellular pH regulation in human preimplantation embryos. *Hum Reprod* 2000;15(4):896–904.

20. Swain JE. Media composition: pH and buffers. *Methods Mol Biol* 2012;912:161–75.

21. Swain JE, Pool TB. New pH-buffering system for media utilized during gamete and embryo manipulations for assisted reproduction. *Reprod Biomed Online* 2009;18(6):799–810.

22. Quinn P, Cooke S. Equivalency of culture media for human in vitro fertilization formulated to have the same pH under an atmosphere containing 5% or 6% carbon dioxide. *Fertil Steril* 2004;81:1502–6.

23. Pool TB. Optimizing pH in clinical embryology. *Clin Embryologist* 2004;7(3):1–17.

24. McNaught AD, Wilkinson A. (eds.) *IUPAC. Compendium of Chemical Terminology The Golden Book*, 2nd edn. Oxford Blackwell Scientific Publications, 1997.

25. Koustas G, Sjoblom C. Epigenetic consequences of pH stress in mouse embryos. *Hum Reprod* 2011;26:i78.

Chapter 2

In vitro maturation of immature human oocytes

Ri-Cheng Chian, Shan-Jun Dai, and Yao Wang

Introduction

At late follicular phase (middle of the menstrual cycle), the preovulatory surge of luteinizing hormone (LH) induces germinal vesicle breakdown (GVBD) and chromosomes progress from metaphase-I (MI) to metaphase-II (MII). The completion of the first meiotic division is characterized by the extrusion of the first polar body (1PB) and formation of the secondary oocyte, both of which contain a diploid chromosome complement. Oocyte maturation is defined as the completion of the first meiotic division from the germinal vesicle (GV) stage to MII stage, with accompanying cytoplasmic maturation necessary for fertilization and early embryonic development. Oocyte maturation is often conceptually divided into nuclear and cytoplasmic maturation. Nuclear maturation is a term that refers to the resumption of meiosis and progression to MII, and cytoplasmic maturation is a term that refers to preparation of oocyte cytoplasm for fertilization and embryonic development [1]. However, these two processes are not completely separated processes. Nuclear maturation is controlled by cytoplasmic maturation. There are many excellent review papers dealing with the mechanism of oocyte maturation [2, 3]. Therefore, here we will not discuss the mechanism of oocyte maturation. In this Chapter, we will focus on the culture condition and its clinical application with immature human oocytes.

Historical aspect of in vitro maturation

Attempts to mature mammalian oocytes in vitro started in the 1930s. Pincus and Enzmann were using a phosphate-buffered Ringer's solution to culture rabbit immature oocytes [4]. This culture medium was supplemented with rabbit serum and extracts of beef pituitary glands as the maturity hormone. The immature rabbit oocytes were cultured at 38 °C in hollow ground slides sealed with paraffin for in vitro maturation (IVM). After obtaining and observing the first two unfertilized human eggs from flushing of excised uterus [5], they tried to culture immature human oocytes with the materials obtained from excision at operation [6]. The human ovaries were collected shortly after excision at operation and placed in Pannet-Copton or Tyrode solution at pH 7.0–7.2. The different sizes of follicles were cut, and the collected immature human oocytes were cultured at 37 °C in small Carrel flasks containing 1 to 2 mL of human serum after different brief treatments. The conclusion was that removal of the ovum from the follicle is sufficient to initiate a nuclear maturation [6].

Culture Media, Solutions, and Systems in Human ART, ed. Patrick Quinn. Published by Cambridge University Press. © Cambridge University Press 2014.

Interestingly, 10 years after the first reporting of in vitro fertilization (IVF) of rabbit in vivo matured oocytes [7], the first in vitro fertilized human oocytes were from in vitro matured oocytes [8]. Nearly 800 human follicular oocytes were isolated from the different sizes of follicles of ovaries derived from patients who underwent laparotomy [9]. The obtained immature oocytes were washed in Lock's solution and incubated for 22 to 27 hours in the serum of the same patients, the oocytes were then exposed to a washed sperm suspension in Lock's solution for 1 hour, and the oocytes were then transferred to fresh serum from a post-menopausal patient, after which cleaved embryos were obtained in vitro [8, 9].

Similar experiments were repeated by Edwards in the 1960s. Ovarian oocytes from mouse, pig, cow, sheep, monkey, and human were cultured in various media: Waymouth's medium, Tissue culture 199 (TC-199) medium, or Hanks's saline supplemented with human and/or calf serum, antibiotics, and various other additives. All media were buffered with bicarbonate (pH 7.2) against 5% carbon dioxide in air [10]. As the culture technique, "Falcon" plastic dishes were used. An important observation was that immature human oocytes from the GV stage to the MII stage needs at least 34–36 hours of incubation in vitro [11]. Afterward, Kennedy and Donahue reported that immature human oocytes can be matured in vitro in a chemically defined media [12, 13], namely F10 medium supplemented with 4 mg of bovine serum albumin (BSA) per milliliter. At the same time, they indicated that the presence of cumulus cells is essential for oocyte maturation in vitro.

Many studies on IVF using in vitro matured human oocytes were carried out in the early days. Edwards *et al.* used Hank's solution supplemented with 15% fetal calf serum (FCS) for immature human oocyte maturation in vitro [14]. After 38 hours in culture, many of the oocytes became mature and these in vitro matured oocytes were used for IVF study. Embryos were produced from in vitro matured oocytes following IVF, but at that time it was impossible to use those embryos for transfer in order to produce a live birth. However, Edwards *et al.* clearly indicated that there may be certain clinical uses for human eggs fertilized by this procedure [14]. Although embryos were produced from preovulatory human oocytes that were aspirated 30–32 hours after injection of human chorionic gonadotropin (hCG) [15], most oocytes obtained were at MI stage. Therefore, the aspirated oocytes needed to be incubated for 1–4 hours in Ham's F10, or Waymouth's medium, or TC-199 medium supplemented with some follicular fluid for final maturation before insemination. This meant that human embryos produced in vitro were from in vitro matured oocytes rather than in vivo matured oocytes. Nevertheless, the first live birth of IVF was from in vivo matured oocytes rather than in vitro matured oocytes [16].

The first successful IVM births were from immature oocytes collected at cesarean section for oocyte donation [17], in which the immature oocytes were matured in TC-199 medium supplemented with up to 50% follicular fluid. The first live birth following IVM using the patient's own immature oocytes was reported by Trounson *et al.* [18]. The immature oocytes were from a patient with polycystic ovarian syndrome (PCOS) and were cultured in TC-199 medium supplemented with 10% FCS. Based on many studies and clinical trials, it has been demonstrated that priming with follicle-stimulating hormone (FSH) and/or hCG prior to immature oocyte retrieval improves oocyte maturation rates and embryo quality as well as pregnancy rates in infertile women with PCOS [19–22]. To date, the clinical pregnancy and implantation rates have reached approximately 35–50% and 15–20%, respectively in infertile women with PCOS [23, 24]. It has been estimated that more than 5000 IVM babies have been born worldwide so far [25, 26].

Oocyte maturation in vitro is profoundly affected by culture conditions. Although simple medium, such as Krebs–Ringer medium supplemented with pyruvate, lactate, and glucose, can support human oocyte maturation in vitro, the complex culture media, such as TC-199 medium, Hank's F10, and Chang's medium buffered with bicarbonate and supplemented with various sera, gonadotropins (FSH and LH), and steroids (estradiol and/or progesterone), have been most widely used in research or clinical application [27]. Apart from the culture conditions, the source of oocytes, especially the size of follicles, may be more important for oocyte maturation, fertilization, and the subsequent embryonic development as well as pregnancy and healthy live births.

Size of follicles

The source of immature oocytes, such as the size of follicles, ovarian phase, priming with gonadotropins (FSH and hCG) before IVM, will affect directly oocyte maturation in vitro. During folliculogenesis, human oocyte grows from 35 μm to 120 μm in diameter [28]. At the end of oocyte growth, the antrum is formed and the oocyte has acquired the capacity to resume meiosis. Most mRNA and protein are synthesized during the period of oocyte growth. It is common belief that the ability to complete maturation to MII and developmental competence is acquired progressively with increasing follicular size. Although it has been reported that human oocytes have a size-dependent ability to resume meiosis from 90 to 120 μm in diameter [29], non-full-size oocytes should not be considered when assessing developmental competence, because the non-full-size oocytes have less products (mRNA and protein) stored in the cytoplasm. Sometimes, small-sized oocytes can be collected from antral follicles, but it is not clear whether those small-sized oocytes are from non-growing oocytes or progressed atretic follicles.

Early studies indicated that the size-dependent ability for meiotic competence depends not only on the size of the follicles and oocytes but also on the stage of the menstrual cycle [30]. It has been confirmed in the human that the oocytes derived from different phases of the menstrual cycle do not affect adversely oocyte maturation in vitro and subsequent fertilization and embryonic development (R. C. Chian, S. H. Yang, J. H. Lim, unpublished data, 2006). It has been demonstrated in animal model studies that the developmental competence of immature oocytes from the small follicles is not immediately affected by the presence of a dominant follicle [31–33].

Priming with FSH alone or both of FSH and hCG before immature oocyte retrieval may promote oocyte maturation in vitro and subsequent embryo development as well as pregnancy outcome [34, 35]. Clearly those IVM results were related directly to the size of follicles. However, the quality of oocytes from the different sizes of follicles in natural cycle and ovarian stimulated cycle may be different due to the microenvironment of follicles. Interestingly, it has been indicated that anti-mullerian hormone (AMH) in serum may be a predictive marker for the selection of patients for oocyte IVM treatment [36]. Therefore, the source of oocytes is the most critical point for oocyte maturation in vitro in terms of oocyte maturation, fertilization, and embryonic development as well as pregnancy rates, not the culture medium.

Culture media

Although numerous data have been accumulated from studies, the current rationale for choosing a specific medium for IVM of immature human oocytes appears to stem largely from adapting methods developed from culturing other cell types. Complex culture media,

TCM-199 medium, Ham's F10 medium, and Chang's medium buffered with bicarbonate and/or HEPES supplemented with various sera, gonadotropins (FSH and LH), growth factors, and steroids, have been most widely used in research and the clinical application of oocyte IVM [27, 37]. All existing media for oocyte maturation in vitro are the base of complex culture media supplemented with different substances.

Energy sources

Different energy substrates can greatly influence oocyte meiotic and cytoplasmic maturation [38, 39]. Lactate, pyruvate, and glucose are the main substrates for energy metabolism in oocytes and embryos. Glutamine can also serve as an energy substrate to improve in vitro nuclear maturation of hamster [40] and rabbit [41] oocytes. Lactate is reversibly converted to pyruvate by lactate dehydrogenase. Pyruvate or oxaloacetate, but not glucose, lactate, or phosphoenolpyruvate, supports the maturation of denuded mouse oocytes through meiosis to MII [42]. Synthesis of pyruvate in cumulus cells from glucose provides evidence that these cells are able to influence the nutritional environment of the maturing oocytes [43].

Oocyte utilization of pyruvate is closely dependent upon cumulus cells, which can convert lactate or glucose into pyruvate to be used by oocytes [44]. Pyruvate directly affects nuclear maturation in mouse oocytes [45]. It has been confirmed that mitochondrial oxidative metabolism is much more important than anaerobic glucose metabolism for energy production in the mammalian oocytes [46]. However, sodium pyruvate in non-serum maturation medium supports and promotes nuclear maturation of bovine cumulus-denuded oocytes [47]. It has been reported that pyruvate alone is insufficient for oocyte cytoplasmic maturation [48].

In early studies the concentration of pyruvate and lactate in the culture medium for embryo development was 0.25 mM and 30 mM, respectively [49, 50]; pyruvate concentration was similar to that found in blood and that of lactate was much higher, because high concentrations of lactate were found in rabbit oviductal fluid and this concentration was increased during the first three days after ovulation [51]. Most IVM media adopted these concentrations of pyruvate and lactate for embryonic development. A deleterious effect of high lactate concentration on early embryonic development has been reported in mouse [52]. Pyruvate alone or pyruvate with lactate can support preimplantation development of mouse embryos until morula stage, but they cannot support the transition to blastocysts without the addition of glucose [53]. Glucose is necessary for embryonic development from morula to blastocyst [54].

Metabolism of glucose through the Embden–Meyerhof pathway is important during bovine oocyte maturation in vitro [55]. The expression pathway of glycolytic metabolism reflects the presence of different mechanisms involved in gene expression/regulation at the transcriptional and translational level and their accumulation during human oocyte maturation [56]. In mice, glucose treatment of cumulus–oocyte complexes produced elevated cyclic AMP (cAMP) concentrations, which were associated with a decreased incidence of GVBD in hypoxanthine-supplemented medium [57, 58]. Although it has been indicated that glucose may have an inhibitory effect on cumulus-free human oocyte maturation during culture in vitro [59], other results indicated that oocyte maturation medium with glucose is beneficial to bovine and human oocyte nuclear and cytoplasmic maturation in vitro [37, 39]. It has been reported that the optimal concentration of glucose in IVM medium for bovine oocyte maturation may be 1 mg/mL [39].

Nitrogen sources

Although amino acids support hamster [40], rabbit [41], porcine [60], and bovine [38] oocyte maturation in vitro, amino acid requirements for oocyte maturation in culture are not fully understood. Essential and/or non-essential amino acids are commonly added to oocyte IVM media. In many species, it has been believed that addition of amino acids to the culture medium is beneficial to oocyte maturation [37, 61, 62]. Supplemental essential amino acids in a simple chemically defined medium are absolutely required for bovine oocyte cytoplasmic maturation to support subsequent embryonic development, and non-essential amino acids with essential amino acids have a synergic effect on bovine oocyte cytoplasmic maturation in vitro [63].

Apart from amino acid use for protein synthesis, they play important roles as osmolytes [64], intracellular buffers [65], heavy metal chelators, and energy sources [61] as well as precursors for versatile physiological regulators, such as nitric oxide and polyamines [66]. It has been shown that the culture medium with amino acids affect glucose metabolism in mouse blastocysts cultured in vitro [67]. Therefore, amino acids may not only act as nitrogen sources for protein synthesis but may also play a role in modifying the metabolic pathway.

In addition, the concentration of amino acids in complex media for somatic cell culture may not be suitable for oocyte maturation in culture. Although there is no direct evidence to prove this hypothesis, it has been shown that a reduced concentration of amino acids in culture medium is beneficial to embryonic development in vitro [68–71].

Vitamins

There is a paucity of information about the effects of vitamins in culture medium on the maturational and developmental competence of immature oocytes. The addition of water-soluble vitamins, particularly inositol, to the embryo culture medium enhances the hatching of rabbit and hamster blastocysts [72, 73]. Vitamins also affect glucose metabolism in mouse [67] and sheep embryos [74]. It has been reported that the presence of vitamins in the oocyte maturation medium is important for subsequent bovine embryonic development [75]. The designed IVM medium containing the essential vitamins showed a better result in terms of nuclear and cytoplasmic maturation of immature human oocytes compared to TC-199 medium [37]. Interestingly, Naruse et al. reported that low concentration of Minimum Essential Medium (MEM) vitamins in IVM medium during porcine oocyte maturation in vitro improves subsequent embryonic development [76]. However, the optimal concentration of vitamins in the IVM medium for human oocyte maturation is needed to be determined.

Antioxidant

Oxygen concentration of female reproductive organs is lower than in the atmosphere [61]. Development is improved in embryos cultured in low oxygen (5–10%) [77]. The beneficial effect of reduced oxygen tension may be due to the decrease of reactive oxygen species (ROS) within the cells. Excess amounts of ROS are known to be major causes of developmental arrest and cell death [78]. The potential deleterious effects of ROS can be eliminated by antioxidant enzyme activities, free radical scavengers, and iron-binding proteins [79, 80]. Antioxidant-related components, such as glutathione, taurine, selenium, apotransferrin, cysteine, cysteamine, and β-mercaptoethanol, are added to IVM medium [81]. Serum contains many factors, including those antioxygen-related components. Therefore, it seems important for serum-free IVM medium to be supplemented with those antioxygen-related components.

Supplements
Proteins

In the 1960s, it was known that a fixed protein source is essential for development of 2-cell stage embryos to develop to blastocyst stage [49, 50]. Initially, BSA or FCS or fetal bovine serum (FBS) was the most commonly used protein source in culture media [82, 83]. Serum is considered crucial for oocyte maturation and may also contain factors essential for human oocyte maturation. The important factors in serum for oocyte maturation could be many growth factors. Patient's own serum supplemented to IVM medium for their own oocyte maturation in vitro may be a good option for IVM treatment in order to obtain a high oocyte maturation rate. In addition, human follicular fluid (HFF) or human peritoneal fluid (HPF) has been used as a supplemental protein source for the maturation medium [17, 84].

Different sources of protein supplement may have different responses for oocyte maturation in vitro and subsequent development as well as the result of pregnancy. We have proven that 10% serum can be replaced by 10% synthetic serum substitute in a designed IVM medium, resulting in approximately 80% maturation rate and more than 90% fertilization rate when the cumulus-free GV oocytes were retrieved from a stimulated IVF and intracytoplasmic sperm injection (ICSI) cycle [37]. The commercially available IVM media from some companies already contain human serum albumin (HSA); therefore, it seems that the extra protein source does not need to be added to those IVM media.

Serum contains complex components, including growth factors, amino acids, and others. Serum fractions of different molecular weights may have different effects on oocyte maturation in culture. Although it is not clear which serum fraction will affect oocyte maturation in vitro, it has been indicated that some fractions contain embryo developmental inhibitory function [85]. Therefore, it seems not certain which component of serum plays an important role in IVM medium during oocyte maturation in vitro. In addition, it has been reported that fatty acid-free BSA might be the optimal supplement to IVM medium due to the higher transcript level of growth factor coding genes accompanied by lower transcript level of heat shock protein 70 kDa (Hsp-70) compared with serum [86, 87]. Indeed, in a designed IVM medium containing gonadotropins (FSH and LH), serum can be replaced by polyvinylpyrrolidone (PVP), resulting in less oocyte DNA fragmentation when the IVM medium was supplemented with 0.3% PVP as serum replacement [88].

Gonadotropins

Oocyte maturation in vitro is gonadotropin-independent. However, most IVM media are supplemented with FSH or LH or a combination of FSH and LH. The effect of gonadotropins and their relative importance for oocyte maturation in vitro and subsequent fertilization and early development is still controversial. Oocyte maturation in vitro is unlikely to undergo the elaborate cascade of endocrine and paracrine molecular signals

A

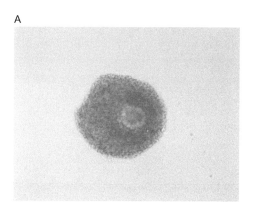

B

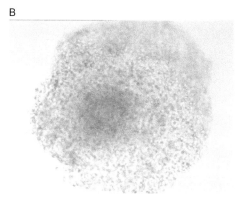

Figure 12.1 Human cumulus–oocyte complex (COC) before and after maturation in culture in a designed IVM medium. (A) The COC was collected immediately from a small follicle (3 mm in diameter) without gonadotropin priming; (B) the same COC was cultured in IVM medium for 24 hours. Note the size of COC expansion before and after maturation in culture (two photos with the same magnification ×200). See plate section for color version.

that occurs during oocyte maturation in vivo [89–92]. Although Gilchrist and Thompson indicated that today's IVM system is unphysiological [93], clinical practice resulted in an acceptable pregnancy rate with the current IVM system supplemented with gonadotropins [23, 24, 33]. While the idea to use FSH and LH is based on the physiological role of FSH and LH in oocyte maturation in vivo, it is most likely that the effects of FSH and LH on oocyte maturation are mediated through cumulus and granulosa cells (Figure 12.1), because it is believed that there are no FSH and LH receptors on oocytes. Nevertheless, it has been reported that mRNA for FSH and LH receptors are present in mouse and human oocytes, zygotes, and preimplantation embryos at different stages [94, 95].

Different concentrations of FSH and LH in IVM medium have been used. The optimal condition for oocyte maturation should be similar to the physiological concentration of gonadotropins in follicular fluid which contains fully mature oocytes [19–21, 23, 24, 33]. In addition, exposure of immature oocytes to a different ratio of FSH:LH during maturation in vitro may result in different developmental competence. Exposure of immature human oocytes to a 1:10 ratio of FSH:LH resulted in significantly higher developmental competence evidenced by increased development to the blastocyst stage in vitro compared with FSH alone or no gonadotropins [96]. However, an animal model study indicated that the ratio of FSH:LH is not important for oocyte maturation and subsequent embryonic development [97].

Mechanism studies of oocyte maturation, especially with a mouse model, indicated that it may not be necessary to supplement IVM medium with LH [2, 58, 98]. It is believed that the epidermal growth factor (EGF) receptor is a central nexus in propagating the LH signal from the granulosa cells, through the cumulus cells to the oocyte [99, 100]. This signal transduction pathway may not be the only way to control oocyte maturation. The increased production of pyruvate and lactate from the cumulus and granulosa cells occurs in response to LH [101, 102]. Therefore, the beneficial effect of LH on the oocytes during IVM involves many possible factors that affect oocyte nuclear and cytoplasmic maturation. Furthermore, it is possible that IVM medium supplemented with physiological concentration of gonadotropins (FSH and LH) stimulates steroid secretion from the cumulus and granulosa cells to affect oocyte maturation.

Steroids

Estradiol and progesterone are mediators of normal mammalian ovarian function. The actions of estradiol and progesterone on oocyte maturation might be mediated rapidly through a non-genomic mechanism via cell membrane proteins as described in *Xenopus* [103]. Estradiol may be important not only in regulating oocyte maturation, but may also be involved in subsequent embryonic development [104]. Interestingly, there is evidence to support the hypothesis that concentrations of progesterone in follicular fluid are closely associated with human oocyte maturity [105].

Considering the effect of estradiol in IVM medium, the consensus appears to be that a concentration of 1.0 µg/mL should be used, which is the concentration in the follicular fluid of pre-ovulatory follicles shortly after the LH peak in cattle [106]. The presence of estradiol in IVM medium had no effect on the progression of human oocyte maturation but improved the subsequent fertilization and cleavage rates [104]. Evidence has revealed that Ca^{2+} release mechanisms are modified during oocyte maturation [107]. When immature oocytes were cultured in vitro, they acquired the capacity to undergo a single large oscillation of intracellular Ca^{2+} [108]. However, subsequent sustained oscillations were not observed in some immature oocytes, indicating that these oocytes failed to develop a fully competent Ca^{2+} signaling system during maturation in vitro. Steroids may be involved in modification of oocytes during maturation, acting via non-genomic effects, which are referred to as "oocyte membrane maturation." Currently, less attention is paid to "oocyte membrane maturation" [109].

There seems to be a negative effect of progesterone on bovine oocyte cytoplasmic maturation when it is added to IVM medium with gonadotropins (FSH and LH) and estradiol (R. C. Chian, J. T. Chung, unpublished data, 2008). IVM medium supplemented with physiological concentrations of FSH and LH stimulates estradiol and progesterone secretion from the cumulus and granulosa cells [110, 111]. Therefore, it may not be necessary to add steroids, particularly to IVM medium when gonadotropins and cumulus and granulosa cells are present.

Growth factors

There are several growth factors in follicular fluid that contains fully mature oocytes. EGF and transforming growth factor beta (TGFβ) and members of the TGFβ superfamily (TGFβ, inhibin, and activin) are involved in the pathway of regulation of oocyte maturation. It is clear that cAMP, which is synthesized in the oocyte by constitutively active G-protein-coupled receptors, is also involved [112]. High levels of intra-oocyte cAMP keep the oocyte meiotically arrested by suppressing maturation-promoting factor (MPF) activity by stimulating cAMP-dependent protein kinase A (PKA). The oocyte possesses a potent type 3 phosphodiesterase (PDE3), an enzyme that degrades cAMP [113]. Growth differentiation factor 9 (GDF9) and bone morphogenetic protein 15 (BMP15) exist in the oocyte and are involved in oocyte maturation in a species-specific manner [114]. All these signals are mediated by the EGF receptor and EGF-like peptide cascade in the cumulus and granulosa cells to control oocyte maturation [115].

EGF alone and associated with gonadotropins induces cumulus expansion and promotes nuclear and cytoplasmic maturation of immature oocytes during culture in vitro [116]. The concentrations of EGF in IVM medium are different from different reports, but it is most likely used at 10.0 ng/mL. It seems that EGF's action is mediated by the cumulus and granulosa cells, because maturation of denuded oocytes was not affected by the

Table 12.1. Composition of a designed IVM medium

Inorganic salt	mg/L
$CaCl_2$	200.0000
KCl	400.0000
$MgSO_4$	98.0000
NaCl	6800.0000
$NaHCO_3$	1250.0000
$NaH_2PO_4 \cdot H_2O$	125.0000
Amino acids	**mg/L**
L-Alanine	8.9000
L-Arginine	126.4000
L-Asparagine	13.2000
L-Aspartic acid	13.3000
L-Cystine	24.0000
L-Glutamic acid	14.7000
L-Glutamine	292.0000
Glycine	7.5000
L-Histidine·HCl·H_2O	42.0000
L-Isoleucine	52.4000
L-Leucine	52.4000
L-Lysine·HCl	72.5000
L-Methionine	15.1000
L-Phenylalanine	33.0000
L-Proline	11.5000
L-Serine	10.5000
L-Threonine	47.6000
L-Tryptophan	10.2000
L-Tyrosine	36.0000
L-Valine	46.8000
Vitamins	**mg/L**
Biotin	0.0010
D-Ca pantothenate	1.0000
Choline chloride	1.0000
Folic acid	1.0000
i-Inositol	2.0000

Table 12.1. (*cont.*)

Vitamins	mg/L
Nicotinamide	1.0000
Pyridoxal·HCl	1.0000
Riboflavin	0.1000
Thiamine·HCl	1.0000

Other components	mg/L
D-Glucose	1000.0000
Sodium pyruvate	110.0000
Sodium DL-lactate	205.0000
Cysteamine HCl	22.7200
EGF	0.0010
Estradiol	1.0000
FSH	75.0000 IU
LH	75.0000 IU
Human serum albumin	3000.0000
Penicillin G	50.0000 units
Streptomycin	50.0000 µg

presence of EGF in IVM medium [117, 118]. Therefore, a designed IVM medium can be supplemented with EGF directly when cumulus–oocyte complexes are cultured for maturation in vitro [23, 93, 119–121]. Interestingly, it has been reported that EGF has a negative effect on marmoset monkey oocyte maturation in vitro in the presence of low gonadotropins, but contrastingly, partially protects oocytes from the negative effects of high gonadotropins, suggesting that the effects of EGF are highly dependent on the concentration of gonadotropins in IVM medium [122].

As mentioned above, serum contains many factors, including growth factors. Therefore, it may not be necessary to add EGF to IVM medium when serum supplement is added to IVM medium for oocyte maturation in vitro [23]. Many commercially available IVM media are ready to use, in which serum is not included in the IVM medium. In this case, it is not clear whether EGF should be added to IVM medium or not, but it seems better to supplement the IVM medium with EGF when serum is not present. However, it has to be noted that the active half-lives of gonadotropins and growth factors are short in IVM medium. Therefore, gonadotropins and growth factors should be supplemented to IVM medium just before use. A designed IVM medium is shown in Table 12.1.

Development of IVM systems

For human infertility treatment with IVM technology, it seems no breakthrough has been made yet by improving the IVM medium itself. Although there are some "new" ideas or approaches proposed with animal models for IVM of immature oocytes that resulted in high blastocyst formation and fetal production [2, 123], there is no report that indicates the ideas or approaches can be applied to human infertility treatment. Maybe, the ideas or approaches are acceptable within the animal industry to use cell cycle-modulating agents or spindle formation inhibitors during oocyte IVM, but usage of these agents for clinical application with human oocyte maturation in vitro should be carefully discussed for its safety issue before adaption of the methodology.

Summary

IVM of immature human oocytes is an old topic, but recently its application to infertility treatment resulted in acceptable clinical pregnancy and live birth rates. Immature human oocytes can be matured in vitro spontaneously after being released from follicles. However, the source of immature oocytes is the most critical point for oocyte maturation in vitro in terms of oocyte maturation, fertilization, and embryonic development as well as pregnancy and live birth rates. Culture conditions, particularly IVM medium, affect oocyte maturation and oocyte quality. The optimal IVM medium for oocyte maturation in vitro should be similar to the physiological condition in follicular fluid which contains fully mature oocytes.

References

1. Cha KY, Chian RC. Maturation in vitro of immature human oocytes for clinical use. *Hum Reprod Update* 1998;**4**:103–20.

2. Gilchrist RB. Recent insights into oocyte-follicle cell interactions provide opportunities for the development of new approaches to in vitro maturation. *Reprod Fertil Dev* 2011;**23**:23–31.

3. Sirard MA. Follicle environment and quality of in vitro matured oocytes. *J Assist Reprod Genet* 2011;**28**:483–8.

4. Pincus G, Enzmann EV. The comparative behaviour of mammalian eggs in vivo and in vitro. I. The activation of ovarian eggs. *J Exp Med* 1935;**62**:665–75.

5. Pincus G, Saunders B. Unfertilized human tubal ova. *Anat Record* 1937;**69**:163–9.

6. Pincus G, Saunders B. The comparative behaviour of mammalian eggs in vivo and in vitro. VI. The maturation of human ovarian ovarian ova. *Anat Record* 1939;**75** (4&Suppl):537–45.

7. Pincus G, Enzmann EV. Can mammalian eggs underdo normal development. *Proc Natl Acad Sci U S A* 1934;**20**:121–2.

8. Rock J, Menkin MF. In vitro fertilization and cleavage of human ovarian eggs. *Science* 1944;**100**:105–7.

9. Menkin MF, Rock J. In vitro fertilization and cleavage of human ovarian eggs. *Am J Obstet Gynecol* 1948;**55**:440–52.

10. Edwards RG. Maturation in vitro of mouse, sheep, cow, pig, rhesus monkey and human ovarian oocytes. *Nature* 1965;**208**:349–51.

11. Edwards RG. Maturation in vitro of human ovarian oocytes. *Lancet* 1965;**286**:926–9.

12. Kennedy JF, Donahue RP. Human oocytes: maturation in chemically defined media. *Science* 1969;**164**:1292–3.

13. Kennedy JF, Donahue RP. Binucleate human oocytes from large follicles. *Lancet* 1969;**7598**:754–5.

14. Edwards RG, Bavister BD, Steptoe PC. Early stages of fertilization in vitro of human oocytes matured in vitro. *Nature* 1969;**221**:632–5.

15. Edwards RG, Steptoe PC, Purdy JM. Fertilization and cleavage in vitro of preovulatory human oocytes. *Nature* 1970;**227**:1307–9.

16. Steptoe PC, Edwards RG. Birth after the reimplantation of a human embryo. *Lancet* 1978;**312**:366.

17. Cha KY, Koo JJ, Ko JJ, *et al.* Pregnancy after in vitro fertilization of human follicular oocytes collected from nonstimulated cycles, their culture in vitro

and their transfer in a donor oocyte program. *Fteril Steril* 1991;**55**:109–13.

18. Trounson A, Wood C, Kausche A. In vitro maturation and fertilization and developmental competence of oocytes recovered from untreated polycystic ovarian patients. *Fertil Steril* 1994;**62**:353–62.

19. Chian RC, Buckett WM, Too LL, Tan SL. Pregnancies resulting from in vitro matured oocytes retrieved from patients with polycystic ovary syndrome after priming with human chorionic gonadotropin. *Fertil Steril* 1999;**72**:639–42.

20. Chian RC, Gulekli B, Buckett WM, Tan SL. Priming with human chorionic gonadotropin before retrieval of immature oocytes in women with infertility due to the polycystic ovary syndrome. *N Engl J Med* 1999;**341**:1624–6.

21. Chian RC, Buckett WM, Tulandi T, Tan SL. Prospective randomized study of human chorionic gonadotropin priming before immature oocyte retrieval from unstimulated women with polycystic ovarian syndrome. *Hum Reprod* 2000;**15**:165–70.

22. De Vos M, Ortega-Hrepich C, Albuz FK, *et al.* Clinical outcome of non-hCG-primed oocyte in vitro maturation treatment in patients with polycystic ovaries and polycystic ovary syndrome. *Fertil Steril* 2011;**96**:860–4.

23. Chian RC, Buckett WM, Tan SL. In-vitro maturation of human oocytes. *Reprod Biomed Online* 2004;**8**:148–66.

24. Chian RC, Lim JH, Tan SL. State of the art in in-vitro oocyte maturation. *Curr Opin Obstet Gynecol* 2004;**16**:211–19.

25. Suikkari AM. In vitro maturation: its role in fertility treatment. *Curr Opin Obstet Gynecol* 2008;**20**:242–8.

26. Chian RC, Uzelac PS, Nargund G. In Vitro maturation of human immature oocytes for fertility preservation. *Fertil Steril* 2013;**99**:1173–81.

27. Trounson A, Anderiesz C, Jones GM, *et al.* Oocyte maturation. *Hum Reprod* 1998;**13** (Suppl 3):52–62.

28. Gougeon A. Regulation of ovarian follicular development in primates: facts and hypotheses. *Endocr Rev* 1996;**17**:121–55.

29. Durinzi KL, Saniga EM, Lanzendorf SE. The relationship between size and maturation in vitro in the unstimulated human oocyte. *Fertil Steril* 1995;**63**:404–6.

30. Tsuji K, Sowa M, Nakano R. Relationship between human oocyte maturation and different follicular sizes. *Biol Reprod* 1985;**32**:413–17.

31. Smith LC, Olivera-Angel M, Groome NP, Bhatia B, Price CA. Oocyte quality in small antral follicles in the presence or absence of a large dominant follicle in cattle. *J Reprod Fertil* 1996;**106**:193–9.

32. Chian RC, Chung JT, Downey BF, Tan SL. Maturational and developmental competence of immature oocytes retrieved from ovaries at different phases of folliculogenesis: bovine model study. *Reprod Biomed Online* 2002;**4**:129–34.

33. Chian RC, Buckett WM, Abdul-Jalil AK, *et al.* Natural cycle in vitro fertilization combined with in vitro maturation of immature oocytes is an alternative approach in infertility treatment. *Fertil Steril* 2004;**82**:1675–8.

34. Fadini R, Dal Canto MB, Renzini MM, *et al.* Predictive factors in in-vitro maturation in unstimulated women with normal ovaries. *Reprod Biomed Online* 2009;**18**:251–61.

35. Fadini R, Dal Canto MB, Renzini MM, *et al.* Effect of different gonadotropin priming on IVM of oocytes from women with normal ovaries: a prospective randomized study. *Reprod Biomed Online* 2009;**19**:343–51.

36. Fadini R, Comi R, Renzini MM, *et al.* Anti-mullerian hormone as a predictive marker for the selection of women for oocyte in vitro maturation treatment. *J Assist Reprod Genet* 2011;**28**:501–8.

37. Chian RC, Tan SL. Maturational and developmental competence of immature human oocytes matured in vitro. *Reprod Biomed Online* 2002;**5**:125–32.

38. Rose-Hellekant TA, Libersky-Williamson EA, Bavister BD. Energy substrates and amino acids provided during in vitro maturation of bovine oocytes alter acquisition of developmental competence. *Zygote* 1998;**6**:285–94.

39. Chung JT, Tan SL, Chian RC. Effect of glucose on bovine oocyte maturation and subsequent fertilization and early embryonic development in vitro. *Biol Reprod* 2002;**66**(Suppl):177.

40. Gwatkin RBL, Haidri AA. Requirements for the maturation of hamster oocytes in vitro. *Exp Cell Res* 1973;**76**:1–7.

41. Bae IH, Foote RH. Utilization of glutamine for energy and protein synthesis by cultured rabbit follicular oocytes. *Exp Cell Res* 1975;**90**:432–6.

42. Biggers JD, Whittingham DG, Donahue RP. The pattern of energy metabolism in the mouse oocyte and zygote. *Proc Natl Acad Sci U S A* 1967;**58**:560–7.

43. Leese HJ, Barton AM. Pyruvate and glucose uptake by mouse ova and preimplantational embryos. *J Reprod Fertil* 1984;**72**:9–13.

44. Leese HJ, Barton AM. Production of pyruvate by isolated mouse cumulus cells. *J Exp Zool* 1985;**234**:231–6.

45. Kim H, Schuetz AW. Regulation of nuclear membrane assembly and maintenance during in vitro maturation of mouse oocytes: role of pyruvate and protein synthesis. *Cell Tissue Res* 1991;**265**:105–12.

46. Gandolfi F, Milanesi E, Pocar P, *et al.* Comparative analysis of calf and cow oocytes during in vitro maturation. *Mol Reprod Dev* 1998;**49**:168–75.

47. Geshi M, Takenouchi N, Yamauchi N, Nagai T. Effects of sodium pyruvate in nonserum maturation medium on maturation, fertilization, and subsequent development of bovine oocytes with or without cumulus cells. *Biol Reprod* 2000;**63**:1730–4.

48. Zheng P, Wang H, Bavister BD, Ji W. Maturation of rhesus monkey oocytes in chemically defined culture media and their functional assessment by IVF and embryo development. *Hum Reprod* 2001;**16**:300–5.

49. Brinster RL. Studies on the development of mouse embryos in vitro. II. The effect of energy source. *J Exp Zool* 1965;**158**:59–68.

50. Brinster RL. Studies on the development of mouse embryos in vitro. IV. Interaction of energy source. *J Reprod Fertil* 1965;**10**:227–40.

51. Mastoianni L, Wallach RC. Effect of ovulation and early gestation on oviduct secretion in the rabbit. *Am J Physiol* 1961;**200**:815–18.

52. Cross PC, Brinster RL. The sensitivity of one-cell mouse embryos to pyruvate and lactate. *Exp Cell Res* 1973;**77**:57–62.

53. Brown JJG, Whittingham DG. The role of pyruvate, lactate and glucose during preimplantation development of embryos from F1 hybrid mice in vitro. *Development* 1991;**112**:99–105.

54. Brinster RL. Uptake and incorporation of amino acids by the preimplantation mouse embryos. *J Reprod Fertil* 1971;**27**:329–38.

55. Krisher RL, Bavister BD. Enhanced glycolysis after maturation of bovine oocytes in vitro is associated with increased developmental competence. *Mol Reprod Dev* 1999;**53**:19–26.

56. Mouatassim SEL, Hazout A, Bellec V, Menezo Y. Glucose metabolism during the final stage of human oocyte maturation: genetic expression of hexokinase, glucose phosphate isomerase and phosphofructokinase. *Zygote* 1999;**7**:45–50.

57. Downs SM. The influence of glucose, cumulus cells, and metabolic coupling on cATP levels and meiotic control in the isolated mouse oocyte. *Dev Biol* 1995;**167**:502–12.

58. Downs SM. Regulation of G2/M transition in rodent oocytes. *Mol Reprod Dev* 2010;**77**:566–85.

59. Cekleniak NA, Combelle CMH, Ganez DA, *et al.* A novel system for in vitro maturation of human oocytes. *Fertil Steril* 2001;**75**:1185–93.

60. Ka HH, Sawai K, Wang WH, Im KS, Niwa K. Amino acids in mammalian medium and presence of cumulus cells at

fertilization promote male pronulear formation in porcine oocytes matured and penetrated in vitro. *Biol Reprod* 1997;**57**:1478–83.

61. Bavister BD. Culture of preimplantation embryos: facts and artifacts. *Hum Reprod Update* 1995;**1**:91–148.

62. Hoshi H. In vitro production of bovine embryos and their application for embryo transfer. *Theriogenology* 2003;**59**:675–85.

63. Rezaei N, Abdul-Jalil AK, Chung JT, Chian RC. Role of essential and non-essential amino acids contained in maturation medium on bovine oocyte maturation and subsequent fertilization and early embryonic development in vitro. *Theriogenology* 2003;**59**:497.

64. Biggers JD, Lawwitts JA, Lechene CP. The protective action of betaine on the deleterious effects of NaCl on preimplantation mouse embryos in vitro. *Mol Reprod Dev* 1993;**34**:380–90.

65. Edwards LJ, Williams DA, Gardner DK. Intracellular pH of the mouse preimplantation embryo: amino acids act as buffers of intracellular pH. *Hum Reprod* 1998;**13**:344–8.

66. Wu G, Morris SM Jr. Arginine metabolism: nitric oxide and beyond. *Biochem J* 1998;**336**:1–17.

67. Lane M, Gardner DK. Amino acids and vitamins prevent culture-induced metabolic perturbations and associated loss of viability of mouse blastocysts. *Hum Reprod* 1998;**13**:991–7.

68. Summers MC, Bhatnagar PR, Lawitts JA, Biggers JD. Fertilization in vitro of mouse ova from inbred and outbred strains: complete preimplantation embryo development in glucose-supplemented KSOM. *Biol Reprod* 1995;**53**:431–7.

69. Summers MC, McGinnis LK, Lawitts JA, Raffin M, Biggers JD. IVF of mouse ova in a simplex optimized medium supplanted with amino acids. *Hum Reprod* 2000;**15**:1791–801.

70. Biggers JD, McGinnis LK, Raffin M. Amino acids and preimplantation development of the mouse in protein-free potassium

simplex optimized medium. *Biol Reprod* 2000;**63**:281–93.

71. Summers MC, Biggers JD. Chemically defined media and the culture of mammalian preimplantation embryos: historical perspective and current issues. *Hum Reprod Update* 2003;**9**:557–82.

72. Kane MT, Bavister BD. Vitamin requirements for development of eight-cell hamster embryos to hatching blastocysts in vitro. *Biol Reprod* 1988;**39**:1137–43.

73. Fahy MM, Kane MT. Inositol stimulates DNA and protein synthesis, and expansion by rabbit blastocysts in vitro. *Hum Reprod* 1992;**7**:550–2.

74. Gardner DK, Lane M, Spitzer A, Batt PA. Enhanced rates of cleavage and development for sheep zygotes cultured to the blastocyst stage in vitro in the absence of serum and somatic cells: amino acids, vitamins, and culturing embryos in groups stimulate development. *Biol Reprod* 1994;**50**:390–400.

75. Abdul Jalil AK, Rezaei N, Chung JT, Tan SL, Chian RC. Effect of vitamins during oocyte maturation on subsequent embryonic development in vitro. *48th Annual Meeting CFAS* 2002;TP-24:49.

76. Naruse K, Kim HR, Shin YM, *et al.* Low concentrations of MEM vitamins during in vitro maturation of porcine oocytes improves subsequent pathenogenetic development. *Theriogenology* 2007;**67**:407–12.

77. Thompson JG, Sympson AC, Pugh PA, Donelly PE, Tervit HR. Effect of oxygen concentration on in-vitro development of preimplantation sheep and cattle embryos. *J Reprod Fertil* 1990;**89**:573–8.

78. Johnson MH, Nasr-Esfahani MH. Radical solutions and cultural problems: could free oxygen radicals be responsible for the impaired development of preimplantation mammalian embryos in vitro? *Bioessays* 1994;**16**:31–8.

79. Nasr-Esfahani MH, Aitken RJ, Johnson MH. Hydrogen peroxide levels in mouse oocytes and early cleavage stage embryos developed in vitro or in vivo. *Development* 1990;**109**:501–7.

80. Nasr-Esfahani MH, Johnson NH. How does transferring overcome the in vitro block to development of the mouse preimplantation embryo? *J Reprod Fertil* 1992;**96**:41–8.

81. Deleuze S, Goudet G. Cysteamine supplementation of in vitro maturation media: a review. *Reprod Domest Anim* 2010;**45**:e476–82.

82. Kane MT, Headon DR. The role of commercial bovine serum albumin preparation in the culture of one-cell rabbit embryos to blastocyst. *J Reprod Fertil* 1980;**60**:469–75.

83. Younis AI, Brackett BG, Fayrer-Hosken RA. Influence of serum and hormones on bovine oocyte maturation and fertilization in vitro. *Gamete Res* 1989;**23**:189–201.

84. Cha KY, Do BR, Chi HJ, *et al*. Viability of human follicular oocytes collected from unstimulated ovaries and matured and fertilized in vitro. *Reprod Fertil Dev* 1992;**4**:695–701.

85. Ogawa T, Ono T, Marrs RP. The effect of serum fractions on single-cell mouse embryos in vitro. *J In Vitro Fert Embryo Transf* 1987;**4**:153–9.

86. Warzych E, Wrenzycki C, Peippo J, Lechniak D. Maturation medium supplements affect transcript level of apoptosis and cell survival related genes in bovine blastocysts produced in vitro. *Mol Reprod Dev* 2007;**74**:280–9.

87. Warzych E, Peippo J, Szydlowski M, Lechniak D. Supplements to in vitro maturation media affect the production of bovine blastocysts and their apoptotic index but not the proportions of matured and apoptotic oocytes. *Anim Reprod Sci* 2007;**97**:334–43.

88. Chung JT, Tosca L, Huang TH, Niwa K, Chian RC. The effect of polyvinylpyrrolidone on bovine oocyte maturation in vitro and subsequent fertilization and embryonic development. *Reprod Biomed Online* 2007;**15**:198–207.

89. Ashkenazi H, Cao X, Motola S, *et al*. Epidermal growth factor family members: endogenous mediators of the ovulatory response. *Endocrinology* 2005;**146**:77–84.

90. Norris RP, Freudzon M, Mehlmann LM, *et al*. Luteinizing hormone causes MAP kinase-dependent phosphorylation and closure of connexin 43 gap junctions in mouse ovarian follicles: one of two paths to meiotic resumption. *Development* 2008;**135**:3229–38.

91. Norris RP, Ratzan WJ, Freudzon M, *et al*. Cyclic GMP from the surrounding somatic cells regulates cyclic AMP and meiosis in the mouse oocyte. *Development* 2009;**136**:1869–78.

92. Vaccari S, Weeks JL, Hsieh M, Menniti FS, Conti M. Cyclic GMP signalling is involved in the luteinizing hormone-dependent meiotic maturation of mouse oocytes. *Biol Reprod* 2009;**81**:595–604.

93. Gilchrist RB, Thompson JG. Oocyte maturation: emerging concepts and technologies to improve developmental potential in vitro. *Theriogenology* 2007;**67**:6–15.

94. Patsoula E, Loutradis D, Drakakis P, *et al*. Expression of mRNA for the LH and FSH receptors in mouse oocytes and preimplantation embryos. *Reproduction* 2001;**121**:455–61.

95. Patsoula E, Loutradis D, Drakakis P, *et al*. Messenger RNA expression for the follicle-stimulating hormone receptor and luteinizing hormone receptor in human oocytes and preimplantation-stage embryos. *Fertil Steril* 2003;**79**:1187–93.

96. Anderiesz C, Ferraretti A, Magli C, *et al*. Effect of recombinant human gonadotrophins on human, bovine and murine oocyte meiosis, fertilization and embryonic development in vitro. *Hum Reprod* 2000;**15**:1140–8.

97. Choi YH, Carnevale EM, Seidel GE Jr., Squire EL. Effects of gonadotropins on bovine oocytes matured in TCM-199. *Theriogenology* 2001;**56**:661–70.

98. Albertini DF, Sanfins A, Combelles CM. Origins and manifestations of oocyte maturation competencies. *Reprod BioMed Online* 2003;**6**:410–15.

99. Hsieh M, Lee D, Panigone S, *et al*. Luteinizing hormone-dependent activation

of the epidermal growth factor network is essential for ovulation. *Mol Cell Biol* 2007;**27**:1914–24.

100. Reizel Y, Elbaz J, Dekel N. Sustained activity of the EGF receptor is an absolute requisite for LH-induced oocyte maturation and cumulus expansion. *Mol Endocrinol* 2010;**24**:402–11.

101. Hillensjo T. Oocyte maturation and glycolysis in isolated preovulatory follicles of PMS-injected immature rats. *Acta Endocrinol* 1976;**82**:809–30.

102. Billig H, Hedin L, Magnusson C. Gonadotrophins stimulate lactate production by rat cumulus and granulosa cells *Acta Endocrinol* 1983;**103**:562–6.

103. Bayaa M, Booth RA, Sheng Y, Liu XJ. The classical progesterone receptor mediates *Xenopus* oocyte maturation through a nongenomic mechanism. *Proc Natl Acad Sci U S A* 2000;**7**:12607–12.

104. Tesarik J, Mendoza C. Nongenomic effects of 17β-estradiol on maturing human oocytes: relationship to oocyte developmental potential. *J Clin Endocrinol Metab* 1995;**80**:1438–43.

105. Seibel MM, Smith D, Dlugi AM, Levesque L. Periovulatory follicular fluid hormone levels in spontaneous human cycles. *J Clin Endocrinol Metab* 1989;**68**:1073–7.

106. Dieleman SJ, Kruip TA, Fontijne P, de Jong WH, van der Weyden GC. Changes in oestradiol, progesterone and testosterone concentrations in follicular fluid and in the micromorphology of preovulatory bovine follicles relative to the peak of luteinizing hormone. *J Endocrinol* 1983;**97**:31–42.

107. Mehlmann LM, Kline D. Regulation of intracellular calcium in the mouse egg: calcium release in response to sperm or inositol trisphosphate is enhanced after meiotic maturation. *Biol Reprod* 1994;**51**:1088–98.

108. Herbert M, Gillespie JI, Murdoch AP. Development of calcium signalling mechanisms during maturation of human oocytes. *Mol Hum Reprod* 1997;**11**:965–73.

109. Li YR, Ren CE, Zhang Q, Li JC, Chian RC. Expression of G protein estrogen receptor (GPER) on membrane of mouse oocytes during maturation. *J Assist Reprod Genet* 2013;**30**:227–32.

110. Chian RC, Ao A, Clarke HJ, Tulandi T, Tan SL. Production of steroid hormones from human cumulus and granulosa cells treated by different concentrations of gonadotropins during culture in vitro. *Fertil Steril* 1999;**71**:61–6.

111. Yamashita Y, Kawashima I, Gunji Y, Hishinuma M, Shimada M. Progesterone is essential for maintenance of Tace/Adam17 mRNA expression, but not EDF-like factor, in cumulus cells, which enhances the EGF receptor signalling pathway during in vitro maturation of porcine COCs. *J Reprod Dev* 2010;**56**:315–23.

112. Mehlmann LM, Jones TL, Jaffe LA. Meiotic arrest in the mouse follicle maintained by a Gs protein in the oocyte. *Science* 2002;**297**:1343–5.

113. Tsafriri A, Chun SY, Zhang R, Hsueh AJ, Conti M. Oocyte maturation involves compartmentalization and opposing changes of cAMP levels in follicular somatic and germ cells: studies using selective phosphodiesterase inhibitors. *Dev Biol* 1996;**178**:393–402.

114. Galloway SM, McNatty KP, Cambridge LM, *et al.* Mutations in an oocyte-derived growth factor gene (BMP15) cause increased ovulation rate and infertility in a dosage-sensitive manner. *Nat Genet* 2000;**25**:279–83.

115. Fan HY, Liu Z, Shimada M, *et al.* MAPK3/1 (ERK1/2) in ovarian granulosa cells are essential for female fertility. *Science* 2009;**324**:938–41.

116. De La Fuente R, O'Brien MJ, Eppig JJ. Epidermal growth factor enhances preimplantation developmental competence of maturing mouse oocytes. *Hum Reprod* 1999;**14**:3060–8.

117. Lorenzo PL, Illera MJ, Illera JC, Illera M. Enhancement of cumulus expansion and nuclear maturation during bovine oocyte maturation in vitro by the addition of epidermal growth factor and insulin-like growth factor. *J Reprod Fertil* 1994;**101**:697–701.

118. Wang WH, Niwa K. Synergetic effects of epidermal growth factor and gonadotropins on the cytoplasmic maturation of pig oocytes in a serum-free medium. *Zygote* 1995;**3**:345–50.

119. Chian RC. In-vitro maturation of immature oocytes for infertile women with PCOS. *Reprod Biomed Online* 2004;**8**:547–52.

120. Gilchrist RB, Lane M, Thompson JG. Oocyte secreted factors: regulators of cumulus cell function and oocyte quality. *Hum Reprod Update* 2008;**14**:159–77.

121. Gilchrist RB, De Vos M, Smitz J, Thompson JG. IVM media are designed specially to support immature cumulus-oocyte complexes not denuded oocytes that have failed to respond to hyperstimulation. *Fertil Steril* 2011;**96**:e141.

122. Tkachenko OY, Delimitreva S, Isachenko E, *et al.* Epidermal growth factor effects on marmoset monkey (*Callithrix jacchus*) oocyte in vitro maturation, IVF and embryo development are altered by gonadotrophin concentration during oocyte maturation. *Hum Reprod* 2010;**25**:2047–58.

123. Albuz FK, Sasseville M, Lane M, *et al.* Simulated physiological oocyte maturation (SPOM): a novel in vitro maturation system that substantially improves embryo yield and pregnancy outcome. *Hum Reprod* 2010;**25**:2999–3011.

Chapter

13

Oocyte and embryo cryopreservation media

Diana Patricia Bernal, Ching-Chien Chang,
and Zsolt Peter Nagy

Introduction

The main goal of cryopreservation of cells, gametes, or embryos is to preserve the specimen in a state of suspended animation, with the hope that it can be reanimated after a certain period of time to continue its normal development. Cryopreservation procedures are designed to minimize damages caused by formation and growth of ice crystals [1]; however, the challenge of a successful cryopreservation is to be able to cool and recover cells from the ultra-low temperatures at which no changes in metabolism and structures are stable over time. Cryopreservation occurs when cryoprotectants or antifreeze solutions are added to the solution surrounding the cell, and then cooled at a certain rate. The biophysical changes caused by the transition of water to ice during cooling are the main cause of damage rather than the low temperature per se. As ice crystals grow, there is a significant osmotic stress, this "freeze–dehydration" was one of the first harmful consequences identified in cell cryobiology that causes several hazardous events including changes in ultrastructure of cell membranes, loss or fusion of membranes, and organelle disruption. In order to avoid cryo-damages, the cooling and warming protocol must be tailored according to the cell characteristics. Therefore, the compositions and modifications of cryomedia are very important to the success of cryopreservation.

Types of cryopreservation
Equilibrium procedures: "slow freezing"

The controlled slow freezing method was established by Whittingham et al. [2] and has been in use since then [3–5]. The general principle is based on the exposure of specimens to a $\geq 10\%$ solution of cryoprotectants, and then they are cooled at a controlled rate to subzero temperatures below $-30\,°C$ and plunged into liquid nitrogen at $-196\,°C$ for long-term storage. For thawing purposes specimens are warmed to physiological temperatures at a rate compatible with the rate at which they were initially cooled, and finally the cryoprotectant is removed [5]. In order to preserve viability, cells need to be dehydrated before ice crystals start propagating into the cell where the cryoprotectant agent (CPA) plays a crucial role [6]. Initially the temperature is lowered to below $0\,°C$ (from $-4\,°C$ to $-9\,°C$). At this point, "ice nucleation," a process also called "seeding," is induced to initiate extracellular ice formation in a controlled fashion. After achieving the initial phase of dehydration during the CPA exposure at subzero temperatures, specimens are cooled to temperatures at which

Culture Media, Solutions, and Systems in Human ART, ed. Patrick Quinn. Published by Cambridge University Press. © Cambridge University Press 2014.

extracellular ice may be formed. To avoid insufficient dehydration (risk of cryo-injury from ice formation) or overexposure to cryoprotectants (risk of cytotoxicity), the optimal rate of cooling is cell-type specific, and it depends on CPA and water permeability of the cell membrane. For human oocytes and embryos, the optimal cooling rate is thought to be between 0.3 °C/min and 1 °C/min which is almost 1/100th of the optimal rate for red blood cells [7]; then specimens are seeded around −7 °C to avoid excessive super cooling, this period of slow cooling ends once the temperature has fallen between -30 °C/min and −80 °C/min, then the cells are stored under lower temperatures in dewars, usually below −130 °C/min [1, 7].

Non-equilibrium procedure "vitrification – rapid cooling protocols"

All successful oocyte cryopreservation methods have one common objective: to avoid ice-crystal formation. The prevention of ice-crystal formation can also reduce the impact of cryo-damages during cryopreservation. The non-equilibrium procedure, vitrification, is a process that produces a glass-like solidification by which water is prevented from forming ice crystals due to the viscosity of highly concentrated cryoprotectant cooled at an extremely rapid rate [8]. The glass-like solidification during the non-equilibrium procedure/vitrification is the phase transition process from liquid to solid. The non-equilibrium procedure was first applied to cryopreserve embryos and oocytes in the 1980s [9, 10] but it was not used until several years ago in the human in vitro fertilization (IVF) field [11–13]. This protocol provides an alternative way to cryopreserve embryos and oocytes other than slow cooling. In general, the advantages of this method are it is simple and rapid and there is low cryo-damage. However, there are still some concerns about this method, such as the toxicity of the solution [7], fracture damage, and osmotic shock [14].

Components of cryopreservation solutions

Carrier solution

This consists of solution ingredients that do not contain CPAs. Its role is to provide basic support for cells at temperatures near to the freezing point. Usually it contains salts, osmotic agents, pH buffers, and sometimes nutritive ingredients or apoptosis inhibitors. All these ingredients are usually present at near-isotonic concentration (300 mOsm) so cells neither shrink nor swell when held in carrier solution; the most common are HEPES-based buffer and phosphate-based solution. It is very important to know that the concentration of the carrier solution is always constant as empirical addition of CPA solution to a carrier solution would dilute the carrier ingredients [15].

Intracellular CPAs, also called "permeating CPAs"

The permeating CPAs are small molecules that can penetrate cell membranes to form hydrogen bonds with water molecules, therefore preventing formation of ice crystals [15]. Usually the small molecules are non-ionic with a high solubility in water in all proportions which could also reduce the freezing point of water to subzero temperatures [16]. These chemical compounds can diffuse through cellular membranes of oocytes and embryos, permeate the cell, and equilibrate within the cytoplasm, replacing the intracellular water without over-dehydrating the cell; penetrated CPAs solidify at lower temperatures than water and thus subsequently reduce the amount of intracellular ice formation at that given temperature [17].

Commonly used permeating CPAs are:

BG: butylene glycol
PrOH: propanediol
PG: propylene glycol
DMSO: dimethyl sulfoxide
Gly: glycerol
EG: ethylene glycol
Met: methanol

Extracellular (non-permeating) CPAs

The extracellular CPAs can increase osmolarity of the extracellular space, which results in cellular dehydration and reduces intracellular ice-crystal formation. Besides, the extracellular CPAs are often included in media for warming or thawing of cells to help to prevent traumatic cell expansion during the process of rehydration. These extracellular CPA compounds are usually high-molecular-weight polymers [15], which do not pass through the membrane of the cells, stabilize cell membranes during the post-thaw phase, and increase the viscosity of the solution. Polymers, such as Ficoll, dextran, polyvinylpyrrolidone, hyaluronic acid, polyvinyl alcohol, polyethylene glycol, and proteins (human or bovine serum albumin), and sugars (i.e., sucrose and trehalose) raise the total solute concentration of a solution without increasing the toxicity of the solution [1].

Commonly used non-permeating CPAs are:

Sucrose
Trehalose
PVP: polyvinylpyrrolidone
Fic: Ficoll
Dex: dextran
PEG: polyethylene glycol

Ice blockers (optional ingredient)

Ice blockers are compounds that directly block ice growth by selective binding with ice or binding to contaminants that trigger ice formation; they can enhance conventional CPAs by interacting with ice or a surface that resembles ice. Some examples are low-molecular-weight polyvinyl alcohol, polyglycerol, and biological antifreeze proteins [15, 18].

Physics of water and CPA

The addition of salts and other solutes to pure water lowers the temperature at which ice forms or melts. There is no limit to how low the freezing/melting point can be reached by solutes, because high concentrations may never form ice but rather will solidify into an ice-free (vitreous) state. The formation and growth of ice crystals can be modified by compounds such as antifreeze proteins, ice blocking agents, and cryoprotectants [1]. In order to preserve cell viability, the cells need to be dehydrated before ice starts to propagate intracellularly [6]. During the cooling process, the presence of CPA in the cryopreservation solution starts generating an osmotic gradient that extracts water from the intracellular environment; therefore, permeable CPAs can penetrate across the cell membrane and interact with biomolecules inside the cell, acting as "water replacements"[6]. Due to the

Table 13.1. Properties of commonly used CPAs

CPA	Molecular weight (g/mol)	Density (g/cm^3)	Melting point (°C)
Ethylene glycol	62.17	1.1132	−12.9
Propylene glycol	76.09	1.036	−59
DMSO	78.13	1.1004	19
Glycerol	92.09	1.261	17.8
Propanediol	76.09	1.0597	−28
Methanol	32.04	0.7918	−98
PVP	2500	1.2	150 to 180
Sucrose	342.3	1.587	186

fact that CPAs permeate the cell membrane slower than water, the loss of intracellular water is faster than the gain of CPAs inside the cell, which causes a change in cell volume over time, producing a typical shrink–swell curve (Table 13.1) [6].

Combination of CPAs

Most cryopreservation solutions used for oocytes and embryos are made up in a physiological solution, adding intracellular CPAs (PrOH, DMSO, EG, Gly) and extracellular CPAs (sucrose, trehalose) with a protein which improves handling characteristics and membrane stability and can reduce toxicity. Several companies produce different formulae of cryopreservation solutions in order to facilitate the availability of the techniques for laboratories and achieve more consistent outcomes. Tables 13.2 and 13.3 show the cryopreservation solutions which are commercially available for slow freezing and vitrification, respectively.

Cooling and warming rates

The conditions under which oocytes or embryos are exposed to CPA are very important, knowing that cell membrane permeability increases at higher temperature; when CPAs are loaded at 37 °C, the rate of exchange of water and CPA between the intra- and extracellular spaces increases and the shrink–swell contraction response is reduced in comparison to dehydration carried out at room temperature [35]. The rate of cooling is dependent on the volume of liquid to be cooled and the surface area of the device used. The smaller the container is, the lower the solute concentration required for vitrification. To maximize the rate of cooling, many devices have been introduced to vitrify embryos and oocytes, including Cryotop [11], Cryotip, Cryoloop [36], Cryoleaf [13], Open Pulled Straws [37].

Mechanism of action

The development of a successful cryopreservation protocol is complex with multiple variables involved in the process. We have to consider those variables including cell-specific sensitivity, cell size, membrane permeability, and lipid contents from different cell types. Besides the variables such as membrane permeability in selecting suitable CPAs,

Table 13.2. Most used commercial solutions for slow freezing

Cryopreservation protocol	Procedure	Media	Composition*	Use for	Company
Slow freezing	Freezing	G-FreezeKit Blast [19]	MOPS + Glycerol + Sucrose 100 mM Sucrose + 5% Glycerol 200 mM Sucrose + 10% Glycerol Protein free	Blastocyst	Vitrolife
	Thawing	G-Thaw Kit Blast [20]	MOPS + Glycerol + Sucrose 200 mM Sucrose + 10% Glycerol 100 mM Sucrose + 5% Glycerol 100 mM Sucrose Protein free		
	Freezing	Freeze-Kit1 [21]	PBS + Human Serum Albumin 1,2 Propanediol 0.1 M Sucrose	Cleavage	
	Thawing	Thaw-Kit1 [22]	PBS + Human Serum Albumin 1,2 Propanediol 0.1 M, 0.5 M and 0.2 M Sucrose		
	Freezing	OocyteFreeze [23]	Plasma Protein Factor 1,2 Propanediol Sucrose	Oocytes	Medicult/ Origio
	Thawing	OocyteThaw [24]	Plasma Protein Factor 1,2 Propanediol Sucrose		
	Freezing	Embryo Freezing Pack [25]	1,2 Propanediol Sucrose Synthetic Serum Replacement	Zygotes and cleavage embryos	
	Thawing	Embryo Thawing Pack [26]	1,2 Propanediol Sucrose Synthetic Serum Replacement		

Table 13.2. (cont.)

Cryopreservation protocol	Procedure	Media	Composition*	Use for	Company
	Freezing	Sydney IVF Cryopreservation Kit K-SICS-5000 [27]	Human Serum Albumin 12 mg/mL Propanediol Sucrose HEPES buffered	Zygotes and cleavage embryos	Cook Medical
	Thawing	Sydney IVF Thawing Kit K-SITS-5000 [27]	Human Serum Albumin 12 mg/mL 1,2 Propanediol Sucrose HEPES buffered		
	Freezing	Sydney IVF Blastocyst Cryopreservation Kit K-SIBF-5000 [27]	Human Serum Albumin 12 mg/mL Glycerol Sucrose HEPES buffered	Blastocysts	Cook Medical
	Thawing	Sydney IVF Blastocyst Thawing Kit K-SIBT-5000 [27]	Human Serum Albumin 12 mg/mL Glycerol Sucrose HEPES buffered		
	Freezing	Quinn's Advantage Embryo Freeze Kit	1.5 M Propanediol + 0.1 M Sucrose 12 mg/mL Human Serum Albumin	Zygotes and cleavage embryos	Sage IVF
	Freezing	Quinn's Advantage Blastocyst Freeze Kit	9% Glycerol 0.2 M Sucrose 12 mg/mL Human Serum Albumin	Blastocyst	
	Thawing	Quinn's Advantage Embryo Thaw Kit	0.5 M and 0.2 M Sucrose 12 mg/ ml Human Serum Albumin	Zygotes, cleavage and blastocyst	

* Please note that some commercially available formulations do not disclose concentrations of the components.

Table 13.3. Most used commercial solutions for vitrification

Cryopreservation Protocol	Procedure	Media	Composition*	Use for	Company
Vitrification	Cooling	Medicult Vitrification Cooling [28]	12 mg/mL Human Serum Albumin 1,2 Propanediol Sucrose Ethylene glycol	Zygotes, cleavage and blastocyst	Medicult/ Origio
	Warming	Medicult Vitrification Warming [28]	Sucrose 12 mg/mL Human Serum Albumin		
	Cooling	Sage Vitrification Kit [29]	MOPS 15% EG + 15% DMSO + 0.6 M Sucrose 12 mg/mL Human Albumin	Zygotes, cleavage and blastocyst	Sage IVF
	Warming	Sage Vitrification Warming Kit [29]	MOPS 1.0 M and 0.5 M Sucrose 12 mg/mL Human Albumin		
	Cooling	Blastocyst Vitrification Kit K-SIBV-5000 [27]	Human Serum Albumin 20 mg/mL HEPES buffered 16% Ethylene glycol 16% DMSO 0.68 M Trehalose	Blastocysts	Cook Medical
	Warming	Blastocyst Warming Kit K-SIBW-5000 [27]	HEPES 0.33 M Trehalose 0.2 M Trehalose		
	Cooling	Vitrification Freeze Solutions [30]	HEPES buffered based M199 15% EG + 15% DMSO + 0.5 M Sucrose 20% Serum Substitute Suplement	Oocytes and embryos	Kitazato/ Irvine
	Warming	Vitrification Thaw Solutions [30]	HEPES buffered based M199 1.0 M and 0.5 M Sucrose 20% Serum Substitute Suplement		

Table 13.3. (cont.)

Cryopreservation Protocol	Procedure	Media	Composition*	Use for	Company
	Cooling	RapidVit Cleave [31]	EG + Propanediol + Ficoll + Sucrose MOPS Human Albumin Serum	Cleavage	Vitrolife
	Warming	RapidWarm Cleave [32]	MOPS Human Albumin Serum Sucrose		
	Cooling	RapidVit Blast [33]	EG + Propanediol + Sucrose MOPS Human Albumin Serum	Blastocyst	
	Warming	RapidWarm Blast [34]	MOPS Human Albumin Serum Sucrose		

* Please note that some commercially available formulations do not disclose concentrations of the components.

concentration of CPAs, temperature at exposure, time of exposure, and the sequence of CPA addition and removal from cells are very important to achieve successful cryopreservation. The ultimate goal of cryopreservation is to avoid or to limit the damage of ice crystal formation resulting from the phase transition of water inside or around cells.

The principle ideas can be outlined by four points below:

1. Replace intracellular water with permeating CPAs
2. Reduce intracellular water with non-permeating CPAs
3. Use high molecular compounds to stabilize membrane during osmotic changes and to modify the vitrification tendencies
4. Minimize toxicity.

There are various types of vitrification solutions, the most common are usually binary (two main CPAs), and the purpose of having more than one CPA in a vitrification solution is to lower the overall molarity at which vitrification occurs; where lowering the molarity is a strategy to reduce the toxicity of the vitrification solution. The mode of action of solutes during cryopreservation is likely to be multifactorial, and is not yet clearly understood; briefly, the cryoprotectants action on a combination of parameters based on the ability to modulate hydrogen bonding and interact with water molecules and the volume occupied by a molecule of the solute. Extracellular CPAs are polyhydroxylic and do not diffuse into the intracellular space, being unable to cross the cell membrane. In this case, cellular dehydration is not accompanied by replacement of part of the intracellular water by these CPAs, instead osmotic equilibrium is obtained by simple concentration of intracellular solutes [6]. Additional modes of action of CPAs have been suggested relating to intermolecular interactions between the agents and biologically important micro molecules, describing the propensity for solutes to interact with proteins either by preferential binding or preferential exclusion from the surface. Agents that are preferentially excluded act to stabilize proteins thermodynamically under conditions where other stresses occur. CPAs such as DMSO may interact electrostatically with phospholipid bilayers. Sucrose and trehalose have also been shown to stabilize membranes during hypertonic exposure as ice crystals grow by interacting with polar head groups of phospholipids [38]. Nash *et al.* described the property of CPAs used in sufficiently high concentrations to produce complete inhibition of ice formation during vitrification/cooling processes; where such vitrification process require very high CPA concentrations often in mixtures, and high cooling rates in order to achieve the glassy matrix at low temperatures [38].

Glass state or ice-free cryopreservation below the glass transition temperature is becoming very popular. It appears that cryoprotectant toxicity is one of the most important barriers to successful vitrification, since the vitrification requires a higher concentration of CPAs to prevent the formation of ice crystals. Cytotoxicity could be caused by osmotic shocks or biochemical modifications on cells, and both forms of damage are simply affected by the concentration of the CPAs and the rate of CPA permeation. CPA cytotoxicity has been shown to increase with time of exposure, temperature, and concentration, which constitutes a challenge in developing cryopreservation protocols, playing an important role in the survival of cells during cooling and warming processes, specifically in vitrification where higher concentrations are needed in order to achieve a glassy matrix [39]. To improve the vitrification process, several investigators have chosen to use cocktail solutions combining CPAs to achieve the necessary concentrations; usually the combination of permeating and non-permeating CPAs has been shown to decrease the total concentration necessary for a successful vitrification, improving the viability and function of the cells preserved [39]. Thus far, there is not a clear standard to evaluate the cytotoxicity of CPAs for embryos and oocytes, even though cytotoxicity has been speculated as a major concern when CPAs are used to cryopreserve embryos and oocytes. Therefore, to clarify clearly the cytotoxicity of the CPAs for embryo and oocyte cryopreservation has become one of the major topics in the field of cryobiology.

Conclusions

The key to the success of oocyte and embryo cryopreservation is to handle appropriately the manner in which water interacts inside and around the cells during the freezing/cooling and thawing/warming processes. Even though there are very many variables other than cryopreservation media involved in the development of the cryopreservation, the improvement of cryopreservation media has always been a top priority in the field of cryobiology. Because the biological characteristics vary among species or cell types, variables such as cell size and membrane permeability are pertinent factors in selecting suitable CPAs, concentration of exposure, temperature at exposure, time of exposure, and the sequence of CPA addition and removal from cells. Successful embryo and oocyte cryopreservation has been achieved and applied clinically; however, continued investigation will still provide tremendous opportunities to improve efficiency of embryo and oocyte cryopreservation.

References

1. Shaw JM, Jones GM. Terminology associated with vitrification and other cryopreservation procedures for oocytes and embryos. *Hum Reprod Update* 2003;**9**(6):583–605.

2. Whittingham DG, Leibo SP, Mazur P. Survival of mouse embryos frozen to -196 degrees and -269 degrees C. *Science* 1972;**178**(59):411–14.

3. Leibo SP. Cryobiology: preservation of mammalian embryos. *Basic Life Sci* 1986;**37**:251–72.

4. Mazur P. Equilibrium, quasi-equilibrium, and nonequilibrium freezing of mammalian embryos. *Cell Biophys* 1990; **17**(1):53–92.

5. Leibo SP. Cryopreservation of oocytes and embryos: optimization by theoretical versus empirical analysis. *Theriogenology* 2008;**69**(1):37–47.

6. De Santis L, Coticchio G. Theoretical and experimental basis of slow freezing. *Reprod Biomed Online* 2011;**22**(2):125–32.

7. Gosden R. Cryopreservation: a cold look at technology for fertility preservation. *Fertil Steril* 2011;**96**(2):264–8.

8. Rall WF, Fahy GM. Ice-free cryopreservation of mouse embryos at -196 degrees C by vitrification. *Nature* 1985;**313** (6003):573–5.

9. Trounson A. Preservation of human eggs and embryos. *Fertil Steril* 1986;**46**(1):1–12.

10. Chen C. Pregnancy after human oocyte cryopreservation. *Lancet* 1986;**1** (8486):884–6.

11. Kuwayama M, Vajta G, Kato O, Leibo SP. Highly efficient vitrification method for cryopreservation of human oocytes. *Reprod Biomed Online* 2005;**11**(3):300–8.

12. Mukaida T, Takahashi K, Kasai M. Blastocyst cryopreservation: ultrarapid vitrification using cryoloop technique. *Reprod Biomed Online* 2003; **6**(2):221–5.

13. Chian RC, Huang JY, Tan SL, *et al.* Obstetric and perinatal outcome in 200 infants conceived from vitrified oocytes. *Reprod Biomed Online* 2008;**16**(5):608–10.

14. Kasai M. Simple and efficient methods for vitrification of mammalian embryos. *Anim Reprod Sci* 1996;**42**:67–75.

15. Wowk B. How cryoprotectants work. *Cryonics* 3rd Quarter 2007;**28**:3–7.

16. Leibo SP, Pool TB. The principal variables of cryopreservation: solutions, temperatures, and rate changes. *Fertil Steril* 2011;**96**(2):269–76.

17. Chian R-C, Quinn P. (eds). *Fertility Cryopreservation.* Cambridge, Cambridge University Press. 2010;271.

18. Naitana S, Ledda S, Loi P, *et al.* Polyvinyl alcohol as a defined substitute for serum in vitrification and warming solutions to cryopreserve ovine embryos at different stages of development. *Anim Reprod Sci* 1997;**48**(2–4):247–56.

19. Vitrolife. G-FreezeKit Blast. Product Insert 2009. p. 2.

20. Vitrolife. G-ThawKit Blast. Product Insert 2009. p. 2.

21. Vitrolife. Freeze-Kit 1. Product Insert 2009. p. 2.

22. Vitrolife. Thaw-Kit 1. Product Insert 2009.

23. Media OM. OocyteFreeze™. Product Insert 2010. p. 2.

24. Media OM. OocyteThaw™. Product Insert 2010.

25. Media OM. Embryo Freezing Pack. Product Insert 2010. p. 2.

26. Media OM. Embryo Thawing Pack. Product Insert 2010.

27. Medical C. www.cookmedical.com 2010.

28. Media OM. MediCult Vitrification Media. 2010. p. 2.

29. Fertilization SIV. Sage Vitrification Solution. Product Catalog 2010. p. 2.

30. Kitazato. Cryotop Safety Kit 2010.

31. Vitrolife. RapidVit Cleave. Product Insert 2009. p. 2.

32. Vitrolife. RapidWarm Cleave. Product Insert 2009.

33. Vitrolife. RapidVit Blast. Product Insert 2009. p. 2.

34. Vitrolife. RapidWarm Blast. Product Insert 2009. p. 2.

35. Paynter SJ, O'Neil L, Fuller BJ, Shaw RW. Membrane permeability of human oocytes in the presence of the cryoprotectant propane-1,2-diol. *Fertil Steril* 2001; 75(3):532–8.

36. Lane M, Bavister BD, Lyons EA, Forest KT. Containerless vitrification of mammalian oocytes and embryos. *Nat Biotechnol* 1999;17(12):1234–6.

37. Vajta G, Holm P, Kuwayama M, *et al.* Open Pulled Straw (OPS) vitrification: a new way to reduce cryoinjuries of bovine ova and embryos. *Mol Reprod Dev* 1998; 51(1):53–8.

38. Fuller BJ. Cryoprotectants: the essential antifreezes to protect life in the frozen state. *Cryo Letters.* 2004;25(6): 375–88.

39. Lawson A, Ahmad H, Sambanis A. Cytotoxicity effects of cryoprotectants as single-component and cocktail vitrification solutions. *Cryobiology* 2011; 62(2):115–22.

Chapter

14

International regulation of ART media

Theresa Jeary

History of assisted reproductive technology (ART) and its regulation

Since the first live birth following in vitro fertilization (IVF) treatment, of Louise Brown, in Oldham, Greater Manchester in 1978, assisted reproductive technologies (ART) have provided treatments for many types of infertility found in women and men. The use of ART occurs in many countries around the world and it is now beyond doubt that this approach provides a realistic option for infertile people wishing to form a family. It is estimated that in some European countries up to 5% of all births are now due to ART [1], so it is evident that ART has made a significant impact on the lives of many infertile and subfertile couples.

While the subject of ART is a highly emotive one, raising many moral and ethical questions, the early start of monitoring of both efficacy and safety of these procedures has resulted in a high degree of public acceptance of the techniques used and a reassurance in the general public, that the IVF technique is reasonably safe for both mother and child [2].

In the early days of IVF, enthusiasm amongst ART scientific teams across the world was contagious; with the sharing of learning points such as some tiny item for the recipe or some small detail which allowed this or that step of progress. At the time, of course, there were no regulations governing reproductive medicine, instead the emphasis focused on the moral and ethical aspects of the technology and impact on the mother and child.

Historically, one of the major problems in IVF from the outset has been the culture conditions and culture media. Few media fulfilled the requirements for successful blastocyst development, at least not with the right time dynamics and for such reasons short in vitro culture was recommended (1–3 days). Typically, most laboratories made their own media, based on information shared across IVF laboratories, with the effectiveness of media formulation evaluated against success rates for blastocyst development and subsequently, live birth rates [3]. With very limited regulatory guidance during the early years of IVF, bovine serum was used in most media; the use of bovine serum has since been replaced with human serum albumin for safety reasons. In recent years, the emergence of biotechnology companies experienced in the development of laboratory reagents and media, with a focus on providing IVF media to the market, has led to a demand for clear regulatory guidance for the quality assurance and quality control of these products.

Culture Media, Solutions, and Systems in Human ART, ed. Patrick Quinn. Published by Cambridge University Press. © Cambridge University Press 2014.

Considering that it is now 35 years since the first live birth following IVF treatment, it is surprising that the classification and regulation of media used in the IVF process within the European Union (EU) was only clarified as recently as May 2008. This chapter looks at the regulation of ART media in Europe and the USA and details the requirements for approval in each of these regions.

Challenges for the regulation and classification of IVF media

IVF and ART media devices cover a wide range of products and a wide range of in vitro procedures, involving sperm, oocytes, eggs, blastocysts, and embryos. The intended use of IVF media may range from maintenance of the physiological homeostasis required to support and promote fertilization in vitro, to the maintenance of the physiological homeostasis of the cells during the cryopreservation process and the minimization of cellular damage during the freezing process. IVF media products are comprised of a cocktail of physiological inorganic salts, energy sources, amino acids, and proteins and there is a range of different formulations available. Some media manufacturers include the broad-spectrum antibiotic gentamicin sulfate, to prevent microbial contamination of the media based on historical information. Others include human serum albumin, to act as a chelating agent for heavy metals that may be present in minute quantities in the microenvironment and also as a surfactant to facilitate embryo and gamete manipulation by preventing them from sticking to glass or tissue culture ware.

There has been a number of challenges relating to the classification of these products:

1. Across the globe there are various approaches to the classification of these products and, therefore, the regulation varies widely between regional areas, making the route to market for IVF media manufacturers complicated if they wish to sell globally.

2. Many IVF media manufacturers have developed from a background in laboratory media preparation, with only the minority having expertise in medical device development.

3. The intended use of IVF media products does not strictly comply with either the medical device or medicinal product definition. The definitions for medical device and medicinal products are similar globally. Available guidance for the definition and regulatory control of IVF media products is a relatively new development.

4. The concept of "intended by the manufacturer to be used for human beings" has been difficult to justify. The definition of a human being and the stage at which human life begins is a very sensitive topic. The definition of when human life begins varies globally and even across the EU member states, depending on religious beliefs and legal definition, for example in the UK an embryo is not legally considered a human being; therefore, as the media are intended to be used on cells/embryos the indication for use is not for the human body. From a legal perspective, such IVF media products could not meet the definition of either a medical device or medicinal substance.

5. Another confusing factor regarding the appropriate regulatory route for the control of IVF media is that a number of IVF media products also contain substances, which if used separately can be considered to be medicinal products, such as antibiotics and human serum albumin. Therefore they are high-risk combination products.

The lack of a clear regulatory route and clarity on classification of IVF media has led to an inconsistent approach for the classification and regulation of IVF media globally. Table 14.1

Table 14.1. Summary of regulatory approval requirements for IVF media in major markets

Country	Classification	Requirements for regulatory approval
Europe	Class IIb, rule 3 or Class III, rule 13 medical device depending on the formulation	CE certification by Notified Body. Consultation with a Competent Authority/EMA for ancillary medicinal substances
USA	Class II medical device	Regulated by the FDA as a medical device with special conditions under the 510k Pre-market notification scheme
Japan	Laboratory reagent	No formal regulatory review or approval at present
Australia	Class III medical device	Regulated by the Australian Therapeutic Goods Authority (TGA)
China	No official designation as a medical device	Regulatory approval by the Chinese Regulator (CFDA) is required to apply for hospital tenders

CFDA = China Food and Drug Administration; EMA = European Medicines Agency; FDA = Food and Drug Administration.

summarizes the global approach to IVF media regulation and the different approaches adopted for the regulation and approval of IVF media.

The certification pathway for approval of IVF media in the two largest jurisdictions, that is, Europe and the USA, shall be detailed in this chapter. Guidance is available for the process required for approval in the emerging markets of China and Australia and at present both these countries' models follow a very similar route for approval to those used in the USA and EU, respectively.

Regulation of ART media in Europe

Historically, within the EU, some countries have regulated these products as medical devices whilst other member states placed no restriction on the usage of non-CE marked IVF media products. This resulted in an uneven and inconsistent approach across the EU, leading to calls for clarification from the borderline working group from manufacturers and Notified Bodies.

Considering the history and wide variation in approach, the issue of the regulation of IVF media used in the ART process has been a matter of discussion at a European level for a substantial period of time, and guidance on the regulatory process for IVF media has only been recently provided.

The following summarizes the current guidance regarding the classification of IVF media as a medical device under Directive 93/42/EEC and outlines the key stages for CE certification.

Classification of IVF media under the Medical Device Directive

To provide a clear regulatory route and classification of IVF media products a review was conducted by the Medical Devices Expert Group's classification and borderline working group and assessed against the definitions available. The Medical Devices Expert Group's classification and borderline working group came to a determination on the regulation of such products in May 2008 and confirmed that IVF media products can be classified as medical devices. The consensus on these products has been published in the "Manual on Borderline and Classification in the Community Regulatory Framework for Medical Devices," a copy of which may be obtained from the European Commission's website reference http://ec.europa.eu/enterprise/sectors/medical-devices/documents/borderline.

In essence this agreement indicates that in general IVF/ART products may be qualified and regulated as medical devices provided that they meet the definition of a medical device as laid out in Directive 93/42/EEC, taking into consideration the principal intended action and intended purpose of the product. The concept of "used for human beings" has been interpreted in the broadest sense as the whole IVF/ART procedure and related products would be seen as (indirectly) "(. . .) used for human beings for the purpose of (. . .) replacement or modification of (. . .) a physiological process" by promulgating pregnancy [4]. Therefore, the definition of medical devices can include IVF/ART products. Due to the variety of products that can be classified as medical devices, the advice from the borderlines group is that classification must be assessed on a case-by-case basis, taking into account all product characteristics; however, this consensus agreement indicates that in general IVF media will be considered as Class III medical devices under classification rule 13, as stated in Annex IX of the Medical Device Directive 93/42/EEC.

Examples of IVF products which could be qualified as medical devices, along with a preliminary classification, are as follows:

- Devices, such as washing, separating, sperm immobilizing, cryoprotecting solutions, which are liable to act with close contact on the inner or outer cells during the IVF/ART are likely to be considered as Class IIb medical devices, in particular by analogy of rule 3, that is, these products are considered to present the same level of risk as non-invasive devices intended for modifying the biological or chemical composition of blood, other body liquids, or other liquids intended for infusion into the body.
- Devices manufactured utilizing animal tissues or derivatives rendered non-viable are considered as Class III medical devices according to rule 17.
- Devices incorporating, as an integral part, (1) a human blood derivative or (2) a substance which, if used separately, can be considered to be a medicinal product, as defined in Article 1 of Directive 2001/83/EC, and which is liable to act on the human body with action ancillary to that of the devices, are considered as Class III medical devices according to rule 13. The assessment of the ancillary nature of the pharmacological, immunological, or metabolic action of any medicinal product contained in IVF/ART products should be done on a case-by-case basis, taking also into account the purpose of the inclusion of this substance into the product. Although it should be noted that case-by-case analysis should always be performed when considering classification, it was agreed that media intended for use in the IVF process to support the growth/storage of the embryo may generally be considered to be Class III medical devices *and* in case of doubt where taking into account all product characteristics, and provided that the concerned product meets both definitions of a medicinal product and of a medical device, Article 2(2) of Directive 2001/83/EC could apply.

Following the May 2008 clarification on IVF media classification, additional guidance was sought, regarding the requirement for consultation for media containing antibiotics (e.g., gentamicin sulfate) with European Competent Authorities. Many such media formulations contain an antibiotic with the intended function of preservation of the media from potential sources of microbial contamination during the manipulation stages of the procedure. In seeking a clear decision on the regulatory pathway for the antibiotic-containing media devices, an argument was presented that concluded that the level of antibiotic included in such formulations would not be liable to act on the mother, based on several factors such as the amount of antibiotic contained in the media, amount of media used per IVF procedure, the amount of media potentially administered to the female, the site of administration, and the physiological conditions of this site of administration of the media. Following a review of the arguments provided, it was advised that IVF media products containing antibiotics should be classified as Class III devices under rule 13, thus requiring a drug consultation in accordance with the Medical Device Directive.

The ruling on the classification of these media products raised many concerns at the time amongst IVF media manufacturers, who wished to place their devices on the market in the EU, for several reasons;

- Many Competent Authorities required IVF media sold in their jurisdiction to have CE certification immediately following the Borderline Group's decision, which considering the length of time for CE certification and completion of the consultation process was impossible for many manufacturers to achieve.
- The decision confirmed that IVF media manufacturers would be required to comply with the expectations of a drug consultation and provide the necessary evidence to show control of the antibiotic or human serum albumin and its inclusion within the media. Given that the antibiotic has historically been considered a media preservative, many manufacturers did not have the required level of information to satisfy the requirements of a drug consultation Competent Authority review.

CE certification process in Europe

Historically, across the EU there has not been a "level playing field" for all involved in the process of the regulation of IVF media. Some Notified Bodies issued CE certification well in advance of the borderline decision of May 2008, while other were left unable to provide a certification service due to the lack of a regulatory pathway.

Following the issuance of the guidance, the CE certification route is now clear for IVF media manufacturers. The CE certification process can appear to be complicated and daunting for manufacturers at the outset, as there is a misperception and fear from many about the involvement of a medicines agency in the process.

Increasing amounts of guidance have been made readily available on the pathway to market for such combination devices as the area of device–drug combinations has grown. To avoid any issues with certification of device-drug combination products, it is advised that medical device manufacturers who are uncertain of the requirements and process engage the services of a European Notified Body who has expertise with combination devices and also that they actively engage and communicate with their chosen Notified Body in the early stages of their device development process.

The most challenging CE certification process for IVF media devices is for those that contain an ancillary medicinal substance, such as an antibiotic or an ancillary human blood derivative. To obtain CE certification for such devices in addition to the Notified Body's review of the device aspects, the Notified Body is also required to conduct two separate medicinal substance consultations, one with a European Competent Authority or the European Medicines Agency (EMA) for the antibiotic and one with EMA for the ancillary human blood derivative. The following section details the key stages involved in the CE certification process for such IVF media devices and outlines some of the key requirements to achieve certification in Europe.

Notified Body responsibility and assessment

The medical device industry is widely diverse and highly innovative and covers a wide range of products, from simple bandages to highly sophisticated life-supporting equipment; therefore, the medical devices sector plays a crucial role in the diagnosis, prevention, monitoring, and treatment of diseases and the improvement of the quality of life of people suffering from disabilities. In Europe the regulation and approval for sale of devices is provided by a Notified Body.

Notified Bodies are designated to carry out conformity assessment according to an appropriate directive. For medical device regulation the Notified Body is designated its scope and status by the Competent Authority in its Member State and the notification of this body is the act whereby the Member State informs the Commission and other Member States that a body fulfills the relevant requirements. Lists of Notified Bodies and the tasks for which they have been notified and their identification number are freely available off the Nando (New Approach Notified and Designated Organisations) website [5].

The responsibility of the Notified Body for medical device certification is:

- To check that the manufacturer has followed its declared procedures and those required by the Directive
- To monitor the manufacturer's system for producing their Declaration of Conformity.

The manufacturer through their Declaration of Conformity takes ultimate responsibility for device safety and product liability and the manufacturer is also responsible for selection of the Route to Conformity for its devices. In the EU the following routes to conformity are available:

1. Follow the procedure relating to the EC Declaration of Conformity set out in Annex II (Full Quality Assurance System), which includes Annex II.3 (Quality Assurance System) and Annex II.4 (Design Examination). It should be noted that the same Notified Body should be used for the Annex II.4 and the Annex II.3 certification process.
2. Follow the procedure relating to the EC Type Examination set out in Annex III (EC Type Examination) coupled with either
   - the procedure relating to the EC Verification set out in Annex IV (EC Verification) or
   - the procedure relating to the EC Declaration of Conformity set out in Annex V (Production Quality Assurance).

In general, most manufacturers select the Full Quality Assurance route to conformity as the Type Examination process requires the Notified Body to ascertain and certify that a representative sample of the production covered and fulfills the relevant provisions of the Directive. The EC Type Examination route requires the testing of batches of the devices to achieve certification, which in the case of IVF media could be an expensive and difficult process due to the lack of a harmonized standard for the testing of such devices. For the purposes of this publication only, the requirements of conformity to the Full Quality Assurance route shall be presented and discussed; this requires assessment to both Annex II.3, examination of the Quality Assurance System and Annex II.4, which involves the examination of the design of the product.

Examination of the Quality Management System

As IVF media has been classified as meeting the definition of a medical device, a Quality Management System appropriate to the medical device industry, such as ISO 13485, is an acceptable standard to follow for the Quality Management System. It is important that manufacturers of such devices also build into their system controls to assure that the quality of medicinal substances contained within their devices is maintained throughout the manufacturing process. The key areas for assessment include: incoming inspection; controls and warehousing; manufacturing controls and procedures; test laboratory controls and procedures; controls to minimize cross-contamination; facilities; procedures for training; and procedures for customer complaints, vigilance, and post-market surveillance. Considering the inclusion of ancillary medicinal substances within many IVF media devices, it would be standard practice that the assessor who conducts the examination of the Quality Management System will have the competency to conduct an assessment of a device–drug combination and also have some experience of medicinal product regulation and the concept of Good Manufacturing Practice requirements.

For devices that contain a human blood derivative, the administrative provisions of Annex II of the Medical Device Directive requires that the manufacturer informs the Notified Body of the release of each batch of devices containing the ancillary human blood derivative to the EU and also requires that the Notified Body is provided with the official certificate, as issued by a State laboratory, concerning the release of the batch of human blood derivative used in that device. It is important that the Quality Management System of the device manufacturer has an adequate procedure to comply with this requirement.

Examination of the design of the device

The Notified Body examination of the design of the medical device includes confirmation that the device conforms to relevant provisions of Essential Requirements of the Medical Device Directive by verifying:

- The conclusions of risk analysis
- The applicable Essential Requirements have been addressed, such as:
  - The device does not compromise the clinical condition of patients
  - The risks are acceptable when weighed against the benefits to the patient
- The relevant standards applied or other solutions have been adopted to meet the Essential Requirements
- The conclusions of the clinical evaluation, which, due to the restricted use of human embryos for research purposes, result in a general lack of prospective randomized clinical trial data relating to the effects of media culture on embryo viability.

In addition to the Notified Body assessment of the above and in accordance with Annex I, Essential Requirement 7.4 of the Medical Device Directive, the quality, safety, and usefulness of the ancillary medicinal substance or ancillary human blood derivative must be verified by analogy with the methods specified in Annex I of Directive 2001/83/EC, which is the European Directive governing the regulation of medicinal products.

As Notified Bodies do not have the competency for Directive 2001/83/EC the verification of the quality and safety of the ancillary medicinal substance must be conducted by a European Competent Authority, while the quality and safety of the ancillary human blood derivative must be conducted by EMA. The Notified Body requests the consultation of the appropriate Medicines authority and the consultation is conducted in parallel to the Notified Body's review of the device aspects.

Competent Authority involvement and requirements

In Europe, each Member State has its own Competent Authority which is the government agency responsible for the regulation and control of medicinal products in their respective Member States. Currently (2013) there are in total 27 EU Member States. The European Economic Area countries of Norway, Iceland, and Liechtenstein are also recognized by the EU (EEA-EFTA states).

In addition to the national Competent Authorities there is a decentralized body of the EU, the EMA, which is located in London. The main responsibility of EMA is the protection and promotion of public and animal health, through the evaluation and supervision of medicines for human and veterinary use. EMA is responsible for the scientific evaluation of applications for *European marketing authorizations* for both human and veterinary medicines submitted under the *centralized procedure*. Under the centralized procedure, companies submit a single marketing-authorization application to the Agency. Once granted by the European Commission, a centralized (or "Community") marketing authorization is valid in all EU and EEA-EFTA states (Iceland, Liechtenstein, and Norway). All medicines for human and animal use derived from biotechnology and other high-tech processes, and human blood derivatives must be approved via the centralized procedure. The same applies to all advanced-therapy medicines and human medicines intended for the treatment of HIV/AIDS, cancer, diabetes, and neurodegenerative diseases. EMA has *six scientific committees*, composed of members of all EU and EEA-EFTA states, some including patients' and doctors' representatives who conduct the main scientific work of the Agency:

- the Committee for Medicinal Products for Human Use (CHMP)
- the Committee for Medicinal Products for Veterinary Use (CVMP)
- the Committee for Orphan Medicinal Products (COMP)
- the Committee on Herbal Medicinal Products (HMPC)
- the Paediatric Committee (PDCO)
- the Committee for Advanced Therapies (CAT).

Due to the increased risk of the transmission of infections from human-derived ingredients, it is mandatory that EMA be consulted for such devices and the consultation process for ancillary human blood derivatives in IVF media is conducted via the centralized procedure in accordance with Regulation (EC) 726/2004 (1), by the Committee for Medicinal Products for Human Use (CHMP).

Documentation requirements

For IVF media containing both an ancillary antibiotic and ancillary human blood derivative, there are three separate modules of documentation which are required to be submitted by the manufacturer to the Notified Body, as follows;

- Design Dossier for the Device Aspects
- Medicinal Dossier for the Quality and Safety aspects of the ancillary antibiotic
- Medicinal Dossier for the Quality and Safety aspects of the ancillary human blood derivative

The details required for each module shall be discussed below in further detail.

Design Dossier

The Design Dossier is the technical documentation to provide evidence of compliance of the device to the Essential Requirements and contains the following elements:

- Device description, product specifications and classification
- Essential Requirements checklist
- Risk analysis and output of the risk management process
- Product Verification and Validation
- Design and Manufacturing Information
- Labeling and Instructions for Use
- Results of Clinical Evaluations
- Declaration of Conformity.

Guidance on the format and content of the Design Dossier is available from NB-MED/ 2.5.1/Rec 5 and the Global Harmonisation Task Force reference SG1(PD)/N011R20.

Medicinal Dossier for the Quality and Safety aspects of the ancillary antibiotic

The medicinal dossier for the ancillary medicinal substance should contain information on the following aspects:

- Quality aspects: CTD Module 3, which can be further divided into

  - Quality aspects for the ancillary medicinal substance itself
  - Quality aspects of the incorporation of the ancillary medicinal substance in the medical device
- Non-clinical data on the ancillary medicinal substance: CTD Module 4
- Clinical data for the device: CTD Module 5.

Guidance on the format of these modules is available in MEDDEV 2.1.3/rev 3 and the use of the Common Technical Document (CTD) format. While use of the CTD format is not mandatory it is advisable to follow the guidance as this is the format assessors at the Competent Authorities see on a routine basis for medicinal product submissions.

The CTD format is concerned with the presentation of the application dossier and was first published in 1998. It provides guidance for the compilation of dossiers for applications for European marketing authorizations and is applicable for the centralized procedure and national procedures, including mutual recognition and decentralized procedures. CTD provides a template for an appropriate format for the data that are required for medicinal product applications across the International Conference on Harmonisation (ICH) regions of the EU, the USA, and Japan.

Medicinal Dossier for the Quality and Safety aspects of the ancillary Human blood derivative

For the EMA consultation for the ancillary human blood derivative the Medicinal Dossier is similar to that for the ancillary medicinal substance, and is compiled of the following modules:

- Quality aspects: CTD Module 3, which can be further divided as
  - Quality aspects for the ancillary human blood derivative itself and
  - Quality aspects of the incorporation of the ancillary human blood derivative in the medical device
- Non-clinical data on the ancillary human blood derivative: CTD Module 4
- Clinical data for the device: CTD Module 5.

The IVF media manufacturer must also have the information contained within and access to Module 3 of the Plasma Master File (PMF). The requirement is outlined in the EMA guidance document EMA/CHMP/578661/2010. This requirement should be considered early in the device development process and is an important factor when evaluating and selecting the supplier of the ancillary human blood derivative. A copy of Module 3 of the PMF must be included with the consultation documentation submission and a letter of access for the PMF Module 3 is not permitted. Failure to comply with this requirement will result in the rejection of the application at the validation stage of the EMA process.

The requirement to have full access to Module 3 of the PMF is based on the risks associated with the inclusion of a biological component and the threat of transfer of blood-borne diseases from the blood donor to the device recipient. This requirement comes from legislation on products containing ancillary human blood derivatives, and the need for control of the product and control of the manufacturing process for biologics and the concern for public health. As part of the EMA review of the quality and safety of the ancillary human blood derivative the quality and manufacturing process used for the human blood derivative in its entirety must be assessed, so detailed information relating to viral inactivation studies and the validation of the manufacturing processes used is required. It is also important to remember that through the inclusion of the medicinal substances within the device, the device manufacturer takes responsibility for the safety of the medicinal substances incorporated into their device, so it is pertinent that knowledge of any safety concerns regarding the medicinal substance and the source of this material is required to be held by the device manufacturer.

Process and timelines

Following submission of the documentation package from the manufacturer to the Notified Body, the Notified Body is required to complete a review of the usefulness of the ancillary medicinal substances and submit a report of the Notified Body review to the relevant Competent Authority and to EMA for the ancillary human blood derivative.

On receipt of the documentation from the Notified Body, the Competent Authority and EMA conduct a validation of the submission documentation prior to the start of the procedure. This validation process is to ensure the necessary sections and forms have been provided and that the Notified Body's usefulness report is also included.

The timeline for completion of the Competent Authority/EMA assessments is 210 days after the receipt of valid documentation. In parallel to the consultation process for the ancillary medicinal substances, the Notified Body conduct their review of both the Quality Management System and device aspects. On completion of all review elements, and on the provision that positive opinions have been provided by all parties, then the Design Examination Certificate may be issued by the Notified Body to the manufacturer, who places the CE mark on the devices covered by the scope of certification. If a negative opinion is given by EMA on the human blood derivative review then certification is not permitted and the manufacturer must complete an additional consultation to address the deficiencies raised. Lastly, the Notified Body advises the Competent Authority and EMA of its final decision regarding the certification of the devices covered by the application.

It is a condition of approval, in accordance with Annex II, paragraph 8 of the Medical Device Directive, that the manufacturer informs the Notified Body of the release of batches of all devices containing ancillary human blood derivatives and provides an official certificate concerning the release of the batch of human blood derivative used in the batches issued by a State laboratory or a laboratory designated for that purpose by a Member State in accordance with Article 114(2) of Directive 2001/83/EC.

Regulation of ART media in the USA

The Food and Drug Administration (FDA) is the government agency within the United States Department of Health and Human Services responsible for the regulation and approval of medicines and medical devices. The FDA is responsible for protecting the public health by assuring the safety, effectiveness, and security of human and veterinary drugs, vaccines and other biological products, medical devices, the nation's food supply, cosmetics, dietary supplements, and products that give off radiation.

The FDAs website, http://www.fda.gov, provides detailed guidance for manufacturers for the process to obtain approval for their products.

Classification of ART media in the USA

In accordance with Title 21 Code of Federal Regulations (CFR), Part 884, subpart G, reproductive media and supplements are defined as products that are used for assisted reproduction procedures. Media include liquid and powder versions of various substances that come in direct physical contact with human gametes or embryos (including water, acid solutions used to treat gametes or embryos, rinsing solutions, sperm separation media, supplements, or oil used to cover the media) for the purposes of preparation, maintenance, transfer, or storage. Supplements are specific reagents added to media to enhance specific properties of the media (e.g., proteins, sera, antibiotics, etc.). Such products are classified as Class II devices requiring special controls, such as mouse embryo assay information, endotoxin testing, sterilization validation, design specifications, labeling requirements, biocompatibility testing, and clinical testing.

Approval process in the USA

Medical devices are subject to the *general controls* of the *Federal Food Drug & Cosmetic (FD&C) Act* which are contained in the procedural regulations in Title 21 CFR Part 800–1200. These controls are the baseline requirements that apply to all medical devices necessary for marketing, proper labeling, and monitoring of performance once the device is on the market.

The basic regulatory requirements that manufacturers of medical devices distributed in the USA must comply with are:

- Establishment registration
- Medical Device Listing
- Premarket Notification 510(k), unless exempt, or Premarket Approval (PMA)

- Investigational Device Exemption (IDE) for clinical studies
- Quality System (QS) regulation
- Labeling requirements
- Medical Device Reporting (MDR).

Detailed guidance on these requirements is available from the FDA website.

To place the device on the market, a Marketing Clearance from the Center for Devices and Radiological Health (CDRH) must be obtained. The manufacturer must also establish and follow the Quality Systems (QS) regulation before and during the 510(k) process. The Quality Systems for FDA-regulated products (food, drugs, biologics, and devices) are known as current good manufacturing practices (cGMPs).

cGMP requirements for devices are detailed in Part 820 (21 CFR Part 820) of these regulations. Class II, Class III, and certain Class I devices are subject to design control requirements of the quality system regulation during the design phase of product development.

The classification of the device identifies the marketing process for FDA clearance and the options available to allow the sale of devices in the USA are either:

- Premarket Notification (510(k)) or
- Premarket Approval (PMA)

The Premarket Notification (510(k)) is the submission made to the FDA to demonstrate that the device to be marketed is safe and effective by proving *substantial equivalence* to a legally marketed US device (predicate device) that is not subject to Premarket Approval (PMA). A claim of substantial equivalence does not mean the device(s) must be identical. Substantial equivalence is established with respect to: intended use, design, materials, performance, safety, effectiveness, labeling, biocompatibility, standards, and other applicable characteristics. In the case for IVF media, the Premarket Notification (510(k)) route is the pathway routinely used, due to the existence of many substantially equivalent devices available.

Content and format of a Traditional 510(k) Notification

The information required in a Traditional 510(k) submission is identified in *21 CFR 807.87* and detailed guidance on the recommended format for submission is available on the FDA website reference *"Format for Traditional and Abbreviated 510(k)s"*. Key elements of a Traditional 510(k) include, but are not limited to:

- *Indications for Use*
- *510(k) Summary* or *510(k) Statement*
- Standards Data Report for 510(k)s – *FDA 3654*, which should be included if the 510(k) documentation includes references to national or international standard
- Items required under *21 CFR 807.87* include:
  - The name of device, include the trade or proprietary name, and device classification
  - Description of the device, include device specifications and reference applicable guidance documents, special controls, or standards
  - Detailed comparison with a *predicate device(s)*, indicating similarities and/or differences accompanied by data, as appropriate; intended use of the device
  - Proposed label, labeling, and advertisements for the device and directions for use

- Information on sterilization, biocompatibility, and expiration date
- A description of the tests and the results obtained are essential. Reasonable and sufficient details of all test procedures and results should be submitted to FDA
- Performance data to help demonstrate the substantial equivalence of the device to one or more legally marketed devices (predicate device). The data may include test results from engineering, bench, design verification, human factors, and animal testing, and clinical studies and clinical trials. Tests should be conducted on all sizes and models of the device in a manner as similar as possible to how the device will be used. The results of testing and methodology/parameters used for testing should be included.

Summary and conclusions

The last quarter of the twentieth century witnessed several major advances in reproductive medicine. Since the birth of Louise Brown in 1978, nearly one million babies have been born worldwide as the result of ART. It is therefore clear that ART has made a significant impact on the lives of many infertile and subfertile couples. However, it has also been the source of great disappointment to those couples for whom ART has proven unsuccessful and to many more infertile people around the world who have no access to these technologies.

The regulation of IVF media used in the ART process varies widely across the globe but is also coming under increasing scrutiny by regulators as the public seek assurances on the quality and safety of the procedure and materials utilized. ART clinics also strive for greater predictability and improved success rates to reduce stress on the couples undergoing these procedures; therefore, it is vital that the quality of a key component in the process such as the media is of a high and consistent quality.

The regulatory approval process for IVF media has become more defined in recent years with consensus for classification achieved in Europe in 2008 allowing IVF media manufacturers a clear pathway to EU markets. While the EU process for market access may appear complicated and lengthy for those not familiar with CE certification, there is a large amount of available guidance and many knowledgeable bodies capable of conformity assessment for these devices.

Acknowledgements

Thanks to Natalie Birnie at BSI for her editorial guidance and support in review of my manuscripts.

References

1. Vayena E, Rowe PJ, Griffin DP. (eds.) *Current Practices and Controversies in Assisted Reproduction. Report of a meeting on "Medical, Ethical and Social Aspects of Assisted Reproduction" held at WHO Headquarters in Geneva, Switzerland 17–21 September 2001.* Geneva, World Health Organization, 2002. http://www.who.int/reproductivehealth/publications/infertility/9241590300/en/index.html (accessed June 13, 2013).

2. Cohen J, Trounson A, Dawson K, *et al.* The early days of IVF outside the UK, *Human Reprod Update,* 2005;**11**(5): 439–60.

3. Jones GM, Figueiredo F, Osianlis T, *et al.* Embryo culture, assessment, selection and transfer. In: Vayena E, Rowe PJ, Griffin DP, eds. *Current Practices and Controversies in Assisted Reproduction. Report of a meeting on "Medical, Ethical and Social Aspects of Assisted Reproduction" held at WHO Headquarters in Geneva, Switzerland, 17–21 September 2001.* Geneva, World

Health Organization. 2002;177–209. http://www.who.int/reproductivehealth/publications/infertility/9241590300/en/index.html (accessed June 13, 2013).

4. Manual on Borderline and Classification in the Community Regulatory Framework for Medical Devices Version 1.15 (06–2013) http://ec.europa.eu/consumers/sectors/medical-devices/documents/borderline/index_en.htm (accessed June 12, 2013).

5. Nando (New Approach Notified and Designated Organisations) Information System http://ec.europa.eu/enterprise/newapproach/nando/index.cfm (accessed June 10, 2013).

Chapter

15

Culture of embryos in dynamic fluid environments

André Monteiro da Rocha and Gary Daniel Smith

Introduction

The 2010 Nobel Prize in Medicine was awarded to Dr. Robert Edwards in recognition of his efforts toward development of human in vitro fertilization (IVF); which gave rise to the birth of the world's first IVF-baby Louise Brown in 1978 [1] and millions of births since. In fact, laboratory growth of mammalian embryos in culture media with defined components was described almost 30 years before the first successful human IVF cycle [2–4]. These studies set foundations for refinements of media composition based on mammalian embryo requirements [5–12] and they were important for the determination of IVF conditions in various species.

Several culture media were developed and have been in use since the establishment of modern embryo culture; however, the static nature of systems for embryo culture remains unaltered. Usually, media for embryo culture are restrained in a culture dish placed into an incubator with a controlled atmosphere [13]. The static environment clearly sustains mammalian embryo development; nevertheless, it does not mirror the environment experienced by oocytes and preimplantation embryos within the body.

The oviduct is the environment in which fertilization and early embryo development take place. It is a tubular organ with an internal lining of ciliated and secretory epithelia arrayed on a cryptic lumen. Additionally, this organ has an active smooth muscle layer [14]. Together, the epithelial ciliary movement and the peristaltic contractions of the smooth muscle layer create a pulsatile and turbulent flow that transports early embryos to the uterus [14].

The human oviduct is a low energy fluid environment in comparison to the fluid environment of the vascular system; however, oviductal flow can disrupt substrate, metabolite, and biomolecule gradients present at the embryo surface as well as provide gentle mechanostimuli for the embryo. These features of the oviduct environment are absent in traditional static culture systems, yet the recent conjugation of embryo culture and bioengineering techniques has resulted in fabrication of devices to create dynamic fluid environments [15–18] currently being evaluated for safety and efficiency of embryo production.

This chapter reviews present technology available to recapitulate dynamic fluid in vivo processes in the IVF laboratory and future applications of similar environments in systems coupling embryo culture and selection assisted by real-time time-lapse photography and substrate/metabolite/secretory product analysis.

Culture Media, Solutions, and Systems in Human ART, ed. Patrick Quinn. Published by Cambridge University Press. © Cambridge University Press 2014.

Fluid dynamics and shear stress

Early efforts to control fluid dynamics in an attempt to mimic physiological conditions resulted in significant medical advances in areas of medicine such as hemodialysis [19] and cardiac surgeries [20, 21]. Indeed, these early attempts were accomplished after development of efficient methods and devices to control fluid dynamics and circumvented hemolysis due to shear stress on red blood cells [19, 22, 23].

Tangential forces exerted by a fluid over a surface produce shear stress (Figure 15.1) [24]. In clinical embryology, shear stress is the result of such forces on the zona pellucida, the surfaces of cells located sub-zona pellucida, or over the cell membrane of hatched blastocysts. Even though systems for embryo culture are predominantly static, significant shear forces can impact embryos when they are moved with pipettes [25].

Modeling the behavior of cells in fluids indicated that stiffness of the surface in contact with the fluid governs surface deformation and object motion [24]. Harder structures are more likely to be lifted by shear force than structures with more "elastic" membranes, which are more likely to suffer deformation [24]. While originally this modeling was not intended to mimic specifically embryo behavior in fluids generating shear forces, one might propose that embryos in various states of development, such as solid morula or late blastocysts, have different elastic properties compared to early cleavage stage embryos, and they might receive and react to shear forces differently.

Aside from the stiffness of oocytes and embryos in different stages of development, they are also enclosed in the zona pellucida, a tridimensional net of glycoproteins with complex supramolecular fibrous architecture that changes over time [26]. The arrangement of extracellular fibers affects the intensities of shear stress on cells and subtle remodeling in fibrous architecture near the cell's surface determines considerable shifts in shear forces [27]. This supposition reinforces the notion that understanding responses of embryos to shear stress during development is complex, a difficult task, and requires further study.

Many cell types are mechanosensitive; meaning that they can perceive shear forces and have a broad range of biological responses from up-regulation of growth-stimulatory or -inhibitory pathways to programmed cell death when facing these forces. For example,

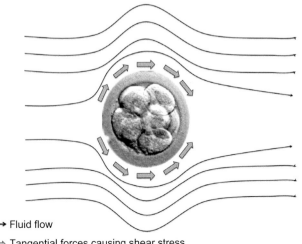

Figure 15.1 Schematic representation of fluid flow generating tangential forces and creating shear stress.

⟶ Fluid flow

⟹ Tangential forces causing shear stress

mesenchymal stem cells derived from human adipose tissue release angiogenic factors under shear forces of $10 \, dyn/cm^2$ [28]. Force of the same intensity is able to produce protective effects on chondrocytes, while increases over this limit of force direct cells into a phenotype that recapitulates osteoarthritis [29].

Mediators and responses to shear forces were thoroughly studied in cellular components of the vascular system. Components of the cytoskeleton act as mechanotransductors and initiate cascades of phosphorylation, which ultimately activate transcription factors and regulate gene expression [30–33]. However, mechanisms and pathways of mechanotransduction for other cell types, such as oocytes and/or blastomeres, have not been investigated in depth and are not completely understood.

Biological resilience to shear stress is tissue and cell dependent [34]. Vascular and blood cells subjected to high energy fluid dynamic environments experience physiological ranges of shear force from 1 to $10 \, dyn/cm^2$ [35, 36] and the threshold force for red blood cells is $1500 \, dyn/cm^2$ [23]. Currently, the shear force experienced by oocyte and embryos in the female reproductive tract is unknown. However, oocytes and preimplantation embryos encounter the tubal fluid dynamic environment before entering the uterus and undergoing implantation; yet, compared to the vascular system, this is a low energy fluid dynamic environment with an estimated flow speed of 6.5–29 μm/s with pulses from 5 to 20 Hz [37]. Thus, preimplantation embryos might not withstand high shear forces in comparison to cellular components of the vascular system.

It has been demonstrated that preimplantation embryos can sense and react to shear stress [38]. As in other cell types, phosphorylation and activation of mitogen-activated protein kinase (MAPK) pathways seems to play an important role in the response to mechanical stimuli [30–33, 38]. Mouse embryos undergo programmed cell death if shear forces of $\sim$1.2 dyn/cm^2 are applied over a 12-hour period [38]. Additionally, the percent of embryos undergoing cell death depended on the combination of intensity of shear force and duration; in other words, high shear stress for short periods might be as detrimental as long exposures to low shear stress [38].

In general, human embryos produced after IVF undergo periods of culture between 72 and 120 hours before transfer to the uterus. Therefore, efforts toward integrating bioengineering devices with culture techniques to provide fluid dynamic environments for embryo growth should consider extensive modeling and designing to produce dynamic environments with shear forces during the period of culture that are not detrimental to embryos.

Application of fluid dynamics in the IVF laboratory

Production of dynamic fluidic environments to tackle multiple tasks in the IVF laboratory has been foreseen and discussed during the last decade. A reasonable number of theoretical and review articles on this matter have been published [16, 39–43]. The lack of commercially available devices for dynamic fluid embryo culture might explain why only a small number of reports on these processes in IVF laboratories have been published [18, 44, 46–50]. The following sections address the use of dynamic fluid environments for sperm preparation and embryo culture.

Dynamic fluid systems for sperm preparation

Semen preparation is a mandatory step in infertility treatments through IVF and intracytoplasmic sperm injection (ICSI). Current techniques of semen preparation rely on centrifugation forces or incubation of semen for prolonged times. These preparation methods have been used for many decades, yet their use can cause DNA damage and sublethal structural damage [51, 52]. Concerns regarding detrimental effects of sperm genomic damage have increased in recent years and it has been suggested that sperm DNA fragmentation is related to embryonic developmental failures and losses of preimplantation embryos after paternal genome activation [53]. Consequently, the development of sperm preparation techniques that minimize risk of genomic damage is necessary.

Principles of microfluidics have been proposed to create a gravity-driven microfluidic sperm sorter. This device was described in 2003 for selection of motile spermatozoa, isolation of motile sperm from seminal plasma, and enhancement of morphologically normal sperm without submitting these cells to centrifugation forces or to prolonged incubation [49, 54]. Although, this device is not commercially available, detailed instructions on how to produce it in house and operate this gravity-driven microfluidic sperm sorter are available [55].

Gravity-driven sperm sorters operate through generation of two parallel microfluidic streams that flow side-by-side without appreciable mixing. Medium forms one stream and the other stream contains seminal plasma, motile sperm, non-motile sperm, and non-gamete cellular debris. Within this device laminar flow creates an interface or meniscus between the two fluid streams that can only be crossed by motile sperm (Figure 15.2). This simple processing procedure is able to yield high rates of sperm showing normal morphology, motility, and low rates of sperm DNA fragmentation [49, 56]. Initial prototypes are limited in their processing volume and final yield, thus precluding their use for sperm preparation for intrauterine insemination. Future modifications of parallel processing could circumvent this limitation. With this caveat, the microfluidic sperm-processing device can provide high quality sperm for standard IVF [57] and ICSI [49]. The impact of this type of sperm selection on human fertilization rates and embryo quality is currently being evaluated by numerous laboratories.

Dynamic fluid environments for embryo culture

Dynamic fluid environments for embryo culture can be obtained with the adaptation of components of traditional culture systems, or through the creation of devices to control fluid flow and pulsatility of the environment. These devices and their mode of dynamic fluid generation are addressed below.

Dynamic fluid environments adapted from traditional static embryo culture systems

At a simplistic level, traditional static culture systems consist of a plastic dish containing media in which the embryos grow in an incubator with a controlled humidified atmosphere. This environment provides little opportunity for disrupting the gradient of biomolecules that can form around an embryo when nutrients are used and waste products are produced [18, 58, 59].

These gradients can be interrupted if the platform holding the embryo culture-ware is moved. Agitation of components of traditional culture systems were reported over 40 years ago for mouse embryo culture, but these studies were not designed to do a pairwise comparison of static and dynamic fluid environments [45]. Recently, the effect of tilting a supporting platform with traditional culture-ware on human embryo development was compared to a static system [46]. A computer-controlled system was programmed to

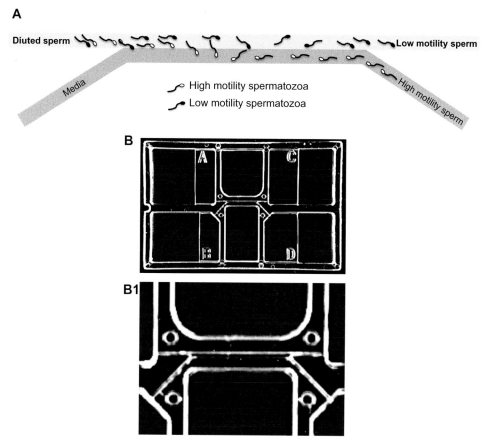

Figure 15.2 (A) Schematic representation of sperm sorting with a microfluidic device. Diluted sperm and media are driven through microchannels by gravity and they create two parallel flows. Spermatozoa with high motility are able to cross the interface between the two flows and are collected in an appropriate well downstream, but the spermatozoa with low motility do not cross the interface and are collected into another well along with non-motile debris. (B) Gravity-driven sperm sorter device transilluminated to enhance the visibility of the microchannels. (B1) Details of the microchannels.

attain a 10° incline with 1°/s increase; in this fashion, embryos were moved at 300 μm/min (Figure 15.3) [46]. The pattern of platform tilting induced shear forces of 1.5×10^{-4} dyn/cm^2 on the embryos. The effects of this simple dynamic fluid culture system were tested on murine and human embryos. The percent of embryos reaching the blastocyst stage was similar among the two culture systems, yet the number of blastomeres in embryos grown under tilting conditions was greater than that obtained in the static culture system [46]. Similar effects of tilting embryo culture systems were also reported for porcine embryos [44]. Further studies to determine the impact of a dynamic fluid environment obtained through platform tilting on implantation and pregnancy rates in animal model systems and/or with human embryos are wanting.

Fluid dynamics and embryo stimulation through vibration

Vibration is one of several methods available to disrupt the static condition of fluid components of cell culture systems (Figure 15.4). In addition, different types of cells are

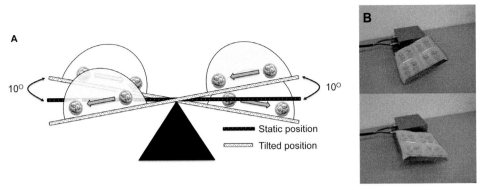

Figure 15.3 (A) Schematic representation of a tilting platform to produce embryo movement and disruption of the static condition of the embryo culture environment. Embryos roll on the bottom of the culture medium drop when the platform is tilted. (B) Images of a tilting embryo culture system operating outside of an embryo incubator (Figure courtesy of Dr. Keiji Naruse).

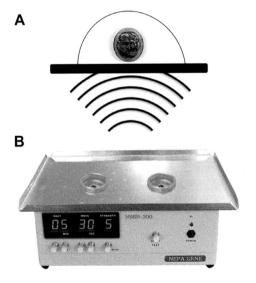

Figure 15.4 (A) Schematic representation of a dynamic fluid environment for embryo culture obtained with a vibrating platform. The platform holding the culture dish vibrates to agitate the embryo and disrupt chemical gradients around the embryo. (B) Image of a vibrating platform holding dishes for embryo culture (Figure courtesy of NepaGene, Japan).

able to sense vibratory stimulation and to react through proliferation and alteration of gene expression [60–62]. Whether oocytes or embryos sense vibratory stimulation has yet to be determined. However, in the tubal environment preimplantation embryos are exposed to vibratory waves ranging from 5 to 20 Hz [37]. Similar vibratory frequencies were recently used to disrupt the static conditions of in vitro maturation (IVM) of pig oocytes and culture conditions of pig embryos generated by somatic nuclear transference [63]. Vibration (20 Hz) for 5 seconds every 60 minutes during pig oocyte IVM enhanced the production of blastocysts [63], but vibratory culture of embryos generated by somatic nuclear transference originated from oocytes matured under static conditions did not seem to show an effect [63].

Nevertheless, a study with human embryos mirroring the partial success of vibrating pig oocytes was conducted in slightly different conditions (44 Hz, for 10 seconds every

60 minutes) [64]. The authors reported impressive increases in the rate of blastocyst formation and pregnancy rates after culture of embryos in this vibratory regimen. Currently, many questions exist as to how and why such excellent results can be obtained with vibratory culture of human embryos. It will be exciting to see where this line of research goes in the future.

Controlled fluid dynamics

Controlled fluid dynamics can be obtained with the utilization of several technologies and devices. Methods to generate controlled fluid dynamics include gravity gradient, syringe pumps, and peristaltic pumping with Braille displays [15–18]. The shape of the embryo housing area in conjunction with the method used to generate fluid dynamics collectively impact development of shear forces the embryo is exposed to, the exposure to refresh media, and the wash out of embryo waste and autocrine factors [18].

A proof-of-concept article demonstrated the ability of pressure gradients of 1 Pa/mm to generate flow of culture media of 100 nL/s with a speed varying from 1 to 2 mm/s throughout a network of microchannels [15]. This microfluidic movement was able to roll embryos over the bottom of the microchannels with half of the speed of the fluid [15].

Gravity gradients were used to create a device for cumulus cell removal and embryo culture [16]. Removal of cumulus cells was fully accomplished in this device and the percentage of blastocysts was increased in relation to static culture systems. Unfortunately, experiments employed a suboptimal culture medium in evaluating microfluidic effects on embryo development, and experiments to detect the efficiency of this system in optimal conditions were not performed [16].

Syringe-driven fluid movement to create a high (0.5 μL/h) and low (0.1 μL/h) culture media flow demonstrated that low microfluidic flow resulted in increased production of blastocysts, while higher flow of media decreased this production in relation to static controls [17]. Once again, suboptimal media for embryo culture were employed in this study, but this study demonstrated that mammalian embryo development could be influenced by changing the dynamic fluid environment. The devices created for both studies comprised microchannels with barriers to hold the embryos in one place and prevent removal of embryos from the microchannels [65, 66]. This type of construction is able to generate significant localized shear forces on the embryos as further demonstrated in mesh modeling [18], which can bring about biological effects on preimplantation embryos. Some other reports on the operation of devices with a single microchannel and barrier also indicated a slight augmentation on the production of blastocysts [48, 67], but again impact of shear forces generated in single microchannels was not emphasized. Finally, evidence that these devices increase implantation and pregnancy rates is still wanting.

Braille displays can be used to produce computer-controlled displacement of thin membranes lining the bottom of a microfluidic channel [68]. The software programmed and orchestrated actions of Braille pins can create a peristaltic effect to deliver different patterns of pulsatile frequencies and flow rates of media [68]. This mode of generating microfluidic flow finds several applications in cell biology and culture such as controlled release of factors to single colonies of stem cells and embryo culture [18, 69].

Initial efforts to utilize Braille pin peristaltic pumping of media for embryo culture was unsuccessful because of significant media osmotic shifts that occurred due to evaporation across thin flexible membranes needed for Braille pin actuation of media flow [70].

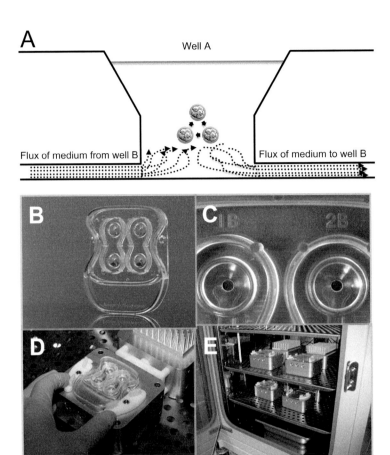

Figure 15.5 (A) Partial schematic representation of a dynamic culture microfunnel device. The device comprises two wells in each side (well A and well B – not shown in the diagram) linked by microchannels laying on top of Braille pins that press into the microchannel, displacing medium, and producing fluid flow in the microchannel between the microfunnel wells. The fluid streams into the well and produces a gentle turbulence that moves the embryos and disrupt chemical gradients. A similar set of Braille pin movements removes medium from the well. (B) Appearance of a dynamic microfunnel device, (C) enlarged view of the microfunnels. (D) Placement of the dynamic microfunnel cartridge onto the Braille pin display and (E) general appearance of the system inside an incubator (Figures B–E are courtesy of Incept Biosystems).

Sandwiching a low water permeable parylene film between flexible membranes allowed the development of microchannels that were collapsible and conducive to Braille pin displacement of media in microchannels without media osmolality changes and thus development of programmable pulsatile fluid flow for embryo culture [18, 70].

Microfunnels were developed to make placement and removal of embryos practical, simple, and safe (Figure 15.5). Recognizing that clinical utility would require 100% efficiency of embryo recovery, the design of a microfunnel instead of embryo placement in microchannels was selected. In addition, microfunnels were developed with mesh modeling to design a dynamic embryo culture environment with low shear forces more evenly distributed over the embryo surface [18]. Mouse embryos grown in dynamic microfunnels under a pulsatile regimen of 0.1 Hz had a higher number of blastomeres in comparison to embryos produced in static systems of culture. This increase in number of cells translated to higher implantation and pregnancy rates [18].

Enhanced developmental potential of mouse embryos grown in dynamic microfunnels might be due to mechanostimulation of embryos, yet the exact mechanism of mechano-sensitivity and the activation of growth-promoting pathways arising from this type of stimulation are unknown in embryos. Another contributing factor for the enhanced viability of these embryos may be the low dissipation of autocrine/paracrine growth factors and mixing that occurs as a collective result of the microfunnel design, periodic refreshment of media, and the slight rocking motion of the embryos [18].

Translation of results obtained from mice to humans still has to be confirmed and studies approved by Institutional Review Boards are ongoing in different sites in North and South America. Preliminary results indicate that human embryos submitted to dynamic microfunnel culture have lower rates of fragmentation on day 3 of culture than those undergoing traditional static culture [71].

Controlled dynamic fluid systems for embryo culture appear to be beneficial and to increase developmental and reproductive potential of embryos. These systems are not commercially available at the present moment, but their production is well detailed in original reports and a step-by-step guide for production of dynamic microfunnel embryo culture devices is available [72]. Even though tilting, vibratory, and microfluidic devices for embryo culture can be produced in well-equipped research laboratories, their use in clinical settings should be implemented cautiously. Validation of results of embryo development and pregnancy rates should be replicated in different model systems and clinical IVF laboratories. Additionally, approval of these devices for clinical use by regulatory agencies should be granted before their widespread use.

Integration of platforms for dynamic fluid culture and analytical tools

Selection of human embryos for uterine transfer is performed by observation of morpho-logical characteristics of preimplantation embryos after fertilization on days 3 and 5 of in vitro development. Embryo assessment based on morphology is subjective and fallible because it does not result in reliable prediction of implantation or gestation [73]. New automated systems for live-cell imaging might produce more accurate predictions of an embryo's developmental potential [74].

Beyond embryo appearance, identification of a molecular phenotype or fingerprint for embryos with increased developmental potential through characterization of their secre-tome and/or metabolome has been considered with great interest in the past few years [73, 75–79]. In general, equipment and processes to generate proteomic profiles can be prohibitively complicated, which detracts from their standard implementation in clinical IVF laboratories. However, a recent study provided information for the production of a viability index obtained through near-infrared spectrometry of small volumes of media removed from culture [75].

Recently, proof-of-concept articles demonstrated that microfluidic devices could inte-grate cell culture and absorbance readings for the production of photonic devices for in-line analysis of culture media contents [80–82]. Investigators have integrated various types of detection devices to microfluidic chips to monitor oxygen tensions, calcium fluctuations, pH, lactate, and glucose production from single somatic cells and 2-cell embryos [83–86].

Recently, a microfluidic device with deformation-based actuation was created to determine embryo metabolism in real time [87]. This device integrated computer-controlled flow to move nanoliters of spent culture medium into a reagent mixing area for a direct measurement of glucose without potential harmful impact of ultraviolet light on cells contained in the device. Validation of this device demonstrated that it was able to detect increasing concentrations of glucose spiked into the culture medium. Furthermore, single and group culture of murine blastocysts decreased glucose in the culture medium over time in a linear fashion; demonstrating that real-time, live cell monitoring of single embryos metabolism is possible [87]. This device demonstrates promise; however, studies with human embryos should be performed to evaluate clinical relevance and to determine metabolic values indicative of embryo developmental competence and implantation potential.

Conclusion

Traditional embryo culture systems utilize a static environment and fail to recapitulate the dynamic fluid environment of the oviducts. Dynamic fluid culture systems can be generated by several modes and almost all of them seem to be beneficial to embryo development.

Several devices were created during the last decade in an attempt to provide dynamic fluid conditions for embryos. Embryologists willing to design new devices for embryo culture should consider that embryo development occurs in vivo in a low energy fluid dynamic environment and embryos are sensitive to shear forces. Additionally, new devices should be designed to integrate with other technologies to allow greater embryo assessment with less embryo manipulation. Finally, newly created microfluidic devices for embryo culture and real-time detection of embryo metabolism will integrate real-time imaging of embryos to produce information on embryo biosynthesis and morphometrics with less embryo manipulation. This translates into multiple benefits, including better embryo development due to reduced manipulation and greater insight into embryo selection. Combination of these new technologies will increase the clinical embryologist's ability to rank embryos, select embryos with the greatest implantation potential, facilitate more frequent use of elective single embryo transfer, and collectively increase pregnancy rates and births of healthy children.

References

1. Edwards RG. Test-tube babies, 1981. *Nature* 1981;**293**(5830):253–6.

2. Whitten WK. Culture of tubal ova. *Nature* 1957;**179**(4569):1081–2.

3. Whitten WK. Culture of tubal mouse ova. *Nature* 1956;**177**(4498):96.

4. McLaren A, Biggers JD. Successful development and birth of mice cultivated in vitro as early embryos. *Nature* 1958;**182**(4639):877–8.

5. McKiernan SH, Clayton MK, Bavister BD. Analysis of stimulatory and inhibitory amino acids for development of hamster one-cell embryos in vitro. *Mol Reprod Dev* 1995;**42**(2):188–99.

6. Wada T. Evaluation of media, protein supplements and potassium concentration for human in vitro fertilization and embryo transfer by preimplanted mouse embryo development. *Nihon Sanka Fujinka Gakkai Zasshi* 1988;**40**(5):640–6.

7. Whitten WK, Biggers JD. Complete development in vitro of the pre-implantation stages of the mouse in a simple chemically defined medium. *J Reprod Fertil* 1968;**17**(2):399–401.

8. Biggers JD, Whittingham DG, Donahue RP. The pattern of energy metabolism in the mouse oocyte and zygote. *Proc Natl Acad Sci U S A* 1967;**58**(2):560–7.

9. Gardner DK, Pool TB, Lane M. Embryo nutrition and energy metabolism and its

relationship to embryo growth, differentiation, and viability. *Semin Reprod Med* 2000;**18**(2):205–18.

10. Gardner DK. Changes in requirements and utilization of nutrients during mammalian preimplantation embryo development and their significance in embryo culture. *Theriogenology* 1998;**49**(1):83–102.

11. Gardner DK, Lane M. Culture of viable human blastocysts in defined sequential serum-free media. *Hum Reprod* 1998;**13**(Suppl 3):148–59; discussion 60.

12. Lane M, Gardner DK. Differential regulation of mouse embryo development and viability by amino acids. *J Reprod Fertil* 1997;**109**(1):153–64.

13. Reed ML. Communication skills of embryos maintained in group culture— the autocrine paracrine debate. *Clin Embryologist* 2006;**9**:5–19.

14. Muglia U, Motta PM. A new morpho-functional classification of the Fallopian tube based on its three-dimensional myoarchitecture. *Histol Histopathol* 2001;**16**(1):227–37.

15. Glasgow IK, Zeringue HC, Beebe DJ, *et al.* Handling individual mammalian embryos using microfluidics. *IEEE Trans Biomed Eng* 2001;**48**(5):570–8.

16. Beebe D, Wheeler M, Zeringue H, Walters E, Raty S. Microfluidic technology for assisted reproduction. *Theriogenology* 2002;**57**(1):125–35.

17. Hickman DL, Beebe DJ, Rodriguez-Zas SL, Wheeler MB. Comparison of static and dynamic medium environments for culturing of pre-implantation mouse embryos. *Comp Med* 2002;**52**(2):122–6.

18. Heo YS, Cabrera LM, Bormann CL, *et al.* Dynamic microfunnel culture enhances mouse embryo development and pregnancy rates. *Hum Reprod* 2010;**25**(3):613–22.

19. Fleming GM. Renal replacement therapy review: past, present and future. *Organogenesis* 2011;**7**(1):2–12.

20. Gerbode F, Osborn JJ, Melrose DG, *et al.* Extracorporeal circulation in intracardiac surgery; a comparison between two heart-lung machines. *Lancet* 1958;**2**(7041):284–6.

21. Boettcher W, Merkle F, Weitkemper HH. History of extracorporeal circulation: the conceptional and developmental period. *J Extra Corpor Technol* 2003;**35**(3):172–83.

22. Dobell AR, Galva R, Sarkozy E, Murphy DR. Biologic evaluation of blood after prolonged recirculation through film and membrane oxygenators. *Ann Surg* 1965;**161**:617–22.

23. Leverett LB, Hellums JD, Alfrey CP, Lynch EC. Red blood cell damage by shear stress. *Biophys J* 1972;**12**(3):257–73.

24. Song C, Shin SJ, Sung HJ, Chang K. Dynamic fluid–structure interaction of an elastic capsule in a viscous shear flow at moderate Reynolds number. *J Fluids Structures* 2011;**27**:438–55.

25. Xie Y, Wang F, Puscheck EE, Rappolee DA. Pipetting causes shear stress and elevation of phosphorylated stress-activated protein kinase/jun kinase in preimplantation embryos. *Mol Reprod Dev* 2007;**74**(10):1287–94.

26. Familiari G, Heyn R, Relucenti M, Nottola SA, Sathananthan AH. Ultrastructural dynamics of human reproduction, from ovulation to fertilization and early embryo development. *Int Rev Cytol* 2006;**249**:53–141.

27. Pedersen JA, Lichter S, Swartz MA. Cells in 3D matrices under interstitial flow: effects of extracellular matrix alignment on cell shear stress and drag forces. *J Biomech* 2010;**43**(5):900–5.

28. Bassaneze V, Barauna VG, Lavini-Ramos C, *et al.* Shear stress induces nitric oxide-mediated vascular endothelial growth factor production in human adipose tissue mesenchymal stem cells. *Stem Cells Dev* 2010;**19**(3):371–8.

29. Zhu F, Wang P, Lee NH, Goldring MB, Konstantopoulos K. Prolonged application of high fluid shear to chondrocytes recapitulates gene expression profiles associated with osteoarthritis. *PLoS One* 2010;**5**(12):e15174.

30. Chien S. Role of shear stress direction in endothelial mechanotransduction. *Mol Cell Biomech* 2008;**5**(1):1–8.

31. Chien S. Mechanotransduction and endothelial cell homeostasis: the wisdom of the cell. *Am J Physiol Heart Circ Physiol* 2007;**292**(3):H1209–24.

32. Li YS, Haga JH, Chien S. Molecular basis of the effects of shear stress on vascular endothelial cells. *J Biomech* 2005;**38** (10):1949–71.

33. Lehoux S, Tedgui A. Cellular mechanics and gene expression in blood vessels. *J Biomech* 2003;**36**(5):631–43.

34. Hua J, Erickson LE, Yiin TY, Glasgow LA. A review of the effects of shear and interfacial phenomena on cell viability. *Crit Rev Biotechnol* 1993;**13**(4):305–28.

35. Resnick N, Yahav H, Shay-Salit A, *et al.* Fluid shear stress and the vascular endothelium: for better and for worse. *Prog Biophys Mol Biol* 2003;**81**(3):177–99.

36. Wang S, Tarbell JM. Effect of fluid flow on smooth muscle cells in a 3-dimensional collagen gel model. *Arterioscler Thromb Vasc Biol* 2000;**20**(10):2220–5.

37. Paltieli Y, Weichselbaum A, Hoffman N, Eibschitz I, Kam Z. Laser scattering instrument for real time in-vivo measurement of ciliary activity in human fallopian tubes. *Hum Reprod* 1995;**10** (7):1638–41.

38. Xie Y, Wang F, Zhong W, *et al.* Shear stress induces preimplantation embryo death that is delayed by the zona pellucida and associated with stress-activated protein kinase-mediated apoptosis. *Biol Reprod* 2006;**75**(1):45–55.

39. Smith GD, Swain JE, Bormann CL. Microfluidics for gametes, embryos, and embryonic stem cells. *Semin Reprod Med* 2011;**29**(1):5–14.

40. Krisher RL, Wheeler MB. Towards the use of microfluidics for individual embryo culture. *Reprod Fertil Dev* 2010;**22**(1):32–9.

41. Smith GD, Takayama S. Gamete and embryo isolation and culture with microfluidics. *Theriogenology* 2007;**68** (Suppl 1):S190–5.

42. Suh RS, Phadke N, Ohl DA, Takayama S, Smith GD. Rethinking gamete/embryo isolation and culture with microfluidics. *Hum Reprod Update* 2003;**9**(5):451–61.

43. Swain JE, Smith GD. Advances in embryo culture platforms: novel approaches to improve preimplantation embryo development through modifications of the microenvironment. *Hum Reprod Update* 2011;**17**(4):541–57.

44. Koike T, Matsuura K, Naruse K, Funahashi H. In-vitro culture with a tilting device in chemically defined media during meiotic maturation and early development improves the quality of blastocysts derived from in-vitro matured and fertilized porcine oocytes. *J Reprod Dev* 2010;**56** (5):552–7.

45. Hoppe PC, Pitts S. Fertilization in vitro and development of mouse ova. *Biol Reprod* 1973;**8**:420–6.

46. Matsuura K, Hayashi N, Kuroda Y, *et al.* Improved development of mouse and human embryos using a tilting embryo culture system. *Reprod Biomed Online* 2010;**20**(3):358–64.

47. Kim MS, Bae CY, Wee G, Han YM, Park JK. A microfluidic in vitro cultivation system for mechanical stimulation of bovine embryos. *Electrophoresis* 2009;**30** (18):3276–82.

48. Raty S, Walters EM, Davis J, *et al.* Embryonic development in the mouse is enhanced via microchannel culture. *Lab Chip* 2004;**4**(3):186–90.

49. Schuster TG, Cho B, Keller LM, Takayama S, Smith GD. Isolation of motile spermatozoa from semen samples using microfluidics. *Reprod Biomed Online* 2003;**7**(1):75–81.

50. Han C, Zhang Q, Ma R, *et al.* Integration of single oocyte trapping, in vitro fertilization and embryo culture in a microwell-structured microfluidic device. *Lab Chip* 2010;**10**(21):2848–54.

51. Matsuura R, Takeuchi T, Yoshida A. Preparation and incubation conditions affect the DNA integrity of ejaculated human spermatozoa. *Asian J Androl* 2010;**12**(5):753–9.

52. Twigg J, Irvine DS, Houston P, *et al.* Iatrogenic DNA damage induced in human spermatozoa during sperm preparation: protective significance of seminal plasma. *Mol Hum Reprod* 1998;4(5):439–45.

53. Sakkas D, Alvarez JG. Sperm DNA fragmentation: mechanisms of origin, impact on reproductive outcome, and analysis. *Fertil Steril* 2010;93(4): 1027–36.

54. Cho BS, Schuster TG, Zhu X, *et al.* Passively driven integrated microfluidic system for separation of motile sperm. *Anal Chem* 2003;75(7):1671–5.

55. Chung Y, Zhu X, Gu W, Smith GD, Takayama S. Microscale integrated sperm sorter. *Methods Mol Biol* 2006;321: 227–44.

56. Schulte RT, Chung YK, Ohl DA, Takayama S, Smith GD. Microfluidic sperm sorting device provides a novel method for selecting motile sperm with higher DNA integrity. *Fertil Steril* 2007;88 (Suppl 1):S76.

57. Sano H, Matsuura K, Naruse K, Funahashi H. Application of a microfluidic sperm sorter to the in-vitro fertilization of porcine oocytes reduced the incidence of polyspermic penetration. *Theriogenology* 2010;74(5):863–70.

58. Trimarchi JR, Liu L, Porterfield DM, Smith PJ, Keefe DL. A non-invasive method for measuring preimplantation embryo physiology. *Zygote* 2000;8(1): 15–24.

59. Trimarchi JR, Liu L, Porterfield DM, Smith PJ, Keefe DL. Oxidative phosphorylation-dependent and -independent oxygen consumption by individual preimplantation mouse embryos. *Biol Reprod* 2000;62(6):1866–74.

60. Kaupp JA, Waldman SD. Mechanical vibrations increase the proliferation of articular chondrocytes in high-density culture. *Proc Inst Mech Eng H* 2008;222 (5):695–703.

61. Ito Y, Kimura T, Nam K, *et al.* Effects of vibration on differentiation of cultured PC12 cells. *Biotechnol Bioeng* 2011;108 (3):592–9.

62. Wolchok JC, Brokopp C, Underwood CJ, Tresco PA. The effect of bioreactor induced vibrational stimulation on extracellular matrix production from human derived fibroblasts. *Biomaterials* 2009;30(3):327–35.

63. Mizobe Y, Yoshida M, Miyoshi K. Enhancement of cytoplasmic maturation of in vitro-matured pig oocytes by mechanical vibration. *J Reprod Dev* 2010;56(2):285–90.

64. Isachenko V, Maettner R, Sterzik K, *et al.* In-vitro culture of human embryos with mechanical micro-vibration increases implantation rates. *Reprod Biomed Online* 2011;22(6):536–44.

65. Wheeler MB, Walters EM, Beebe DJ. Toward culture of single gametes: the development of microfluidic platforms for assisted reproduction. *Theriogenology* 2007;68(Suppl 1):S178–89.

66. Clark SG, Haubert K, Beebe DJ, Ferguson CE, Wheeler MB. Reduction of polyspermic penetration using biomimetic microfluidic technology during in vitro fertilization. *Lab Chip* 2005;5(11):1229–32.

67. Wheeler MB, Clark SG, Beebe DJ. Developments in in vitro technologies for swine embryo production. *Reprod Fertil Dev* 2004;16(1–2):15–25.

68. Gu W, Zhu X, Futai N, Cho BS, Takayama S. Computerized microfluidic cell culture using elastomeric channels and Braille displays. *Proc Natl Acad Sci U S A* 2004;101 (45):15861–6.

69. Villa-Diaz LG, Torisawa YS, Uchida T, *et al.* Microfluidic culture of single human embryonic stem cell colonies. *Lab Chip* 2009;9(12):1749–55.

70. Heo YS, Cabrera LM, Song JW, *et al.* Characterization and resolution of evaporation-mediated osmolality shifts that constrain microfluidic cell culture in poly (dimethylsiloxane) devices. *Anal Chem* 2007;79(3):1126–34.

71. Alegretti JR, Motta ELA, Serafini P, *et al.* Development of human embryos in a dynamic microfluidic culture system: results from a prospective randomized study. *Hum Reprod* 2011;26(Suppl 1):i38.

72. Heo YS, Jovic A, Cabrera LM, Smith GD, Takayama S. Osmolality control for

microfluidic embryo cell culture using hybrid polydimethylsiloxane (PDMS)-parylene membranes. In: Nahmias Y, Bhatia SN, eds. *Methods in Bioengineering: Microdevices in Biology and Medicine*, 1st edn. Boston, Artech House. 2009;109–27.

73. Bromer JG, Seli E. Assessment of embryo viability in assisted reproductive technology: shortcomings of current approaches and the emerging role of metabolomics. *Curr Opin Obstet Gynecol* 2008;**20**(3):234–41.

74. Wong CC, Loewke KE, Bossert NL, *et al.* Non-invasive imaging of human embryos before embryonic genome activation predicts development to the blastocyst stage. *Nat Biotechnol* 2010;**28**(10):1115–21.

75. Seli E, Vergouw CG, Morita H, *et al.* Noninvasive metabolomic profiling as an adjunct to morphology for noninvasive embryo assessment in women undergoing single embryo transfer. *Fertil Steril* 2010;**94** (2):535–42.

76. Botros L, Sakkas D, Seli E. Metabolomics and its application for non-invasive embryo assessment in IVF. *Mol Hum Reprod* 2008;**14**(12):679–90.

77. Aydiner F, Yetkin CE, Seli E. Perspectives on emerging biomarkers for non-invasive assessment of embryo viability in assisted reproduction. *Curr Mol Med* 2010;**10** (2):206–15.

78. Royere D, Feuerstein P, Cadoret V, *et al.* Non invasive assessment of embryo quality: proteomics, metabolomics and oocyte-cumulus dialogue. *Gynecol Obstet Fertil* 2009;**37**(11–12):917–20.

79. Katz Jaffe MG, McReynolds S, Gardner DK, Schoolcraft WB. The role of proteomics in defining the human embryonic secretome. *Mol Hum Reprod* 2009;**15**(5):271–7.

80. Demming S, Vila-Planas J, Aliasghar Zadeh S, *et al.* Poly(dimethylsiloxane) photonic microbioreactors based on segmented waveguides for local absorbance measurement. *Electrophoresis* 2011;**32** (3–4):431–9.

81. Au SH, Shih SC, Wheeler AR. Integrated microbioreactor for culture and analysis of bacteria, algae and yeast. *Biomed Microdevices* 2011;**13**(1):41–50.

82. Urbanski JP, Johnson MT, Craig DD, *et al.* Noninvasive metabolic profiling using microfluidics for analysis of single preimplantation embryos. *Anal Chem* 2008;**80**(17):6500–7. doi:10.102/ ac8010473.

83. Cheng W, Klauke N, Sedgwick H, Smith GL, Cooper JM. Metabolic monitoring of the electrically stimulated single heart cell within a microfluidic platform. *Lab Chip* 2006;**6**(11):1424–31.

84. Shackman JG, Dahlgren GM, Peters JL, Kennedy RT. Perfusion and chemical monitoring of living cells on a microfluidic chip. *Lab Chip* 2005;**5**(1):56–63.

85. Mehta G, Mehta K, Sud D, *et al.* Quantitative measurement and control of oxygen levels in microfluidic poly (dimethylsiloxane) bioreactors during cell culture. *Biomed Microdevices* 2007; **9**(2):123–34.

86. Mehta K, Mehta G, Takayama S, Linderman J. Quantitative inference of cellular parameters from microfluidic cell culture systems. *Biotechnol Bioeng* 2009;**103**(5):966–74.

87. Heo YS, Cabrera LM, Bormann CL, Smith GD, Takayama S. Real time culture and analysis of embryo metabolism using a microfluidic device with deformation based actuation. *Lab Chip* 2012;**12**:2240–6. doi:10.1039/c2lc21050a.

Time-lapse imaging of embryo development: using morphokinetic analysis to select viable embryos

Markus H. M. Montag, Kamilla S. Pedersen, and Niels B. Ramsing

This chapter is dedicated to Lynette Scott. It was her, who had originally been asked to contribute this chapter and Lynette accepted to do so with her usual enthusiasm and dedication to the field of IVF. Lynette was among the first to apply time-lapse recordings for the assessment of embryo development – initially on the basis of oxygen respiration rate measurements and later using time-lapse imaging to evaluate the time course of early events in human embryo development.

The tragic, unexpected and untimely passing away of Lynette in early 2012 did not allow her to finish this chapter nor any of the multitudes of other research projects she was involved in. We, the authors of this chapter and the editor of this book, would like to express our deep gratitude to the inspiration Lynette gave to us and to the global community of embryologists.

Summary

Identification and selection of a viable embryo for transfer is a clear prerequisite to any efficient and successful in vitro fertilization (IVF) treatment. Fertility clinics rely almost exclusively on a morphological assessment of embryo appearance at a few distinct time-points during development to pick a viable embryo for transfer. However, embryo development is a very dynamic process and critical stages between observations go unnoticed. This chapter discusses some of the shortcomings of current IVF protocols and substantiates how embryo selection could possibly improve based on a kinetic analysis of time-lapse images documenting embryo development. Novel diagnostic possibilities based on time-lapse monitoring (TLM) are discussed and recently published clinical results using such systems are evaluated.

Introduction

Infertility is experienced by approximately 8% of all couples worldwide [1]. It is a growing problem due to increasing maternal age and decreasing semen quality. Assisted reproduction is a growing area of medicine, driven by infertile couples' increasing acceptance of infertility treatments, decreasing tolerance of infertility, and better access to fertility clinics.

The number of fertility treatments performed worldwide is currently estimated at 1.5 million per year with an annual growth rate of about 10% [1]. Despite a considerable

Culture Media, Solutions, and Systems in Human ART, ed. Patrick Quinn. Published by Cambridge University Press. © Cambridge University Press 2014.

international research effort, there are still two prominent shortcomings of current fertility treatments:

- An unsatisfactorily low success rate. On average it is only every fourth or fifth initiated treatment cycle that succeeds and gives rise to a live birth rate of 20% to 25% in most countries in Europe [1] and slightly higher, around 32%, in the USA [2].
- A large number of multiple pregnancies (twins, triplets) from assisted reproductive technology (ART) treatments, which poses a significant medical risk to the mother and offspring and results in additional costs in the healthcare system.

A contributing factor to the low success rate in current IVF procedures is our inability to determine objectively and reliably which embryos from the available cohort are viable and to select one of these embryos for transfer [3–5].

Current selection procedures are mainly based on a morphological evaluation of the embryo at distinct time-points during development followed by an evaluation at the time of transfer using standard microscopy (Figures 16.1 and 16.2). However, these time-points may vary from lab to lab and also within a lab from cycle to cycle. Hence, it is widely recognized that the evaluation procedure needs qualitative as well as quantitative improvements. In search of making morphological evaluation of embryos comparable, ESHRE and Alpha produced a consensus paper recommending time-points that are considered to be crucial for embryo evaluation [6, 7]. However, although the consensus paper is a major step forward, it still relies on a few daily observations and does not attempt to quantify the dynamic morphological changes over time, which is often referred to by the term morphokinetics. Routine clinical use of morphokinetic embryo analysis was not feasible until the recent introduction of commercial time-lapse-based imaging systems. Time-lapse imaging (TLI) provides automated acquisition of images for one or more embryos at preset time

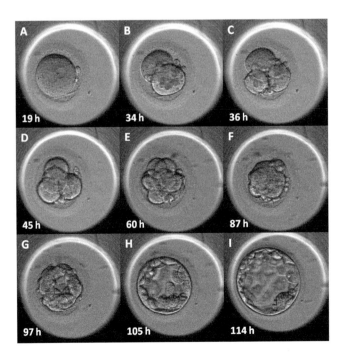

Figure 16.1 Stages of early human embryo development taken from a time-lapse image series showing the embryo at nine representative time-points; (A) oocyte at pronuclear stage at 19 hours; (B) 2-cell stage at 34 hours; (C) 3-cell stage at 36 hours; (D) 4-cell stage at 45 hours; (E) 8-cell stage at 60 hours; (F) morula stage at 87 hours; (G) early blastocyst stage at 97 hours; (H) normal blastocyst stage at 105 hours; (I) expanding blastocyst at 114 hours, prior embryo transfer. The remaining 340 images from that time-lapse series are not shown.

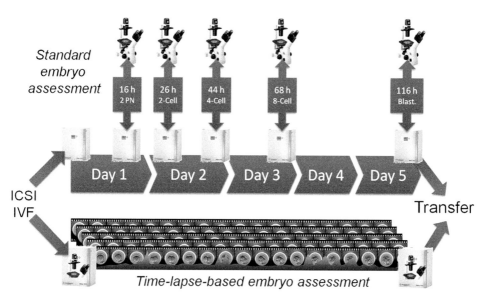

Figure 16.2 Time-lapse-based embryo assessment provides automated image acquisition within a controlled incubation environment. Time-lapse monitoring (TLM) thus eliminated the need for periodic transfer of the embryos to a microscope for evaluation of morphology. These inspections may affect embryo development due to changes in temperature, pH, and O_2 concentration. The figure shows recommended time-points for morphological assessment according to the Alpha-ESHRE consensus work [6, 7]. The embryos may still need to be removed from the time-lapse system for media changes.

intervals (Figure 16.2). The increasing number of publications on time-lapse-based morphokinetic embryo evaluation indicates the importance and clinical potential of this topic.

This chapter will give an overview of different approaches to TLI, including simple incubator inserts acquiring images of a group of embryos cultured over time as well as high-end TLM systems which offer TLI of multiple individual embryos integrated within a built-in incubator. It will further discuss the challenges of current embryo selection and substantiate expectations that improved embryo selection based on morphokinetic analysis of preimplantation embryo development is possible and beneficial.

Approaches to TLI in human embryology

Until the introduction of the first commercial TLI system (EmbryoScope®) in 2009 TLI-based studies were almost exclusively performed under experimental settings and mostly allowed the researcher to follow only one single embryo over a certain time period. Time-lapse was usually done with an inverted microscope that was modified by addition of a heated stage and a microchamber incubation device. In routine IVF laboratories this occupied a complete microscope workstation for the entire observation period.

One of the first studies published by Payne reported the fate of polar body extrusion and pronuclear formation in human oocytes after intracytoplasmic sperm injection (ICSI) [8]. Further experimental work using time-lapse recording of images documenting embryo development revealed the remarkably dynamic nature of embryo development and suggested that the timing of specific developmental events could be used to identify viable embryos in a given treatment [9–13].

Clearly, any routine application of TLI in human IVF requires robust and stable technology certified for IVF. Consequently, novel time-lapse devices were designed for automated routine for clinical use in IVF treatments. The most prominent of the currently available commercial systems can be subgrouped into three different categories.

Incubation chambers built onto existing microscopes

Several companies (e.g., Tokai Hit, Japan) produce incubation chambers that can be placed on the microscope stage of a standard research grade inverted microscope [14, 15]. The incubation chamber provides basic temperature control and the possibility to use premixed incubation gas with a defined composition (e.g., 5% CO_2 and 5% O_2). The prime advantage of such systems is the full range of optical solutions available for research microscopes and the image quality that can be obtained. Some automation is possible with motorized stages and software to acquire sequential images of several embryos from the same patient. However, the system is complicated to set up, time-consuming to operate, and can only handle a single patient at a time. The combined system is not certified for clinical use in IVF and extensive and repetitive exposure to high intensity light from a standard microscope can potentially impair embryo development [16–18]. Such systems have therefore only been used for research purposes, and in veterinary applications.

Image acquisition systems to be placed inside standard incubators

An obvious advantage of an image acquisition insert is the ability to use existing incubators in clinics, where these are already present. However, this is also a risk as the incubators have not been engineered and built to accommodate image acquisition units, and their presence can change internal airflow and induce temperature gradients within the incubator. Embryo-Guard™ was the first commercial attempt to build an image acquisition unit that can be placed inside a standard incubator [19]. However, this never developed into a routine clinical instrument largely because of temperature problems arising from heat produced by motor and camera systems introduced inside the incubator and the system is no longer commercially available (IMT International, personal communication, 2009).

More recent systems have chosen to eliminate all moving parts and have thus employed culture of all embryos in close vicinity and are acquiring a single image of all embryos from a given treatment simultaneously. The advantage of this solution is a relatively simple system with few moving parts and very low heat dissipation inside the incubator. One system is required per patient, and a large incubator can accommodate multiple systems. The disadvantage is a limited optical resolution because of the necessity to photograph a larger area encompassing many embryos. The two current image acquisition inserts have different advantages, notably:

Hoffmann modulation contrast imaging unit for a single patient (PrimoVision™)

This system is based on the well-of-the-well technology [20] that was initially developed to allow for group culture of animal embryos and later adapted for human IVF [21, 22]. One well-of-the-well dish with a capacity for holding 9 to 16 embryos from one patient can be placed in an imaging system that every 5 minutes acquires an image stack of the whole area where the 9 to 16 wells are located. The imaging system itself, which consists of an illumination device and a camera connected to a computer, must be placed into a standard incubator. Publications and recent research have shown the applicability of this system in IVF [22–25].

Dark-field imaging unit with software-based embryo evaluation (Eeva™)

The Eeva™ system is similar to the PrimoVision™ system but acquires time-lapse images under dark-field illumination which differ from the Hoffmann modulation contrast used for embryo evaluation in conventional IVF, but is better suited for digital image analysis. The system uses a software algorithm to classify the embryos in two categories based on their likelihood of developing successfully to the blastocyst stage. The analysis is based on characteristics of the early cleavages from the 1-cell to the 4-cell stage. The software was developed and tested on frozen-thawed human pronuclear stage oocytes that were cultured up to blastocyst [26]. At present the system uses a combination of dark-field illumination and imaging intervals of 5 minutes in one focal plane. Clinical studies using a further developed software version (Eeva™) are ongoing and clinical data may be published in the near future.

Integrated TLI unit combining image acquisition, embryo evaluation, and incubation control

These integrated TLI systems are capable of providing controlled incubation conditions while automatically acquiring images of individual embryos from several patients. In addition, these systems provide a comprehensive digital record of all the treatment information, including the digital images, extensive documentation of the incubation environment, and the treatment outcome information. The two commercial systems that are currently available are:

A modified standard incubator with flexible TLI (InCu-View Live™)

The InCu-View Live™ system consists of a modified standard incubator from Sanyo that hosts a TLI system by Olympus which allows for the incubation and time-lapse analysis of 12 samples with 10 viewpoints (embryos) per sample and 3 focal planes at 15-min intervals using a 10× objective lens. An advantage of the InCu-View Live™ system is the ability to use virtually any culture vessel. The disadvantage of the system is a requirement for time-consuming manual finding of embryos and initiation of the time-lapse process.

A TLM system certified for clinical use in IVF (EmbryoScope®)

The EmbryoScope® was initially developed for oxygen respiration measurements of oocytes [27] and embryos [28, 29]. The further improvement of that system resulted in a stand-alone TLM system, which consists of an integrated unit with a 20× objective lens, an image acquisition system and a benchtop-like temperature controlled incubation chamber with a gas-mixing device including HEPA-filtering and optional UV sterilization. The Embryo-Scope® is certified as a Class IIa medical device and US Food and Drug Administration (FDA) cleared. This device allows for the incubation of 6 EmbryoSlide® culture dishes (equivalent to 6 patients) at a capacity of 12 embryos per slide and an image acquisition interval of 10 minutes per embryo with one image taken at the central focal plane, and up to three images above and three images below the central focal plane. An advantage of this system is its ability to find the embryos in individual micro-wells and initiate image acquisition automatically. Individual numbered incubation wells for each embryo also prevent potential mixing of embryos. A disadvantage is the requirement to use the Embryo-Slide® culture dishes that enable this automatic initiation.

The main differences between the available TLI systems and aspects of TLI

Whereas the Eeva™ system is based on automatic software that predicts the probability of an embryo developing to blastocyst stage, the other systems have integrated evaluation software that presupposes embryo annotation by an embryologist. On the contrary, PrimoVision™ and EmbryoScope® allows development of condition-specific algorithms and the software support model implementation to assist the embryologist in identifying implantation-competent embryos.

An increasing number of recent publications have described various aspects of time-lapse-based embryo selection, which include:

- Safety of clinical routine use of TLI instruments [30, 31]
- Morphokinetic parameters that characterize normal embryo development and in particular the properties of implanting embryos [32–34]
- Factors that may affect timing of human embryo development such as media composition, stimulation protocol, and patient characteristics [35–42]
- Proposed selection criteria and exclusion criteria based on parameters that can only be assessed by TLI [26, 33, 43–45]
- Lessons learned from TLI that can be used to improve standard procedures, for example by optimizing the time-point normally chosen for routine assessment [10, 46, 47].
- Retrospective analyses of outcomes from time-lapse incubations have been compared with concurrent standard incubations in the same clinics [48].

Some of these aspects are summarized in a review article [49].

TLM in clinical IVF

Studies on safety and non-inferiority

TLM integrated with an incubator allows for undisturbed culture conditions, as in contrast to standard IVF, embryos are not removed from the incubator at certain time-points (Figure 16.2).

This, however, has certain implications for routine work and one of the first issues that were discussed relates to the safety of the system, especially with regards to potential negative effects of accumulated light exposure from repeated acquisition of time-lapse images. In standard embryo assessment a dish holding embryos is taken from the incubator once per day and embryo classification is done either at an inverted light microscope or under a stereomicroscope. In contrast, TLI requires light exposure every 5–20 minutes for each individual embryo over the entire culture period of up to 5 days in the case of blastocyst culture. The total integrated light dose has been tested in one TLM device (the EmbryoScope®) and interestingly it was lower compared to a normal standard embryo assessment scheme based on daily annotations (Figure 16.3). This is due to a very short exposure time (15 to 40 ms) for each image and a very low internal light intensity. The system furthermore uses low energy red light (around 635 nm), which is much less likely to cause damage than short-wavelength light.

To evaluate the overall incubation conditions in different time-lapse systems, several studies have been designed to demonstrate non-inferiority of integrated TLM systems compared to standard incubation conditions.

Nakahara and coworkers published the very first study in 2010 [51]. These authors used a standard incubator that was modified with a build-in imaging system that exposed

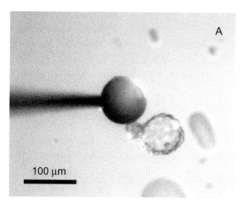
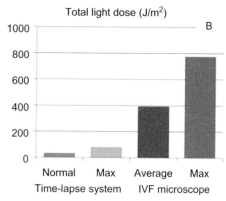

Figure 16.3 Comparison of light exposure within a time-lapse instrument to exposure during standard microscope evaluation. Embryo exposure to light during incubation was measured with a scalar irradiance microsensor with a tip diameter of 100 μm placed within the TLM system at the position of the embryo in the culture dishes. (A) shows the sensor sphere, which measures incident light from all directions and has the same dimensions as the expanding mouse embryo shown next to it. Similar measurements were made with the same sensor on standard microscopes used in fertility clinics. The total exposure time in the time-lapse system during a 3-day culture period and acquisition of 1420 images was 57 seconds, compared to a total microscope inspection time of 167 seconds reported for a standard IVF treatment [50]. As the light intensity measured within the TLM system with the scalar irradiance microsensor was much lower than the light intensity measured in microscopes used in IVF clinics, we found the total light dose during 3 day incubation in the time-lapse system to be 20 J/m^2 ($\approx$ 0.24 μJ/embryo) (normal, time-lapse system, B) as opposed to an exposure of 394 J/m^2 during microscopy in normal IVF treatments ($\approx$ 4.8 μJ/embryo) (average, IVF microscopy, B). Furthermore, the spectral composition of the light in the TLM system was confined to a narrow range centered around 635 nm, and thus devoid of low-wavelength light $\leq$ 550 nm, which has been shown to be inhibitory to embryo development [17, 18] and comprises $\approx$15% of the light encountered in a normal IVF microscope. These light-field evaluations were made in an EmbryoScope™, FertiliTech A/S, Aarhus Denmark as reported in Meseguer *et al.* [44]

embryos every 15 minutes with 0.1 W white light for 80 ms per focal plane. No differences in fertilization rate and the proportion of excellent and good quality embryos on day 3 were found between the TLM and a standard incubator.

Another study found similar blastocyst rates for integrated TLM versus standard incubation in oocyte donation cycles [30]. Fertilized embryos were randomly distributed between a TLM and a standard incubator. Embryo evaluation and selection were based solely on discrete time-points performed by removal of the embryos from the incubation environment (44 hours and 68 hours). No additional information from time-lapse was used for evaluation and selection of embryos. Several parameters were analyzed, for example embryo quality, blastocyst rate, and pregnancy rates. No significant differences were found between the TLM system and the standard incubator for any of the investigated parameters, thus an initial validation of the safety of the TLM. This study was confirmed by another registered clinical trial that compared embryo development in a time-lapse system versus a conventional IVF incubator using a randomization scheme for even distribution of embryos using split cycles [31]. Embryo evaluation was based on discrete time-points and as in the previous study time-lapse information was not utilized for embryo selection. Embryo scoring, selection for transfer and freezing was blinded for the laboratory technician. Progression of embryo development in a standard incubator and in the TLM system was similar, with no significant differences as evaluated by the proportion of embryos with $\geq$ 4 cells on day 2, of embryos with $\geq$ 7 cells on day 3, or of blastocysts on day 5.

In conclusion, all the above studies reported that culture of embryos in a TLM system supports embryo development similarly to culture in a conventional incubator. The physical and mechanical devices in the investigated TLM system have no negative effect on embryo viability, development in vitro, and implantation.

Morphological selection criteria: TLM versus standard embryo assessment

Assessment of embryo viability based on morphological appearance has been an essential part of embryo selection from the very first human IVF treatments and it still is today. A clear correlation between embryo morphology and viability is well established, and extensively documented in the scientific literature [3, 5, 52].

The sequential procedures currently applied in IVF clinics usually rely on three to four observations of embryo morphology to select a viable embryo for transfer. The time-points for making these observations have been chosen to give as much information as possible while avoiding odd working hours (e.g., late evening, night-time, and early morning) [6, 7]. These observations provide a very limited static view of a highly dynamic developmental process. Furthermore, it is widely believed and acknowledged that important events indicative for viability may occur unnoticed between these static observations. Despite that, embryos that are symmetrical and at the most advanced stage of development on the day of transfer are most commonly chosen for transfer.

However, it is generally recognized that even embryos with good morphology may fail to implant while asymmetrical embryos with poor morphology may in some cases succeed. Chromosomal defects, such as aneuploidy (i.e., an abnormal number of chromosomes), have been shown to reduce or eliminate the viability of embryos (see review by Ambartsumyan and Clark [53]). While some of these defects can lead to abnormal embryo morphology, other defects can latently be present in healthy-looking embryos with good morphology at the time of selection for transfer [54–56].

In view of the shortcomings of an approach that traditionally assessed both timings and some morphological criteria such as pronuclear scoring, early cleavage, and blastocyst score on day 5, TLI gives a new insight on some of these selection criteria and reveals the difficulty of applying these at a single static time-point [57].

Early cleavage

An important developmental parameter to consider as an initial quality indicator is "early division" to the 2-cell stage, (i.e., before 25–27 hours post insemination/injection). In this approach, embryos are visually inspected 25–27 hours after insemination to determine if the first cell division has been completed. Several studies have documented a strong correlation between early cleavage and subsequent developmental potential of individual embryos (Figure 16.4) [3, 58, 59].

All studies, including those shown in Figure 16.4, found very strong and highly significant differences in viability and implantation rates between embryos with early cleavage and those that did not cleave early. Only one study found that early cleavage at 25–27 hours cannot be used for embryos from an antagonist stimulation protocol [61].

Several observers pointed out the need for more frequent observation; however, frequent observations, with associated transfers from the incubator to an inverted microscope,

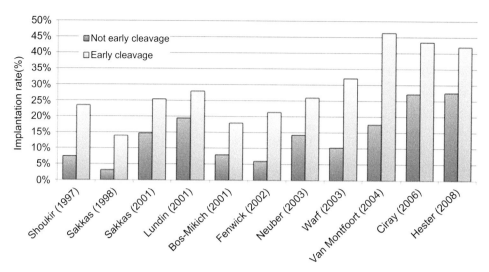

Figure 16.4 Overview of literature in view of implantation rates for early cleaving embryos (EC) and late cleaving embryos (Not EC) using an assessment period of 25–27 hours (figure based on Hesters *et al.* [60]).

induce a physical stress that may have a potential negative impact on embryo development. Frequent observations are also time-consuming and difficult to incorporate in the daily routine of IVF clinics. All the above studies thus relied on a single static observation that only determined if an embryo had already cleaved at a particular time-point or not. These studies did not attempt to determine at what time-point the first cleavage had occurred.

Early cleavage in view of TLM

Different laboratories have been more or less stringent in maintaining a rigorous observation regimen that takes procedural parameters that may affect the timing of the first cell division into account. These parameters include the method of fertilization (IVF, ICSI), the type of culture media used, and the stimulation protocol [10, 61, 62]. The clear advantage of TLI is that the exact onset and duration of the first cell division can be automatically and precisely assessed [63].

Therefore, it is not surprising that time-lapse revealed substantial variability in the onset of early cleavage in human embryos. A retrospective study on parameters that are linked to embryos with known implantation compared to embryos with no implantation reported an optimal window for the first cleavage, comprising 24.3–27.9 hours post ICSI. Embryos with cleavage times in this range had an implantation rate of 31% versus 19% for embryos outside this range [44]. Another study showed that if early cleavage is defined as division prior to 26 hours post ICSI, almost half of the embryos defined as early-cleaved embryos do actually cleave before 25 hours [57].

Too early cleavage and subsequent earlier division cycles is much less common, but it could indicate embryos with chromosomal aneuploidy. For day 3 embryos, Magli and colleagues showed that embryos with too high cell numbers (as well as those with too low cell numbers) at 62 hours post insemination were less likely to be genetically normal (Figure 16.5) [64]. Thus it appears that among a cohort of early cleaving embryos there may be a small fraction that cleave too quickly or show direct cleavage from 1 to 3 cells, and those are likely to be genetically abnormal.

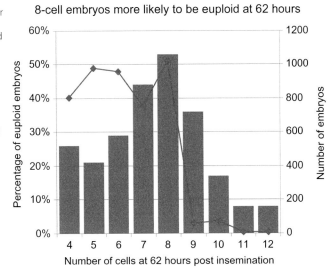

Figure 16.5 Embryos with either a slow or a fast developmental progression on day 3 – expressed by the number of blastomeres – are more prone to an abnormal chromosomal content. Interestingly, almost half of the embryos on day 3 are outside of the expected range of development defined as 6- to 8-cell stage (modified from Magli *et al.* [64]). Bars correspond to percentage of euploid embryos, the curve/diamonds correspond to number of embryos.

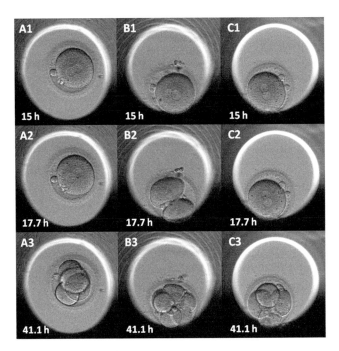

Figure 16.6 Three embryos from one patient are shown (A–C) where the embryo in the middle column (B1) showed fading of the pronuclei at 15.25 hours post ICSI and early cleavage at 17.7 hours (B2). By day 2 the embryo had already advanced to the 8-cell stage (B3; 41.1 hours) whereas the other two embryos showed a normal cleavage pattern with 4 cells on day 2 (A3 and C3).

   Time-lapse image analysis may allow predicting premature embryo cleavage on day 2 based on aberrant observations as early as on day 1. An example from a routine treatment cycle is shown in Figure 16.6 where one embryo showed a fading of the pronuclei already at 15.25 hours after ICSI. The same embryo underwent early cleavage to the 2-cell stage at 17.7 hours and reached the 8-cell stage on day 2 by 41.1 hours. Although this is an extreme example, it points to the importance of very early events like premature pronuclear fading and subsequent unusually early cleavage that may already serve as an indicator for impaired embryo quality despite the morphological appearance looking fine and sometimes passing unnoticed. In view of this the term early cleavage would better be replaced by the term "optimal first cleavage window."

Blastomere size and fragmentation

Over a decade ago, embryos with even-sized blastomeres were shown to exhibit higher implantation rates [65]. Scott and colleagues subsequently published a remarkable demonstration of the reduced viability of uneven-sized embryos [5].

However, it is sometimes difficult to distinguish between blastomeres of uneven size and large fragments that may arise after cell divisions and this is a major hurdle in static observation and systems with low-resolution images. Although a smaller blastomere may contain a nucleus, thus making it better distinguishable from a fragment, this may only be visible for a certain time period during the cell cycle.

Furthermore, the degree of fragmentation is a notoriously difficult parameter to quantify objectively. Computing a quantitative measurement of fragmentation using image analysis is very time-consuming and difficult to perform on a routine basis even at a few discrete time-points per embryo [66].

To complicate matters, previous time-lapse studies have shown that appearance and disappearance of fragments is a dynamic process and can be very dependent upon the observation time-point (Figure 16.7). Qualitative evaluation of time-lapse images revealed that fragments are sometimes reabsorbed, and embryos that appear highly fragmented immediately after cleavage, can appear very differently even half an hour later [10, 14, 67].

Furthermore, the morphological appearance of embryos does change, especially after the completion of a cleavage cycle. It has been shown that embryo grading is subject to change if scoring is done at 38.40 or 42 hours post ICSI and that 33–49% of the embryos are scored different [57].

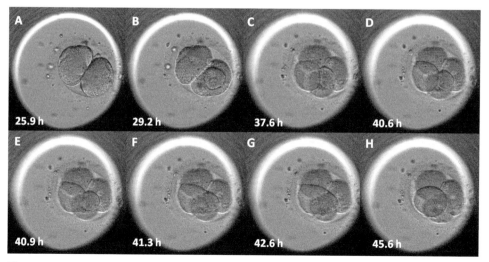

Figure 16.7 Appearance and disappearance of a fragment. In this embryo a fragment appeared at the 2-cell stage (A/B) which persisted for quite some time (C–E) before it merged (F) and finally fused (G) to a blastomere at the 4-cell stage which then rounded up (H).

Advantage of kinetic analysis of embryo morphology with TLM

TLM allows a more clear and informed distinction between uneven-sized blastomeres and the products of fragmentation events as well as investigating any recovery from previous fragmentation. Access to a complete documentation of individual embryo development will enable the embryologist to detect appearance and disappearance of a nucleus in blastomeres of different size. It will further enable fragmentation estimates based on the stable residual fragmentation that is present between cell divisions, as opposed to the pronounced and highly irregular fragmentation that may occur only transiently in connection with cell division events. It is hypothesized that the transient fragmentation that does not lead to permanent loss of cytoplasm, as the fragments are reabsorbed, could be less harmful than persistent fragmentation whereby valuable biomass is permanently lost from the cell [68]. At present we can use this temporal information to select appropriate time-points to evaluate the degree of fragmentation and evenness of blastomere size (i.e., midpoints between cell division).

Finally, it could be speculated that transient fragmentation may be the cause of aneuploidy, in which case transient fragmentation may be equally detrimental. Prolonged cytoplasmic rearrangements connected with cell divisions may thus be an indicator of poor viability.

Multinucleation

Numerous studies have shown that multinucleation impairs embryo viability [5, 68]. It can be argued that multinucleation in a single cell at the 4- or 8-cell stage may not be detrimental, since that particular blastomere may be excluded from the developing embryo, and subsequently degenerate by apoptosis. However, apoptosis will reduce the total available biomass and resources for the developing embryo, which may impair subsequent development, and many embryologists agree that embryos with substantial multinucleation are not likely to be viable. Recent results with embryos with a single multinucleate blastomere may indicate that even a single multinucleate cell may be detrimental [5].

Analyzing multinucleation with TLI

A particular problem with routine static assessment of multinucleation is that the nuclear membrane dissolves prior to cytoplasmic cell division, and only reforms in the daughter cells after the division is completed. It is therefore not always possible to assess multi-nuclearity, when the embryo is only observed at a few defined time-points.

With time-lapse microscopy it is possible to evaluate multinucleation at optimal time-points such as midpoints between cell division events. However, the impact of multinucleation is at present under discussion [69, 70]. An interesting and surprising finding of TLI is that multinucleation at the 2-cell stage appears significantly less detrimental to embryo viability than multinucleation at the 4-cell stage or later. This is surprising as a multi-nucleated blastomere at the 2-cell stage gives rise to a large fraction of progeny cells that could be adversely affected (i.e., 50% of the cells in the developing embryo). However, it has frequently been observed that daughter cells of a multinucleated 2-cell embryo all appeared normal with a single nucleus at the 4-cell stage [69–71].

Further, TLI does sometimes reveal the underlying reason for multinucleation. The embryo shown in Figure 16.8 was characterized by so-called reverse cleavage, which means that at the 4-cell stage the initiation of another cleavage cycle was initiated twice but that

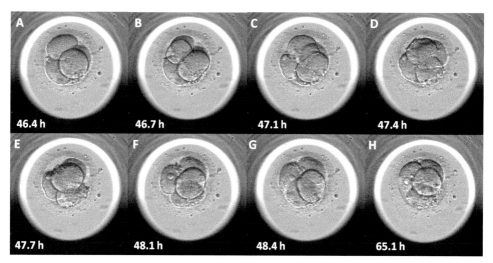

Figure 16.8 Reverse cleavage at the 4-cell stage and multinucleation. This embryo started at the 4-cell stage (A); cleaved to a 5-cell stage (B) but only for a very short time period, as the fifth cell immediately reversed cleavage and fused to another blastomere (C). During further development the embryo initiated another cleavage cycle (D; E) that was again characterized by reverse cleavage (F–H). The embryo showed multinucleation and finally progressed to the 8-cell stage and even reached the blastocyst stage but was not transferred.

blastomere/cell division did not occur. Instead multiple nuclei could be observed after several rounds of reverse cleavage.

Using array comparative genomic hybridization (array-CGH) embryos derived from reverse cleavage were analyzed and reported to be euploid [72]. However, provided that reverse cleavage is associated with a complete replication of all chromosomes from one or more blastomeres, array-CGH will not be able to detect this kind of ploidy. Hence these data need to be confirmed by other chromosomal detection methods that allow distinguishing the presence of a few polyploid blastomeres among euploid ones.

Novel TLM-based selection and de-selection parameters

Besides the established selection parameters outlined above, which can all be more readily and accurately quantified by TLI, there are a number of novel and intriguing parameters that can be assessed exclusively or at least far more efficiently through TLI. These will be presented and discussed in this section.

Time-lapse-based embryo assessment: defining annotation parameters

A central value of TLM is the ability to characterize and quantify the temporal occurrence of key events in embryo development, thus requiring a concise terminology to describe and exchange information about these events. We will thus initially give an overview of the current terminology that has been proposed for morphokinetic parameters in recent publications. The different parameters are depicted in Figure 16.9 and the individual parameters are explained in the figure legend. The list of parameters is not intended to be comprehensive but focuses on those parameters that have been proposed to be useful in embryo quality assessment algorithms.

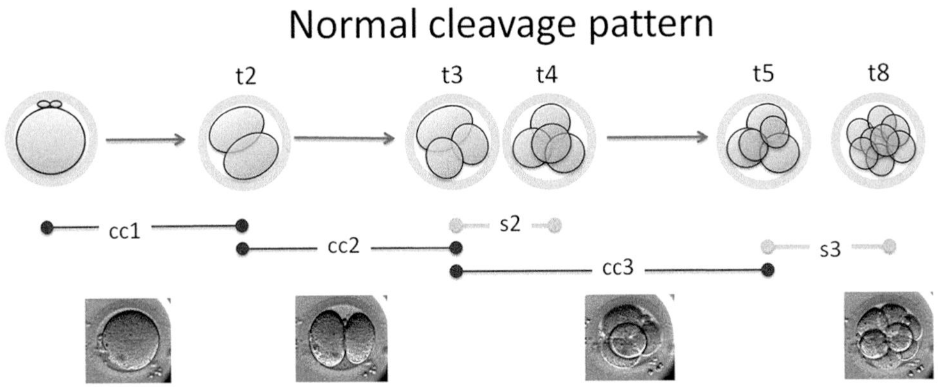

Normal cleavage pattern

Figure 16.9 Graphic representation of parameters describing key events in embryo development. Cleavage times, t2, t3, t4, t5, and t8, are usually measured as the first time-points after cytoplasmic division has been detected and the ensuing daughter cells are completely separated by a confluent cell membrane. The cleavage times are numbered tN, where N refers to the number of cells formed, t2 is the time of completed division to 2 cells, t3 to 3 cells, etc. Cell cycle times, cc1, cc2, and cc3 are the time intervals required for completing of the cell cycles for the fastest developing cell line. cc1 is the unusual first cell cycle from insemination to completion of the first division (i.e., cc1 = t2), cc2 is the second cell cycle: cc2 = t3 − t2, and cc3 is the third cell cycle, which starts with the formation of a third-generation cell at t3 and ends when the first fourth-generation cell is formed at t5: cc3 = t5 − t3. The difference in cleavage timing between progeny in the different cell generations are indicated by the synchrony, sN; the synchrony of the second cell cycle: s2 = t4 − t3 is the difference between cleavage times of the two first blastomeres, s3 = t8 − t5 is the synchrony of the four cleavages going from 4 to 8 cells. It should be noted that low s2 and s3 values indicate asynchronous cell divisions.

Even cell numbers and synchrony of division

An indirect measure of lack of divisional synchrony can be observed if embryos are in the 3-cell or the 5-cell stage at day 2 or day 3, respectively, thus showing uneven cell numbers at the standard observational time-points which most likely reflect delayed development and a pronounced dyssynchrony of cell divisions. However, asynchrony of cell division can only be detected if the embryo has an odd number of cells at the exact time of observation. Unfortunately, the second and third cell divisions (i.e., from 2 cell to 3 cell and then to 4 cell) occur approximately 37–41 hours after fertilization, which in most clinics occurs very early in the morning on day 2 (e.g., before 6 a.m.). Using static observation, very few laboratories – if any – make an attempt to evaluate the synchrony of nucleus disappearance, cytoplasmic division, and nucleus reappearance.

Very convincing data published by Scott and colleagues demonstrated that embryos with an uneven cell number at the standard observational times (i.e., 44 hours and 68 hours after insemination) invariably fail to implant [5]. However, characterizing and quantifying the extent of division asynchrony clearly needs successive observations of the same embryo within a short time period. For the early cleavage stage, it is hypothesized that the two daughter cells arising after the first division should optimally be symmetrical and develop in synchrony. It has been reported that synchronous appearance of nuclei after the first division, and synchrony of subsequent divisions are also significantly associated with pregnancy success and can be an indicator of embryo quality [5, 10]. Asynchronous divisions may indicate genetic abnormalities that are similar to those recorded in arrested embryos [64, 65].

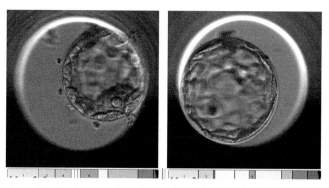

Figure 16.10 Uneven cell numbers and asynchronous division. The bars below the images depict a timeline for embryo development. The numbers (1, 2, 4, or 8) indicate the cell number in the respective periods. The stages with an extended duration due to DNA replication corresponding to 1, 2, 4, or 8 cells are shown in shades of green. Transient stages such as 3, 5, 6, or 7 cells due to lack of synchrony are shown in yellow. Stages of compaction and blastulation are indicated in blue. The blastocyst on the right is more expanded than the left one. However, time-lapse images of the embryo to the left revealed synchronous divisions from the 2-cell stage to the 4-cell stage and a relatively fast progression from the 4- to 8-cell stage. In contrast, the embryo to the right immediately divided from the 2- to the 6-cell stage and spent a long time in the 6- to 7-cell stage prior to reaching the 8-cell stage, which was of short duration. Although the time interval from the onset of the 2-cell stage until the end of the 8-cell stage is identical in both embryos, the one at the left has a better history of even cell numbers and synchronous cleavage cycles. The asynchronous cell division of the right-hand embryo could indicate a lower quality and the embryo to the left should probably be preferred for transfer. See plate section for color version.

TLI of embryo division cycles

TLM reveals that time spent at an "odd" cell state can be significantly different between embryos. In some cases these differences are not visible at the standard observation time-points and conventional evaluation based on static observations will not be able to take these differences into account. Time-lapse observation allows unattended and accurate assessment of the degree of asynchrony (see Figure 16.10).

Duration of cleavages and cell cycles

The duration of the cytoplasmic cleavage and subsequent rearrangements of the individual blastomeres appears to be highly indicative of subsequent viability of bovine embryos [63]. In initial studies, the number of cellular movements was quantified between consecutive image frames in a time-lapse image series. The resulting blastomere activity displayed pronounced peaks at times of cell divisions and could thus be used to determine the timing of cell divisions [73]. Prolonged periods of cellular rearrangements following a cell division event were indicators of poor embryo viability and correlated with poor developmental competence and failure to develop to the expanded blastocyst stage [74].

The duration of the first cell cleavage expressed as the time from the detection of the first indentations in the cytoplasmic membrane to the complete separation of the daughter cells by confluent membranes (i.e., the cytokinesis) was likewise found to correlate with a subsequent ability to develop to expanded blastocysts for human embryos [26]. The authors propose combining a fast cell cleavage (i.e., cytokinesis < 33 minutes) with criteria for cleavage synchrony (i.e., s2 < 5.8 hours) and for cell cycle length (i.e., cc2 between 7.8 and 14.3 hours) to evaluate whether a given embryo is likely to develop successfully to the expanded blastocyst stage.

Related findings were recently reported by Cruz and colleagues for human embryo development [75]. According to the data presented by Cruz and coworkers, the blastocyst formation rate as well as the quality of the blastocyst was strongly dependent on the timing of cleavage to 5 cells in hours after ICSI, (t5), synchronous division (s2), evenness of blastomere size at the 2-cell stage, absence of multinucleation at the 4-cell stage, and on the timing of cleavage events in particular so that they allow time for DNA replication (cc2).

Timing of cleavages and other embryonic events

The timing of the cytoplasmic cleavages appears to be linked to successful implantation as shown in a retrospective analysis on time-lapse data from human embryos [76]. The timing of first, second, and third cleavage, as well as the timing of pronuclear (PN) formation and fading, were analyzed for 159 transferred embryos where the outcome was either 100% implantation (where the number of gestational sacs confirmed by ultrasound match the number of transferred embryos), or 0% implantation. For each event the timing was measured in hours after ICSI. Table 16.1 is a recompilation of the data originally presented by Herrero and colleagues [76]. In this study they classified the embryos according to their morphokinetic timing for the respective parameters based on quartiles. The first and preferred class for each parameter includes embryos with timing in the two central quartiles; and the second category includes embryos with timing in the two outer quartiles, referred to as "outside range" in Table 16.1. It should be noted that cycles with partial implantation (e.g., one gestational sac after transfer of two embryos) are NOT included in

Table 16.1. Percentage of embryos with known implantation that implanted for quartile based ranges of different morphokinetic parameters.

Event	PN formation		PN fading *		First division *		Second division *		Third division *	
Time-range (h)	7.8–11.1	Out-side range	22.3–25.8	Out-side range	24.4–28.2	Out-side range	35.3–40.6	Out-side range	36.0–41.6	Out-side range
100% implantation	15	13	23	12	23	12	13	5	19	7
0% implantation	60	62	55	67	57	67	43	52	45	56
Percentage known to implant	20%	17%	29%	15%	29%	15%	23%	9%	30%	11%
Significance assessed by χ^2 test	NS		P = 0.031		P = 0.039		P = 0.036		P = 0.009	

* Denotes significance (P < 0.05).
NS = not significant.
Data recompiled from Herrero et al. [74].

the analysis as it is not clear which embryo implanted. The "percentage known to implant" is thus substantially smaller than the gross implantation rate for the clinic in the reported time period.

For the events of PN fading, first, second, and third cleavage, the abundance of 100% implanting embryos is significantly higher in the central quartiles category than in the "outside range" category (Chi-square test, $P < 0.05$). In conclusion, the timing of PN fading, and first, second, and third divisions appears to be significantly linked to successful embryo implantation.

Embryo evaluation algorithm

Based on an extension of the data shown in Table 16.1 comprising 247 embryos with known implantation outcome as detected by fetal heart beat (61 implanting and 186 that failed to implant), the same group applied the classification approach by using quartiles for each of the parameters which were previously presented in Figure 16.9. The parameters include: time of division to 2-cell, 3-cell, 4-cell, and 5-cell stage (t2, t3, t4, and t5), the duration of the cell cycles in the 2-cell and 4-cell stage (cc2 = t3 – t2; cc3 = t5 – t3) and the synchrony of division from the 2-cell to the 4-cell stage (s2 = t4 – t3) and from the 4-cell to the 8-cell stage (s3 = t8 – t5) [44]. Based on the correlation with the known implantation data the authors established a hierarchical ranking of their criteria and found that t5 had the highest efficacy to predict for implantation followed by s2 and cc2. This approach was further used to propose a hierarchical classification algorithm to identify the embryos with the highest probability to implant. The primary criterion was the cleavage time to five cells, t5, which should be in the range from 48.8 to 56.6 hours after ICSI; the secondary criterion was a synchronous cell division with s2 < 0.76 hours and a tertiary criterion was where the second cell cycle should be cc2 < 11.9 hours. Exclusion criteria were: direct cleavage from zygote to 3 or more cells (cc2 < 5 hours); multinucleation at the 4-cell stage; and markedly uneven cell size at the 2-cell stage. This model is currently being tested in a prospective multicenter study [77].

De-selection parameters

In addition to positive selection criteria, another major concept that has emerged from TLI studies is the concept of de-selection. One of the most discriminative de-selection parameters appears to be direct cleavage from the zygote stage to the 3-cell stage within less than 5 hours (Figure 16.11). The potential clinical benefit of applying this de-selection marker has been addressed in a retrospective multicentric study [33] where the implantation rate of direct cleaved embryos was reported to be below 2% compared to a known implantation rate of >20% in the control group.

A possible explanation for the poor implantation of directly cleaving embryos is that these embryos may not have enough time to perform a proper DNA replication and in addition may have a spindle or centriole configuration that is abnormal. Consequently, one would expect a higher incidence of chromosomal abnormalities in such embryos and this has been reported in an animal system [78].

Initial data for human embryos have been reported at ESHRE 2012 evaluating chromosomal normality of embryos with direct cleavage. The aneuploidy rate in such an embryo was found to be abnormally high; however, further data are needed to give a definite picture [79].

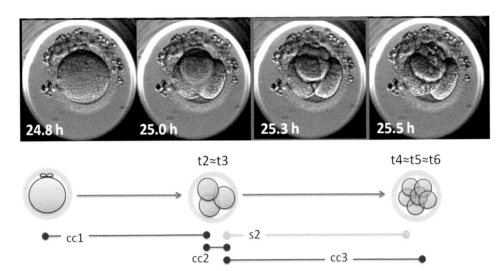

Figure 16.11 A human zygote after pronuclear fading is shown, which cleaved in less than 5 hours directly from the 1-cell to the 3-cell stage. Direct cleavage does not leave time for every blastomere to complete cell cycle-related events such as DNA replication. These embryos are characterized by a very short second cell cycle, cc2 and a very long s2.

Adapting TLI strategies

When starting to use TLI in a laboratory it is initially difficult to find appropriate selection and de-selection markers and to combine them in an appropriate evaluation algorithm. It is thus tempting simply to implement morphokinetic classification criteria reported in the previously mentioned publications in one's own IVF program. However, while such an approach may indeed result in improved success rates, it may also fail to produce better results if the evaluation criteria do not fit to a given subset of patients or even to the entire IVF program, which could be due to differences in operational practice (media, incubation conditions, stimulation, etc.) between different clinics. It should be remembered that any kinetic event is based on fundamental principles of cell biology and physiology. Therefore, it is not surprising that numerous factors can influence the course and timing of cellular functions (Figure 16.12). Some of these factors can be measured and controlled, such as incubation conditions (temperature, pH, oxygen concentration, media, etc.). However, others may escape unnoticed, either because their relationship with embryo development has not yet been established or because underlying complexity impairs the necessary evaluations. A clear relationship between timing of embryo development measured using TLI has already been described for different stimulation protocols [36], laboratory procedures [80], and for different culture media [35].

It is therefore recommended when starting with TLI, to initially adapt and incorporate relatively robust de-selection parameters in a first phase. Criteria such as avoiding transfer of embryos that cleaved directly from the zygote stage to 3 cells or more within less than 5 hours appear generally applicable. In a second phase, when more data from previous treatments in the specific clinic become available, it would be interesting to evaluate potential selection parameters based on the retrospective application of different selection

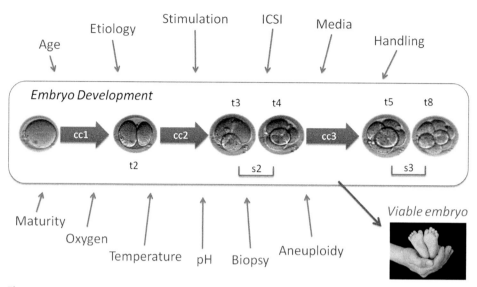

Figure 16.12 Factors that are prone to affect the morphokinetic parameters characterizing human embryo development.

models on the clinic's own data set to discover which model appears to provide the best estimate of embryo viability.

Is there a clinical benefit of TLI?

TLI has been and is still broadening our understanding of basic embryology, and the full benefit of TLI will only be realized as we gradually learn to interpret differences in embryonic development and efficiently use morphokinetic parameters to select the most viable embryo for transfer in any given treatment.

However, any study of possible improvements in the outcome due to TLI is obviously interesting.

One retrospective analysis has recently shown that TLI appears to have had a significant beneficial effect on implantation and pregnancy rates in a large IVF program [48]. This study was based on data from 10 IVF centers comprising 7305 concurrent ICSI treatment cycles. Embryos from 1390 cycles were cultured in a time-lapse system and 5915 in standard incubators. After evaluating and accounting for a wide range of confounding factors it was shown that TLI gave a relative increase of the clinical pregnancy rate of +20% per treatment with oocyte retrieval. The cancellation rate after incubation in the TLI system was significantly lower so when measuring the improvement per transfer it was only +15%. In view of the reported potential for different prognostic factors that are currently being evaluated for raising the success rates in ART, TLI appears definitely to be one of the most effective technologies. This may also explain why TLI is spreading rapidly as a novel technique in fertility centers.

Conclusions

TLI does change the routine in most IVF laboratories. It increases the number of times the embryo morphology may be assessed while avoiding the inevitable stress of performing a standard observation which involves transfer of the embryo from the incubator to a microscope and back. Furthermore, with automated time-lapse image acquisition there is no need for laboratory personnel to be on duty at odd hours to maintain a rigorous observation regimen. Instead, a complete documentation of embryo development for any previous time-point may be evaluated and discussed during normal working hours and at any other time where it may be convenient for the laboratory. It has been reported that due to the fascination of time-lapse images and uncertainty about which parameters are most important to annotate the workload feels higher in the beginning when introducing TLI in a new clinic, as everybody in the lab often gathers around the TLI system in the morning and other convenient time-points during the day. However, once the ease of retrospectively assessing any time-point in the developmental history is accepted, time-lapse does integrate smoothly into the daily routine. Experienced and structured clinics often report the TLI system to be a promising time-saver.

Time-lapse does change the embryologists view on embryos. By dynamic observation of embryo development, factors which affect embryo quality can be systematically assessed and used to select or de-select embryos at different stages of development. Based on the rapidly increasing knowledge base for quantitative embryo assessment we predict that further critical parameters and correlations will be identified in the near future and will help our selection of viable embryos.

References

1. ESHRE. ESHRE ART Fact Sheet. 2012; Available from: http://www.eshre.eu/ESHRE/English/Guidelines-Legal/ART-fact-sheet/page.aspx/1061 (accessed October 2, 2013).

2. SART. Data of the US National Registry. 2012.

3. Neuber E, Rinaudo P, Trimarchi JR, Sakkas D. Sequential assessment of individually cultured human embryos as an indicator of subsequent good quality blastocyst development. *Hum Reprod* 2003;**18**: 1307–12.

4. Ebner T, Moser M, Sommergruber M, Tews G. Selection based on morphological assessment of oocytes and embryos at different stages of preimplantation development: a review. *Hum Reprod Update* 2003;**9**:251–62.

5. Scott L, Finn A, O'Leary T, McLellan S, Hill J. Morphologic parameters of early cleavage-stage embryos that correlate with fetal development and delivery: prospective and applied data for increased pregnancy rates. *Hum Reprod* 2007;**22**:230–40.

6. Alpha/ESHRE. The Istanbul consensus workshop on embryo assessment: proceedings of an expert meeting. *Hum Reprod* 2011;**26**:1270–83.

7. Alpha Scientists in Reproductive Medicine, ESHRE Special Interest Group Embryology. Istanbul consensus workshop on embryo assessment: proceedings of an expert meeting. *Reprod Biomed Online* 2011;**22**:632–46.

8. Payne D, Flaherty SP, Barry MF, Matthews CD. Preliminary observations on polar body extrusion and pronuclear formation in human oocytes using time-lapse video cinematography. *Hum Reprod* 1997;**12**:532–41.

9. Adachi Y, Takeshita C, Wakatsuki Y, *et al.* Analysis of physiological process in early stage of human embryos after ICSI using time-lapse cinematography. *J Mamm Ova Res* 2005;**22**:64–70.

10. Lemmen JG, Agerholm I, Ziebe S. Kinetic markers of human embryo quality using time-lapse recordings of IVF/ICSI-fertilized oocytes. *Reprod Biomed Online* 2008;**17**:385–91. Epub 2008/09/04.

11. Meng L, Jastromb N, Alworth S, Jain J. Remote monitoring and evaluation of early human embryo development by a robotic-operated culture-imaging system. *Fertil Steril* 2009;**91**:S7.

12. Mio Y. Morphological analysis of human embryonic development using time-lapse cinematography. *J Mamm Ova Res* 2006;**23**:27–35.

13. Mio Y, Maeda K. Time-lapse cinematography of dynamic changes occurring during in vitro development of human embryos. *Am J Obstet Gynecol* 2008;**199**(660):e1–5.

14. Hardarson T, Lofman C, Coull G, *et al.* Internalization of cellular fragments in a human embryo: time-lapse recordings. *Reprod Biomed Online* 2002;**5**:36–8.

15. Holm P, Booth PJ, Callesen H. Kinetics of early in vitro development of bovine in vivo- and in vitro-derived zygotes produced and/or cultured in chemically defined or serum-containing media. *Reproduction* 2002;**123**:553–65.

16. Hegele-Hartung C, Schumacher A, Fischer B. Effects of visible light and room temperature on the ultrastructure of preimplantation rabbit embryos: a time course study. *Anat Embryol (Berl)* 1991;**183**:559–71.

17. Oh SJ, Gong SP, Lee ST, Lee EJ, Lim JM. Light intensity and wavelength during embryo manipulation are important factors for maintaining viability of preimplantation embryos in vitro. *Fertil Steril* 2007;**88**:1150–7.

18. Takenaka M, Horiuchi T, Yanagimachi R. Effects of light on development of mammalian zygotes. *Proc Natl Acad Sci U S A* 2007;**104**:14289–93.

19. Arav A, Aroyo A, Yavin S, Roth Z. Prediction of embryonic developmental competence by time-lapse observation and 'shortest-half' analysis. *Reprod Biomed Online* 2008;**17**:669–75.

20. Vajta G, Korosi T, Du Y, *et al.* The Well-of-the-Well system: an efficient approach to improve embryo development. *Reprod Biomed Online* 2008;**17**:73–81.

21. Pribenszky C, Losonczi E, Molnar M, *et al.* Prediction of in-vitro developmental competence of early cleavage-stage mouse embryos with compact time-lapse equipment. *Reprod Biomed Online.* 2010;**20**:371–9.

22. Pribenszky C, Matyas S, Kovacs P, *et al.* Pregnancy achieved by transfer of a single blastocyst selected by time-lapse monitoring. *Reprod Biomed Online* 2010;**21**:533–6.

23. Hlinka D, Dudas M, Rutarova J, Rezacova J, Lazarovska S. Permanent embryo monitoring and exact timing of early cleavages allow reliable prediction of human embryo viability. *Hum Reprod* 2010;**25**:i184.

24. Pribenszky C, Losonczi E, Kuron B, *et al.* Effect of maternal factors and culture conditions on in vitro embryo development – a multicenter retrospective study. *Fertil Steril* 2012;**98**:S168.

25. Semião-Francisco L, Samama M, Ueno J. Time-lapse imaging and the ideal time for embryo cleavage on the third day of development: preliminary results. *Fertil Steril* 2012;**98**:S179.

26. Wong CC, Loewke KE, Bossert NL, *et al.* Non-invasive imaging of human embryos before embryonic genome activation predicts development to the blastocyst stage. *Nat Biotechnol* 2010;**28**:1115–21.

27. Scott L, Ramsing NB. Oocyte and embryo respiration rate measurements in a clinical setting – potential to improve embryo selection? *Clin Embryologist* 2007;**10**:5–9.

28. Tejera A, Herrero J, de los Santos MJ, *et al.* Oxygen consumption is a quality marker for human oocyte competence conditioned by ovarian stimulation regimens. *Fertil Steril* 2011;**96**:618–23.e2.

29. Tejera A, Herrero J, Viloria T, *et al.* Time-dependent O_2 consumption patterns determined optimal time ranges for selecting viable human embryos. *Fertil Steril* 2012;**98**:849–57.e3.

30. Cruz M, Gadea B, Garrido N, *et al.* Embryo quality, blastocyst and ongoing pregnancy rates in oocyte donation patients whose embryos were monitored by time-lapse imaging. *J Assist Reprod Genet* 2011;**28**:569–73.

31. Kirkegaard K, Hindkjaer JJ, Grondahl ML, Kesmodel US, Ingerslev HJ. A randomized clinical trial comparing embryo culture in a conventional incubator with a time-lapse

incubator. *J Assist Reprod Genet* 2012;**29**:565–72.

32. Herrero J, Tejera A, Ramsing N, *et al.* Establishing the optimal time ranges of key events during development using time lapse video cinematography. *Fertil Steril* 2011;**96**:S102.

33. Rubio I, Kuhlmann R, Agerholm I, *et al.* Limited implantation success of direct-cleaved human zygotes: a time-lapse study. *Fertil Steril* 2012;**98**:1453–63.

34. Romano S, Albricci L, Stoppa M, *et al.* Morphodynamic analysis of 100 human embryos with known developmental fate *Hum Reprod* 2012;**27**(Suppl 2):i203.

35. Ciray HN, Aksoy T, Goktas C, Ozturk B, Bahceci M. Time-lapse evaluation of human embryo development in single versus sequential culture media – a sibling oocyte study. *J Assist Reprod Genet* 2012;**29**:891–900.

36. Muñoz M, Cruz M, Humaidan P, *et al.* Dose of recombinant FSH and oestradiol concentration on day of HCG affect embryo development kinetics. *Reprod Biomed Online* 2012; **25**:382–9.

37. Fosas N, Redondo AM, Marina F, *et al.* The number of collected eggs in an egg donor cycle alters the kinetic-patterns of the embryo development. *Hum Reprod* 2012;**27** (Suppl 2):ii188.

38. Redondo AM, Marina F, Molfino F, *et al.* Stimulation cycle longer than 12 days affects the kinetics of embryo division in an egg donor program. *Hum Reprod* 2012;**27** (Suppl 2):ii188.

39. Kirkegaard K, Hindkjaer J, Ingerslev HJ. Effect of oxygen concentration on human embryo development evaluated by time-lapse monitoring. *Fertil Steril* 2013;**99**:738–744.e4.

40. Perez-Cano I, Gadea B, Martínez M, *et al.* Oocyte insemination techniques are related with alterations of the embryo development timing in an oocyte donation model. *Human Reprod* 2012;**27**(Suppl 2): ii202–3.

41. Freour T, Dessolle L, Lammers J, *et al.* Comparison of embryo morphokinetics after IVF ICSI in smoking and non smoking women. *Fertil Steril* 2013;**99**:1944–50.

42. Liebenthron J, Montag M, Köster M, *et al.* Influence of age and AMH on early embryo development realized by time-lapse imaging. *Hum Reprod* 2012;**27** (Suppl 2):ii170.

43. Azzarello A, Hoest T, Mikkelsen AL. The impact of pronuclei morphology and dynamicity on live birth outcome after time-lapse culture. *Hum Reprod* 2012;**27**:2649–57.

44. Meseguer M, Herrero J, Tejera A, *et al.* The use of morphokinetics as a predictor of embryo implantation. *Hum Reprod* 2011;**26**:2658–71.

45. Herrero J, Rubio I, Tejera A, *et al.* Defining poor prognosis markers of implantation for embryo selection by time-lapse. *Fertil Steril* 2012;**98**:S18.

46. Fréour T, Lattes S, Lammers J, *et al.* Reconsidering early cleavage in ICSI cycles according to time lapse criteria. *Hum Reprod* 2012;**27**(Suppl 2):ii164.

47. Aguilar J, Ojeda M, Taboas E, *et al.* Time-lapse analysis allows identifying abnormal fertilization in oocytes out of the standard observation period. *Hum Reprod* 2012;**27** (Suppl 2):ii204.

48. Meseguer M, Rubio I, Cruz M, *et al.* Embryo incubation and selection in a time-lapse monitoring system improves pregnancy outcome compared with a standard incubator: a retrospective cohort study. *Fertil Steril* 2012;**98**:1481–9.e10.

49. Kirkegaard K, Agerholm IE, Ingerslev HJ. Time-lapse monitoring as a tool for clinical embryo assessment. *Hum Reprod* 2012;**27**:1277–85.

50. Ottosen LD, Hindkjaer J, Ingerslev J. Light exposure of the ovum and preimplantation embryo during ART procedures. *J Assist Reprod Genet* 2007;**24**:99–103.

51. Nakahara T, Iwase A, Goto M, *et al.* Evaluation of the safety of time-lapse observations for human embryos. *J Assist Reprod Genet* 2010;**27**:93–6.

52. Racowsky C, Ohno-Machado L, Kim J, Biggers JD. Is there an advantage in scoring early embryos on more than one day? *Hum Reprod* 2009;**24**:2104–13.

53. Ambartsumyan G, Clark AT. Aneuploidy and early human embryo development. *Hum Mol Genet* 2008;**17**:R10–15.

54. Basile N, Bronet F, Nogales MDC, *et al.* Time-lapse technology reveals no difference between embryo quality and the chromosomal status of day 3 embryos. *Fertil Steril* 2012;**98**:S142.

55. Melzer KE, McCaffrey C, Adler A, *et al.* Developmental morphology and continuous time-lapse microscopy (TLM) of human embryos: can we predict euploidy? *Fertil Steril* 2012;**98**:S136.

56. Rienzi L, Capalbo A, Colamaria S, *et al.* Relationship between embryo morphodynamic and molecular karyotype in poor prognosis patients. *Hum Reprod* 2012;**27**(Suppl 2):ii291.

57. Montag M, Liebenthron J, Koster M. Which morphological scoring system is relevant in human embryo development? *Placenta* 2011;**32** Suppl 3: S252–6.

58. Salumets A, Hydén-Granskog C, Mäkinen S, *et al.* Early cleavage predicts the viability of human embryos in elective single embryo transfer procedures. *Hum Reprod* 2003;**18**:821–5.

59. Windt ML, Kruger TF, Coetzee K, Lombard CJ. Comparative analysis of pregnancy rates after the transfer of early dividing embryos versus slower dividing embryos. *Hum Reprod* 2004;**19**:1155–62.

60. Hesters L, Prisant N, Fanchin R, *et al.* Impact of early cleaved zygote morphology on embryo development and in vitro fertilization-embryo transfer outcome: a prospective study. *Fertil Steril* 2008;**89**:1677–84.

61. Yang WJ, Hwu YM, Lee RK, Li SH, Fleming S. Early-cleavage is a reliable predictor for embryo implantation in the GnRH agonist protocols but not in the GnRH antagonist protocols. *Reprod Biol Endocrinol* 2009;7:20.

62. Lechniak D, Pers-Kamczyc E, Pawlak P. Timing of the first zygotic cleavage as a marker of developmental potential of mammalian embryos. *Reprod Biol* 2008;**8**:23–42.

63. Ramsing NB, Callesen H. Detecting timing and duration of cell divisions by automatic image analysis may improve selection of viable embryos. *Fertil Steril* 2006;**86**:S189.

64. Magli MC, Gianaroli L, Ferraretti AP, *et al.* Embryo morphology and development are dependent on the chromosomal complement. *Fertil Steril* 2007;**87**:534–41.

65. Hardarson T, Hanson C, Sjogren A, Lundin K. Human embryos with unevenly sized blastomeres have lower pregnancy and implantation rates: indications for aneuploidy and multinucleation. *Hum Reprod* 2001;**16**:313–18.

66. Hnida C, Ziebe S. Total cytoplasmic volume as biomarker of fragmentation in human embryos. *J Assist Reprod Genet* 2004;**21**:335–40.

67. Van Blerkom J. Translocation of the subplasmalemmal cytoplasm in human blastomeres: possible effects on the distribution and inheritance of regulatory domains. *Reprod Biomed Online* 2007;**14**:191–200.

68. Agerholm IE, Hnida C, Cruger DG, *et al.* Nuclei size in relation to nuclear status and aneuploidy rate for 13 chromosomes in donated four cells embryos. *J Assist Reprod Genet* 2008;**25**:95–102.

69. Aguilar J, Perez M, Ojeda M, *et al.* Early blastomere multinucleation evaluated in 2-cells embryos by time-lapse system is not affecting implantation rate. *Fertil Steril* 2012;**98**:S169–70.

70. Muñoz Ramirez J, Galera Fernandez F, Silván Bueno A, *et al.* Importance of multinucleation at 2-cell stage: study in a time-lapse incubator. *Fertil Steril* 2012;**98**:S169.

71. Azzarello A, Hoest T, Mikkelsen AL. The impact of time-lapse assessment on nuclearity: is multinucleation a proper character for embryo selection. *Hum Reprod* 2012;**27**(Suppl 2):ii103.

72. Hickman CFL, Campbell A, Duffy S, Fishel S. Reverse cleavage: its significance with

regards to human embryo morphokinetics, ploidy and stimulation protocol. *Hum Reprod* 2012;**27**(Suppl 2):ii103.

73. Ramsing NB, Berntsen J, Berntsen JDR, inventors; UNISENSE FERTILITECH,A.S., assignee. Embryo quality determination for in vitro fertilization involves determining timing, duration, spatial distribution and extent of observed cell divisions and associated cellular and organelle movement patent WO2007144001-A2; WO2007144001-A3; EP2035548-A2; IN200900285-P1; CN101495619-A; JP2009539387-W; US2010041090-A1; EP2035548-B1; DE602007008419-E. 16.06.2006.

74. Ramsing NB, Berntsen J, Callesen H. Automated detection of cell division and movement in time-lapse images of developing bovine embryos can improve selection of viable embryos. *Fertil Steril* 2007;**88**:S38.

75. Cruz M, Garrido N, Herrero J, *et al.* Timing of cell division in human cleavage-stage embryos is linked with blastocyst formation and quality. *Reprod Biomed Online* 2012;**25**:371–81.

76. Herrero J, Alberto T, Ramsing NB, *et al.* Linking successful implantation with the exact timing of cell division events obtained by time-lapse system in the embryoscope. *Fertil Steril* 2010;**94**:S149.

77. Meseguer M. Looking at embryo development – clinical results from time-lapse RCT. *Hum Reprod* 2012;**27**(Suppl 2):ii36.1.

78. Somfai T, Inaba Y, Aikawa Y, *et al.* Relationship between the length of cell cycles, cleavage pattern and developmental competence in bovine embryos generated by in vitro fertilization or parthenogenesis. *J Reprod Dev* 2010;**56**:200–7.

79. Davies S, Christopikou D, Tsorva E, *et al.* Delayed cleavage divisions and a prolonged transition between 2- and 4-cell stages in embryos identified as aneuploid at the 8-cell stage by array CGH. *Hum Reprod* 2012;**27** (Suppl 2):ii84.

80. Kirkegaard K, Hindkjaer JJ, Ingerslev HJ. Human embryonic development after blastomere removal: a time-lapse analysis. *Hum Reprod* 2012;**27**:97–105.

Chapter

17

Optimizing culture conditions

Kathleen A. Miller

Introduction

The limiting factor in every in vitro fertilization (IVF) laboratory is its ability to grow "viable competent" embryos. With the increasing emphasis to replace fewer or a single embryo back to our patients at transfer time, the IVF laboratory needs to maintain a culture system and environment that can sustain consistent yields of embryos with high implantation potential. Opinions contrast on whether poor embryo development is prognostic of intrinsic oocyte or sperm factors, stimulation issues, or a suboptimal culture system. Often time the difference between a good laboratory and a great laboratory is attention to detail. Although some details may seem insignificant and even unremarkable, they can accumulate and compound causing significant alterations in the laboratory's ability to create viable embryos capable of producing live births.

How can the IVF laboratory maximize the development of viable embryos and confidently and routinely perform embryo transfer with limited numbers of embryos? Firstly, the IVF laboratory design should reflect a controlled environment imitating in vivo conditions for the collection and culture of oocytes, sperm, and embryos [1]. Secondly, the culture system used in the IVF laboratory should be designed to meet the various and diverse needs of an embryo to develop in vitro and avoid unnecessary stressors to the embryo. When an embryo is stressed in culture, the embryo may grow slowly and fail to progress to the blastocyst stage of development. Additionally, embryos produced under stress may have altered metabolism, gene expression and imprinting, reduced viability, and inability to implant [2]. Thirdly, the laboratory's culture system, which includes the environment, equipment, culture media, and technical staff performance; and the system's utilization should be habitually scrutinized to evaluate its ability to create a cohort of viable embryos capable of producing live births in both fresh and subsequent frozen cycles. Fourthly, avoid the impulse to introduce something new into your culture system to overcome the inability of your culture system to produce viable embryos. Instead of implementing new or different media, oils, supplements, incubators, dishes, and/or gases; focus on reducing stressors that may be influencing the ability of your culture system to produce the most competent viable embryos. Frequently what is considered some of the most insignificant details of a culture system can collectively contribute to the success of developing viable embryos.

What details are important?

Usage of an intact culture media system

The composition of culture media used in the IVF laboratory has evolved over the last 15 years with a prevalent usage of "sequential culture media systems" that comprise a range of media and buffers designed to provide optimized support to each stage of the IVF process, from oocyte isolation through fertilization and embryo cleavage out to the blastocyst stage of development [3]. Now a monoculture medium system, where a single medium is supplemented with all the required components to sustain the embryo for growth to the blastocyst stage, is gaining popularity. The monoculture media system is based on letting the embryo choose when and which nutrients and compounds are needed for suitable development [4]. Although many publications report the ability of embryos to grow to the blastocyst stage in a wide variety of culture media systems, the ability of those blastocyst embryos to implant and produce a live birth is significantly dissimilar among different culture conditions [5].

Great care should be taken to select and validate a culture media system that produces highly competent and implantable embryos through all stages of development. Once a culture system is employed, the laboratory should utilize all the media and reagents consistently from one vendor in an attempt to reduce shock to the embryo induced by the introduction of different base components, buffering systems, or pH culture requirements. Likewise, attention should be paid to the number of manipulations and the length of time out of the incubator an embryo is exposed in each culture system.

Maintaining thermal stability

Thermal control is one of the most important culture system variables in the IVF laboratory and requires close attention and management. Oocytes and embryos are particularly sensitive to alterations in temperature. Temperature fluctuations have been known to disrupt spindle and chromosomal organization of human oocytes and cause chromosomal abnormalities of embryos developing from those oocytes [6, 7]. Although 37 °C is the widely accepted tolerance limit for culturing human embryos, the optimal temperature is still debated and many investigators are still researching the best temperature range for embryo culture performance and outcome [8, 9]. Several IVF laboratories are reporting increased pregnancy rates when embryos are exposed to and manipulated and cultured in thermal environments between 36.5 and 36.9 °C [7, 10].

Since incubators and warming surfaces and devices are prone to drift in and out of calibration during normal operation, the IVF laboratory should use equipment with a steady temperature profile. Equipment with a thermal component should be monitored with an external measuring device with a measurement sensitivity of at least ±0.2 °C accuracy [10–12]. Additionally, the actual microenvironment the oocytes and embryos are manipulated and cultured in should be monitored for thermal stability given that the actual temperature of the heated surface is not reflective of these microenvironments. Hot and cold zones in any piece of equipment thermally controlled should be documented (Figure 17.1).

Most designs of the disposable culture dishes do not allow the base of the dishes to come into direct contact with the heated surface due to an air gap. Since air is a poor conductor of heat and reduces the efficiency of heated surfaces, the actual microenvironment to which

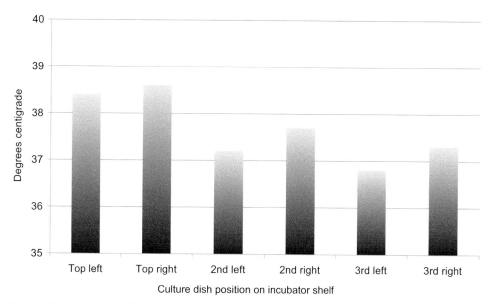

Figure 17.1 Temperature differentials between shelves in Forma 3110 incubator (K. Miller, unpublished).

the oocytes or embryos are exposed to is cooler than the observed temperature of the heated surface. Because temperature loss occurs rapidly and is related to the length of time a culture dish stays out of the incubator; manipulating and observing oocytes and embryos in a temperature and gaseous controlled closed environment, such as an isolette chamber, may contribute to more competent embryos [13–16].

Likewise, having an inadequate number of incubators will result in excessive door openings and fluctuations in the thermal and gaseous phases of the incubators [12, 16, 17]. If at all possible, separate incubators for media equilibration and embryo culture should be used in the laboratory to minimize the embryos' exposure to unnecessary door opening. Several studies have shown that incubators' inability to maintain sufficient thermal and gaseous state control or recovery times of either state can affect the ability of embryos to develop and maintain their competency [18, 19]. A new generation of micro-incubators (0.3 cubic feet) is now available to use for embryo culture and these have been reported to have temperature, humidity, and CO_2 recovery times up to 15 times faster than traditional large volume 6.5 cubic feet incubators [12, 20]. On the horizon, incubators are being developed with time-lapse image capture capabilities that allow for the dynamic and flexible scoring of the developing embryo and allow the embryologist to review and analyze embryos throughout their development without removing them from their incubator environment [21]. Microfluidic technology shows promise in mimicking in vivo conditions, decreasing intervention by laboratory personnel, decreasing gamete and embryo manipulation, and allowing for greater consistency of incubation conditions [22].

Maintaining pH stability

Over the past decade, the optimization of culture media systems has focused on emulating the in vivo environment as closely as possible to the oocyte and embryo's specific stage of development [3]. It is now evident that throughout the developmental processes, human

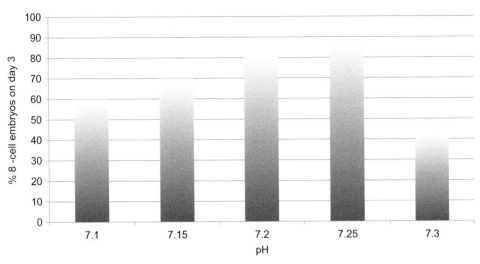

Figure 17.2 Effect of pH on percentage of zygotes developing to 8 cells on day 3 of culture. Based on 96 431 embryos (K. Miller, unpublished).

oocytes and embryos not only have different chemical and nutrient requirements but physical ones as well. Increasing attention is being made to determining and validating the optimum pH values needed to culture oocytes and embryos through the different steps of the IVF process. Several studies have demonstrated that oocytes and embryos require culture environments equilibrated at dissimilar pH values [23, 24]. Typically, oocytes undergoing conventional insemination need a more basic milieu around 7.3–7.4 and several studies have shown in both animal and human models that fertilization rates are compromised if the pH of the fertilization medium falls below 7.2 [3, 25]. Data have also shown that cleavage stage embryos develop better when the pH values of cleavage embryo-specific culture media is at 7.2 (Figure 17.2) and equally cleavage stage embryos develop into higher quality blastocysts when the extended culture medium is at 7.3 (Figure 17.3) [3, 10, 26, 27].

The embryologist is not only faced with the challenges of deciding the target pH which provides the highest fertilization and embryo development rates, but of maintaining the environment to stabilize pH and reduce the fluctuations of pH that may induce stressors to the developing embryos. Minor changes in pH can disrupt many intracellular metabolic processes in the embryo [28, 29]. Although the dogma that overexposure of oocytes and embryos to HEPES-buffered media is toxic is still unrefuted, most embryologists shy away from using bicarbonate-buffered media for all oocyte and embryo manipulations and culture due to the difficulty of keeping these media pH-stabilized outside of the incubator [30]. As previously discussed, the usage of a temperature and gaseous controlled closed environment, such as an isolette chamber, can allow the oocytes and embryos to be manipulated and observed in bicarbonate-based media, reducing or alleviating the toxicity concerns related to using media containing non-bicarbonate buffering systems.

The correct application of a culture media system requires the use of a special environment that is at the very least enriched with carbon dioxide (CO_2), humidity and temperature and maintained in appropriate culture vessels. Media are dynamic entities that react to their climate and atmosphere. Although commercial vendors of culture media have recently been formulating their media products to specific pH values, embryologists are still

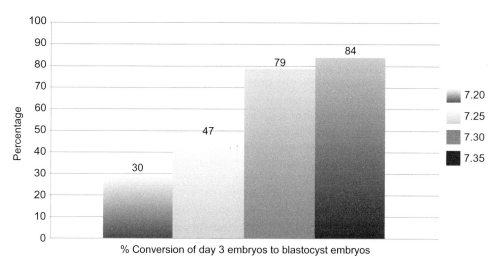

Figure 17.3 Effect of pH on percentage of day 3 embryos developing to blastocysts on day 5/6 of culture. Based on 39 567 embryos (K. Miller, unpublished).

reluctant to fine-tuning the CO_2 concentrations in their incubators to obtain the most precise pH levels [31, 32]. pH should never be adjusted by any other means than titrating CO_2 levels in the laboratory's incubators. Directed daily management of pH values is essential to obtaining the highest outcome levels in the embryology laboratory since every laboratory's environment is different due to many parameters; for example, equipment, culture media, plasticware, temperature, humidity, and/or altitude.

Maintaining osmotic stability and appropriate application and equilibration of culture media and dishes

Essentially today, the culture of embryos in vitro has evolved into the placement of oocytes and embryos into microdroplets of culture media overlaid with culture oil to protect against changes in temperature, humidity, and pH. Although an oil overlay is an essential protective and supportive element to an embryo culture system, culture oil in tandem with plasticware are the least defined components used in embryo culture systems and usually are the source of toxins in the culture systems which can disrupt embryo development [33]. Even though commercially available materials usually arrive with detailed quality control specifications outlining endotoxin levels, pH, osmolality, sterility, and results of a bioassay, IVF laboratories should still conduct their own independent appraisal of materials using set quality control guidelines since the manufacturer is only guaranteeing the integrity of the product at the manufacturing site with no allowance made for shipping irregularities [34, 35]. Confirmation of osmolality and pH of culture media will verify the accuracy of the media preparation process and should be evaluated before media usage. The implementation of several different validation levels of laboratory materials will decrease variation in gamete and embryo development and should successfully avert a total collapse of the culture system.

Culture medium is not inert and reacts rapidly to the climate and atmosphere of its surroundings. Great care should be taken when storing and handling all media solutions used for culturing embryos in the IVF laboratory. Media should be utilized within the manufacturers' reported expiration date and stored refrigerated until usage. Culture media should be opened using aseptic technique in a laminar flow hood and used within 5 days of its first opening. Each patient should have their dishes prepared individually and no more than two microdroplet culture dishes should be prepared at one time so as to avoid evaporation of media during dish preparation. Deviations from established culture dish and media preparation protocols may alter growth conditions and impact subsequent embryo development. Because media osmolality can impact embryo development, the preparation of media and culture dishes should be handled with extreme care and attention. The method of microdrop preparation and the environmental condition under which media and culture dishes are prepared can result in media osmolality shifts that can negatively impact subsequent embryo development. [36].

Embryo culture strategies are diverse and there is no consensus or standardization of culture dish type, open or oil system, media or oil volume and embryo density within the media volume. A culture strategy should be chosen that provides and maintains the most stable environment of temperature, humidity, and pH, is simplistic in function, and develops and supports the most competent embryos. Prior to placing any oocyte or embryo into a culture, culture dishes containing any type of media should be pre-equilibrated for temperature and, if bicarbonate-buffered media are utilized, for pH. Equilibration times should be at least 4 hours although recent studies demonstrated that an 8–10 hour equilibration window was needed to stabilize target pH in culture dishes containing 50 μL microdroplets or 500 μL of culture medium overlayed by culture oil [37]. Culture dishes containing culture media without oil overlay are equilibrated in one hour. Equilibration times should not exceed 18 hours, as the degradation of amino acids, protein sources, vitamins and the antibiotics will begin. Embryos should be changed into fresh medium every 48–72 hours to counteract this breakdown of media components.

When using a bicarbonate-buffered media system it is essential to minimize the amount of time a culture dish is out of the heated gaseous humidified incubator environment. Temperature loss occurs rapidly and is related to the amount of time a culture dish stays out of the incubator. Several studies have shown rapid de-equilibration of both temperature and pH after removal of culture dishes from the incubator and slow re-equilibration [12, 37, 38]. These differences are due to the relative magnitudes of the differential CO_2 contents between the equilibrated medium and air and between the incubator's atmosphere and the partially out-gassed medium [38].

Appropriate manipulation of zygotes and gametes

Oocytes and embryos are extremely sensitive and can sense shear stress. Rough handling of oocytes and embryos during their processing can cause irreparable damage. Shear stress over 1.2 dyn/cm^2 has been reported to cause lethality within 12 hours to blastocyst embryos [39]. Using a pipette that is too narrow or with a jagged edge can also cause damage to the oocyte or embryo [40]. The diameter of the pipette should be slightly larger than that of the oocyte (approximately 130–175 μm), the cleavage embryo (175 μm) or the blastocyst embryo (275–300 μm).

Minimizing embryo observations

Many studies have illustrated a positive correlation with implantation rates when embryo morphological appearances and rate of embryo development are used in tandem to

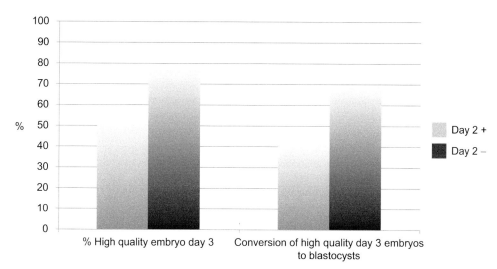

Figure 17.4 Deletion of day 2 observations on day 3 embryo cohort quality and subsequent blastocyst development. based on 9600 embryos (K. Miller, unpublished).

select the highest quality embryos for transfer [41–43]. Despite the development of more sophisticated embryo grading systems, the majority of IVF laboratories worldwide are unable to define and/or trace with certainty the embryos that create live births. Thus, the embryos in their laboratory are subjected to unnecessary observations that generate data never used conclusively to try to select the embryos with the greatest potential to cause a live birth. Studies have shown that improvements in IVF outcome with respect to embryo quality, cryopreservation rate, and possibly implantation rate may result from reduced embryo observations, which contribute to the increased stabilization of the culture environment (Figure 17.4) [44, 45].

Air quality
In IVF laboratories it is well documented that ambient air carries harmful volatile organic compounds (styrenes, formaldehydes, glutaraldehydes, toluene) as well as harmful microbes [46]. Perfumes, deodorants, as well as any odor from the outside environment are potential molecules that deter the development of embryos. The only way to solve this issue is to destroy the harmful molecules. Many studies have shown improvement in embryo quality and reduction of loss rates when air quality was improved in the IVF laboratory. Air can be purified by activated carbon, potassium permanganate, UV and HEPA filtration and sanitization.

Can optimizing culture systems make a difference?
Faced with the possibility of transferring only one embryo in the future due to elective or regulatory pressures attributed to the concerns regarding increased multiple pregnancy rates, IVF laboratories must devote time and attention to the selection and maintenance of appropriate culture systems and equipment. The laboratory should have in place functional quality assurance and improvement programs that enable the monitoring of key laboratory performance indicators. To culture successfully blastocyst embryos that will have high

competency, utilization, and implantation rates and give the clinician and the patient the confidence to transfer only one blastocyst, IVF laboratories must be able to detect laboratory variations beyond the usual and expected before the results manifest into a less than desirable clinical outcome [47]. As more IVF laboratories move forward in their pursuit of improving success rates and lowering multiple births by transferring fewer more competent embryos, attention to fine detail and monitoring relevant laboratory indicators will assist the laboratory in integrating crucial treatment options for patients.

References

1. Practice Committee of American Society for Reproductive Medicine; Practice Committee of Society for Assisted Reproductive Technology. Revised guidelines for human embryology and andrology laboratories. *Fertil Steril* 2008; **90**(5 Suppl):S45–59.

2. Gardner D. Road to single embryo transfer. *Clin Embryologist* 2004;7:1.

3. Quinn P. Media systems used in the assisted reproductive technologies laboratories. In: Patrizio P, Tucker MJ, Guelman V, eds. *A Color Atlas for Human Assisted Reproduction: Laboratory and Clinical Insights.* Philadelphia, Lippincott Williams & Wilkins. 2003;241.

4. Gardner DK, Lane M. Development of viable mammalian embryos in vitro: evolution of sequential media. In: Cibelli J, Lanza RP, Campbell KHS, West MD, eds. *Principles of Cloning.* New York, Academic Press. 2002;187–213.

5. Biggers JD, Racowsky C. The development of fertilized human ova to the blastocyst stage in KSOMAA medium: Is a two-step protocol necessary? *Reprod Biomed Online* 2002;5(2):133–40.

6. Almeida PA, Bolton VN. The effect of temperature fluctuations on the cytoskeletal organisation and chromosomal constitution of the human oocyte. *Zygote* 1995;3:357–65.

7. Wang WH, Meng L, Hackett RJ, Odenbourg R, Keefe DL. Rigorous thermal control during intracytoplasmic sperm injection stabilizes the meiotic spindle and improves fertilization and pregnancy rates. *Fertil Steril* 2002;77:1274–7.

8. Brinster RL. In vitro cultivation of mammalian ova. *Adv Biosci* 1969;4:199–233.

9. Hunter RHF. Temperature gradients in female reproductive tissues and their potential significance. *Anim Reprod* 2009;6:7–15.

10. Higdon HL 3rd, Blackhurst DW, Boone WR. Incubator management in an assisted reproductive technology laboratory. *Fertil Steril* 2008;**89**:703–10.

11. Yeung QS, Briton-Jones CM, Tjer GC, Chiu TT, Haines C. The efficacy of test tube warming devices used during oocyte retrieval for IVF. *J Assist Reprod Genet* 2004;**21**:355–60.

12. Cooke S, Tyler JP, Driscoll G. Objective assessments of temperature maintenance using in vitro culture techniques. *J Assist Reprod Genet* 2002;**19**:368–75.

13. Testart J, Lassalle B, Frydman R. Apparatus for the in vitro fertilization and culture of human oocytes. *Fertil Steril* 1982;**38**:373–5.

14. Khabani A, Tufts K, Craig L, Soules M, Scott L. Cooling and warming rates in microdrops for embryo culture. *Fertil Steril* 2003;**80**:117.

15. Kalan MJ, Francis MM, Lewis DE, *et al.* Temperature fluctuation in culture media in the IVF lab: Is the isolette a better environment than the bench top? *Fertil Steril* 2008;**89**:S21.

16. Kelly PB, Deignan KC, Emerson G, Mocanu E. Assessment of temperature variation during in vitro culturing: a comparison of different IVF micro-environments. *Fertil Steril* 2009;**92**:S234.

17. Sharma L, Tarchala S, Nakagawa J, Perry J, Rawlins R. *Next Generation Quality Control in the IVF Laboratory: Using Data Loggers to Monitor Real Time Incubator Temperature. Technical Bulletin.* California, Marathon Products.

18. Morrison L, Carney S, Portmann M, *et al.* Do busier IVF days from grouped cycles impact pregnancy rates and embryo development? *Fertil Steril* 2005; **84**:S18.

19. Fujiwara M, Takahashi K, Izuno M, *et al.* Effect of micro-environment maintenance on embryo culture after in-vitro fertilization: comparison of top-load mini incubator and conventional front-load incubator. *J Assist Reprod Genet* 2007; **24**:5–9.

20. Lee MA, Grazi R, Seifer DB. Incorporation of the Cook K-Minc – 1000 triple gas incubator and media system into the clinical IVF lab. *Fertil Steril* 2008; **90**:S413–14.

21. Pribenszky C, Losonczi E, Molnar M, *et al.* Prediction of the in-vitro developmental competence of early cleavage-stage embryos with compact time-lapse equipment. *Reprod Biomed Online* 2010;**20**:371–9. doi:10.1016/j. rbmo.2009.12.007.

22. Suh RS, Phadke N, Ohl DA, Takayama S, Smith GD. Rethinking gamete/embryo isolation and culture with microfluidics. *Hum Reprod Update* 2003;**9**(5):451–61.

23. Dale B, Menezo Y, Cohen J, DiMatteo L, Wilding M. Intracellular pH regulation in the human oocyte. *Hum Reprod* 1998;**13**:964–70.

24. Phillips KP, Leveille MC, Claman P, Baltz JM. Intracellular pH regulation in human preimplantation embryos. *Hum Reprod* 2000;**15**:896–904.

25. Miyamoto H, Toyoda Y, Chang MC. Effect of hydrogen-ion concentration on in vitro fertilization of mouse, golden hamster, and rat eggs. *Biol Reprod* 1974;**10**:487–93.

26. Quinn P, Stone BA, Marrs RP. Suboptimal laboratory conditions can affect pregnancy outcome after embryo transfer on day 1 or 2 after insemination in vitro. *Fertil Steril* 1990;**53**:168–70.

27. Ferring Pharmaceuticals. Council for the Advancement of Ovulation Induction and Assisted Reproductive Technology. Marrs RP, Steinkampf MP, chairpersons. The assisted reproductive global monitor.

May council meeting, special meeting reporter, Session 1. 1999.

28. Edwards LJ, Williams DA, Gardner DK. Intracellular pH of the preimplantation mouse embryo: Effects of extracellular pH and weak acids. *Mol Reprod Dev* 1998;**50**:434–42.

29. Nematollahi-mahani SN, Nematollahi-mahani A, Moshkdanian G, Shahidzadehyazdi Z, Labibi F. The role of co-culture systems on developmental competence of preimplantation mouse embryos against pH fluctuations. *J Assist Reprod Genet* 2009;**26**:597–604.

30. Swain J. New pH-buffering system for media utilized during gamete and embryo manipulations for assisted reproduction. *Reprod Biomed Online* 2009;**18**:799–810.

31. Pool TB. Optimizing pH in clinical embryology. *Clin Embryologist* 2004; **7**:1–17.

32. Quinn P, Cooke S. Equivalency of culture media for human in vitro fertilization formulated to have the same pH under an atmosphere containing 5% or 6% carbon dioxide. *Fertil Steril* 2004;**81**:1502–6.

33. Morbeck DE, Khan Z, Barnidge DR, Walker DL. Washing mineral oil reduces contaminants and embryotoxicity. *Fertil Steril* 2010;**94**(7):2747–52.

34. Bavister BD, Andrews JC. A rapid sperm motility bioassay procedure for quality control testing of water and culture media. *J In Vitro Fert Embryo Transf* 1988; **5**(2):67–75.

35. Weiss TJ, Warnes GM, Gardner DK. Mouse embryos and quality control in human IVF. *Reprod Fert Dev* 1992; **4**(1):105–7.

36. Swain JE, Cabrera L, Xu X, Smith GD. Environmental factors and manual manipulations during preparation influence embryo culture media osmolality. *Fertil Steril* 2010;**94**(4):S32.

37. Conaghan J, Steel T. Real-time pH profiling of IVF culture medium using an incubator device with continuous monitoring. *J Clin Embryol* 2008;**11**:15–16.

38. Blake DA, Forsberg AS, Hillensjo T, Wikland M. The practicalities of sequential

blastocyst culture. Presented at ART, Science and Fiction, the Second International Alpha Congress, Copenhagen, September 1999.

39. Xie Y, Wang Y, Zhong W, *et al.* Shear stress induces preimplantation embryo death that is delayed by the zona pellucida and associated with stress-activated protein kinase-mediated apoptosis. *Biol Reprod* 2006;**75**(1);45–55.

40. Xie Y, Wang Y, Puscheck EE, Rappolee DA. Pipetting causes shear stress and elevation of phosphorylated stress-activated protein kinase/jun kinase in preimplantation embryos. *Mol Reprod Dev* 2007;**74**(10);1287–94.

41. Payne D, Flaherty SP, Barry MF, Matthews CD. Preliminary observations on polar body extrusion and pronuclear formation in human oocytes using time-lapse video cinematography. *Hum Reprod* 1997; **12**(3):532–41.

42. Van Royen E, Mangelschots K, De Neubourg D, *et al.* Characterization of a top quality embryo, a step towards single embryo transfer. *Hum Reprod* 1999;**14**:2345–9.

43. Gardner DK, Lane M, Stevens J, Schlenker T, Schoolcraft WB. Blastocyst score affects implantation and pregnancy outcome: towards a single blastocyst transfer. *Fertil Steril* 2000;**73**:1155–8.

44. Khabani A, Shen S, Fujimoto VY, *et al.* Improved embryo quality and rates of cryopreservation with modifications in an in vitro fertilization (IVF) culture system. *Fertil Steril* 2000; **74**:S104.

45. Skiadas CC, Biggers JD, Racowsky C. Correctly classifying viability of day 3 embryos is compromised by evaluations performed on multiple days before transfer. *Fertil Steril* 2009; **92**:S159.

46. Boone WR, Johnson JE, Locke AJ. Control of air quality in an assisted reproductive technology laboratory. *Fert Steril* 1999;**71**:150–4.

47. Mortimer D. Quality management in the IVF laboratory. In: Jansen R, Mortimer D, eds. *Towards Reproductive Certainty.* New York; The Parthenon Publishing Group. 1999;421.

Chapter

18

Low cost IVF

Luca Gianaroli, M. Cristina Magli, and Anna P. Ferraretti

Introduction

It is estimated that more than 80 million couples worldwide suffer from infertility, the reason for which varies greatly among countries basically owing to several factors, both genetic and acquired, which are strictly related to lifestyle differences.

Contrary to the common belief that infertility is a primary problem of Western society, its highest incidence is found in developing countries where it is quoted at rates that very likely are underestimates.

Infertility in developing countries

The most common cause of infertility in developing countries is tubal occlusion secondary to sexually transmitted diseases or pregnancy-related infections, mainly consequent to gonorrhea and chlamydia contagion [1]. These conditions could be efficiently treated with assisted reproductive technologies (ART), which unfortunately are either very expensive or unavailable in developing countries. As a result the large majority of this population has no access to ART and this is in sharp contrast with the extremely negative consequences of infertility, especially for local women. It is well known that in the great majority of developing countries, a woman's status is directly related to motherhood, with infertility being a reason for psychological, social, and economic burden. The magnitude of the problem varies between different geographic areas because of different religious, ethical, and sociocultural influences, but in the most severe realities it can lead to segregation of the woman, to her abandonment, domestic violence, and even suicide [2, 3].

In such conditions, motherhood turns out to be the only manner for women to improve their status within the family and the community, and there is no doubt that ART could represent a favorable option to assist their infertile condition. Unluckily, the access to specific treatments is not open to all people due to many barriers including costs and distance to travel.

In the face of this reality, the concept of low cost in vitro fertilization (IVF) started to take shape in the scientific community and arrived at the practical possibility of offering assisted conception services at minimal cost.

In this respect, two initiatives were especially relevant, namely, the Low Cost IVF Foundation (www.lowcost-ivf.ch) and the ESHRE Task Force on Developing Countries (www.eshre.eu). The non-profit Low Cost IVF Foundation was founded in 2007 by a group

Culture Media, Solutions, and Systems in Human ART, ed. Patrick Quinn. Published by Cambridge University Press. © Cambridge University Press 2014.

of colleagues, Alan Trounson (Melbourne – Australia), Luca Gianaroli (Lugano – Switzerland), Ian Cooke (Sheffield – England), and Outi Hovatta (Stockholm – Sweden), with the aim of promoting the provision of clinical ART services for a cost lower than 200 € that will enable couples, particularly infertile women, to access infertility treatment. Besides implementing clinical IVF at several sites in low-resource countries, the Foundation ensures proper training of the clinicians and scientists involved, as well as education and periodical monitoring of the clinical activities. Working on the same direction, the ESHRE Task Force on Developing Countries has been especially active in promoting debates for the strategic and technical issues involved in making ART more accessible to developing countries.

Affordable ART

Since the birth of the first test-tube baby in 1978, many technical improvements have greatly contributed to increase significantly the reproductive chances of infertile patients. Concomitantly, the cost per cycle has been increasing over the years due to high-tech equipment and complex techniques, making ART an expensive and extended process that is often beyond the reach of the majority of those seeking infertility treatments.

For the successful implementation of infertility care in low-resource settings, several steps must be undertaken including (1) a strategic design of the level of reproductive care, (2) an adequate training of the operators and professionals, and (3) the simplification of procedures to reduce the costs.

Levels of reproductive care should be rationally organized (Figure 18.1) with the first level dedicated to the preliminary work-up, which includes initial examinations to identify fertility problems, semen analysis, and screening for infectious diseases. A second level embracing a smaller number of clinics would comprise sperm preparation for intrauterine insemination (IUI); while a third level including a restricted number of centers would provide the most advanced ART techniques such as IVF and intracytoplasmic sperm injection (ICSI). The advanced level is the most demanding in terms of costs, training, and risks of complications.

A crucial phase for setting up an affordable ART program is represented by adequate training of professionals, both clinicians and scientists, to operate in conditions that often require spirit of adaptation, confronting emergency situations, and having the capacity to solve problems. These demands are tightly dependent on the need to reduce the high costs

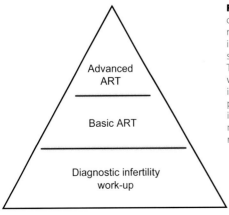

Figure 18.1 Level of reproductive care: distribution of ART centers in a low-resource economy. The first level includes a relatively large number of clinics where patients can have an initial examination to identify fertility problems, including semen analysis and screening for infectious diseases. The second level embraces a smaller number of clinics where sperm preparation can be done for intrauterine insemination. Finally, a restricted number of centers could provide advanced ART techniques including IVF and intracytoplasmic sperm injection (ICSI), which represent the most demanding approaches in terms of costs, training, and risks of complications

that actually represent the key point for the application of standard ART in low-resource settings, where the limited amount of funding is generally directed towards other priorities.

Setting up a program of infertility care in developing countries

The challenge will be to optimize resources by reducing ART costs in relation to the provided benefits, keeping in mind that low cost should not, in any way, imply a compromise on quality. Several aspects in ART could be simplified, from the diagnosis of infertility for the identification of couples that could actually benefit from treatment, to the implementation of simplified technical procedures to be performed in less costly clinical settings. Other important points are the use of minimal equipment acquired at a favorable price and the acquisition of consumables in bulk, as well as the development of strategies that minimize the risks and complications of ART.

There is no doubt that the first step is to select accurately couples that might reasonably benefit from infertility treatment. Logically, when the available funding is not sufficient to treat everyone, a selection must be made according to established criteria that in theory could be based on chances of success, specific costs, and need for motherhood [4].

Data from the literature demonstrate the importance of performing an accurate exploration of the female reproductive tract to increase the chances of live birth [5, 6]. The incidence of intrauterine pathology has been reported to be especially high in infertile patients [7] and for this reason many consider it unacceptable not to implement diagnostic hysteroscopy in the routine exploration of the infertile patient [8]. In this way, major and minor lesions can be detected that can cause or contribute to implantation failure with a consequent negative effect on ART results. Depending on the characteristics of the pathology, major lesions can be treated in an ambulatory setting or referred to the operating room, while for minor lesions the clinical significance is still unclear and results are currently under evaluation [9].

In developing countries, the vast majority of women searching for pregnancy are relatively young with a notably high incidence of surgical pathologies, such as hydrosalpinx and myomas. In consideration of the limited access to ART, diagnostic hysteroscopy should be included in the routine exploration of the infertile patient to identify pathologies that are incompatible with implantation. The currently available equipment is of moderate cost, but certainly proper training of the endoscopist should be performed.

Intrauterine insemination (IUI)

The process of selection means not only to identify patients with a good prognosis for success, but also to address couples to the most suitable treatment.

As mentioned above, IUI could be a good treatment option for selected categories of patients. Although published data show controversial results, the cost-effectiveness of IUI in cases of unexplained infertility or moderate male infertility appears to be higher than IVF [10]. From a technical point of view IUI programs are easy to run and devoid of severe complications, with costs that are greatly lower than IVF/ICSI cycles. In view of these considerations, IUI could be considered as the first-line approach for cases of non-tubal infertility with sperm samples showing parameters close to normozoospermia.

A special application of IUI could be considered for serodiscordant couples. It has actually been documented that in cases of viral infection in the sperm sample, a specific washing procedure and density gradient separation can effectively remove viral particles from the sperm preparation [11, 12]. This approach could be part of a general initiative to counteract HIV transmission in developing countries. It is clear that specialized training of the laboratory staff is mandatory to avoid any risk of cross-contamination or incomplete semen decontamination. The procedure should be only performed in laboratories with dedicated facilities and with access to a reliable viral validation assay. Sample treatment is based on washing to remove the seminal plasma, followed by separation in a discontinuous density gradient; motile spermatozoa are then left to swim-up and recovered for the IUI. Specific conical test tubes have been designed that permit performing the whole treatment in a closed device that can be tightly capped and discarded without having to extract those layers that are potentially contaminated [13]. In this way, various viral particles (human immunodeficiency virus [HIV], hepatitis C virus [HCV], and cytomegalovirus [CMV]) and bacteria (i.e., *Staphylococcus aureus*, *Enterococcus faecalis*, *Escherichia coli*) have been reported to be successfully removed [14].

Hormonal stimulation

Ovarian stimulation protocols are generally complex, long, and expensive, leading to a significant increase in the financial demand on the patient, as well as of certain complications and risks. The use of mild or minimal stimulation protocols could contribute to solving these problems, representing a suitable solution for low-resource countries where priority is given to simple approaches that exclude embryo cryopreservation and try to diminish complications. This implies that IVF doctors (and embryologists) should be prepared to work with fewer oocytes and to maximize their in vivo maturation (meaning that stimulation and oocyte pick-up need to follow optimal timing) and development.

Mild ovarian stimulation usually refers to the use of low-dose gonadotropins in combination with a gonadotropin-releasing hormone (GnRH) antagonist, whilst minimal stimulation refers to the use of clomiphene citrate (CC) in sequential administration followed by low-dose gonadotropins and possibly a GnRH antagonist. CC was especially used in the early days of IVF because of its simplicity of administration (oral), low cost, and acceptable success rates.

To test the applicability of a minimal stimulation protocol as a model to be exported to low cost IVF programs, we set up in our center a program dedicated to patients with good prognosis for pregnancy, namely, young normoovulatory patients at their first ART attempt with tubal infertility or moderate male factor. The finality was to recover the number of oocytes necessary to perform a transfer with no need of cryopreserving spare oocytes or embryos.

Ovarian stimulation was obtained by CC and fixed doses of gonadotropins. Ultrasound monitoring began on the ninth day of the cycle. Embryo transfer was performed on day 2 if ≤ 2 transferrable embryos were available or on day 3 if > 2 embryos were available to allow natural selection of viable embryos in culture.

As presented in Table 18.1, 238 cycles from 112 patients were treated between 2008 and 2010. Cancellation rate due to poor response to stimulation or spontaneous ovulation was 15%. Of the remaining 201 cycles, 112 performed one cycle, 58 two cycles, and 31 three cycles, resulting in a total of 61 clinical pregnancies with a take-home baby rate per patient of 47%. The implantation rate, calculated per fetal heartbeat, was 16.9% per transferred embryo with 9 pregnancies being twins (14.7%) and 2 triplets (3.3%). The high rate of

Table 18.1. Lite IVF: minimal ovarian stimulation with clomiphene citrate and outcome after oocyte pick-up

No. cycles	201
No. patients	112
Maternal age (M±SD), years	33.9±3.1
No. retrieved oocytes (M±SD)	5.3±3.1
No. inseminated	674
No. fertilized (%)	558 (83)
No. embryos (%)	544 (97)
No. transferred cycles (%)	189 (94)
No. transferred embryos (M±SD)	409 (2.2±0.6)
No. clinical pregnancies (%)	61 (32)
No. spontaneous abortions	6
No. ectopic pregnancies	2
Implantation rate/transferred embryo (%)	(16.9)
Take-home baby rate/patient (%)	(47)
OHSS	0

M±SD = mean ± standard deviation; OHSS = ovarian hyperstimulation syndrome.

multiple pregnancies was due to the Italian law on IVF that until the end of May 2009, when it was modified by the Supreme Court, made it compulsory to transfer all the generated embryos [15].

These data suggest that the adopted stimulation using CC is compatible with implantation and delivery, yielding a favorable take-home baby rate and minimizing the risk of ovarian hyperstimulation syndrome (OHSS) occurrence. This approach could be adequate for ART in developing countries being simple, needing a reduced dosage of gonadotropins and fewer days of monitoring. The expected results are lower cost, a decrease in OHSS, and a reduction in multiple pregnancies provided that one or two embryos are normally transferred [16, 17].

Laboratory techniques and equipment

Assisted reproduction laboratory techniques and equipment are expensive and therefore difficult to implement in developing countries [18]. Nevertheless, strategies can be designed to bypass the use of high-technology equipment to reduce significantly the cost of the procedures.

It is well known that gamete/embryo manipulations must be performed in sterile culture-ware, while culture requires chambers gassed with 5–6% carbon dioxide (CO_2) to maintain constant temperature and pH of culture medium.

There are alternative approaches that could significantly reduce the expenses of the program and make it more accessible to low-resourced regions.

- **Sperm preparation**. After liquefaction, the sample can be prepared by the swim-up technique after overlying a milliliter of HEPES-buffered medium on an aliquot of sperm

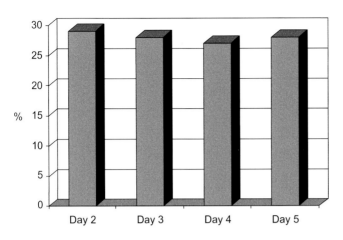

Figure 18.2 Take-home baby rate in 585 cycles according to the day of transfer. All these cycles had at least three embryos on day 2.

in a test tube. In this way the use of a centrifuge is avoided and motile spermatozoa are recovered after 30–60 minutes incubation at 37 °C. The recovered fraction can be used for IUI or for IVF/ICSI.

It is important to specify that in cases of viral infection a centrifuge is necessary to perform the specific washing procedures and density gradient separation that are recommended to remove viral particles from the sperm preparation.

- **Culture medium**. In the early days of IVF, media for embryo culture to day 2 or day 3 post insemination were based on simple salt formulations with added carbohydrate energy sources such as pyruvate, lactate, and glucose, and containing a serum additive. For a long time, these media, T6 [19], HTF [20], and EBSS [21], were used, yielding reasonable pregnancy rates [22]. In the following years, more complex formulations were designed, which are mostly based on the composition of oviduct and uterine fluids. This led to the development of stage-specific sequential media that support each of the three phases of fertilization, cleavage, and blastocysts [23]. Under these conditions, three different culture media are required to reach the blastocyst stage, with the concomitant use of several culture disposables. Nevertheless, for a low cost IVF program, short-term cultures could represent the best option, possibly associated with the use of non-sequential media, including formulations, for example KSOM medium, where the optimization of concentrations permits blastocyst formation [24]. This approach would be more than acceptable especially when considering that there is no proven evidence demonstrating any significant advantage when transferring, in similar categories of patients and under comparable conditions, on day 2, day 3, day 4, or day 5 embryos. Figure 18.2 reports the data from a group of patients treated in our center between 2004 and 2009 that were randomly transferred on different days. In all 585 cycles were considered that had at least three embryos on day 2. The mean maternal age did not differ among the groups and the resulting take-home baby rate was comparable.
- **Submarine incubator**. A classical CO_2 incubator could be replaced by a water bath in which 4-well tissue culture dishes are individually wrapped in waterproof foil bags nearly impermeable to gases such as CO_2, oxygen, and nitrogen and are filled with a premixed gas mixture to create a mini, submarine incubator [25]. Before being admitted to human IVF, the submarine incubator was tested on mouse embryos and the rate of blastocyst formation was comparable to that obtained with conventional culture

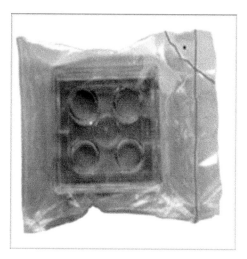

Figure 18.3 A 4-well dish is placed in a foil bag that is heat-sealed (vertical line on the right). The bag is then gently inflated with 5% CO_2 by inserting a 19 G needle in one corner of the bag; the needle is connected to a gas cylinder. A second seal is done internally to the hole and the bag is now ready to be placed in the submarine incubator.

systems [26]. The same Australian group also performed a trial with sibling human zygotes from six patients, which were cultured partly in the submarine incubator and partly in a conventional incubator. The resulting embryo development was comparable, with two resulting pregnancies that were generated after mixed transfers (Jones, personal communication).

According to our proposed protocol for the submarine incubator, two 4-well dishes should be prepared for each patient. The day before oocyte collection, a 4-well dish (referred to as dish A) is set up with 0.5 mL of fertilization medium in each well. A second 4-well dish (referred to as dish B) is set up with a 50 μL drop of fertilization medium under oil in well 1. Each dish is placed in a foil bag that is heat-sealed (Figure 18.3). The bag is then gently inflated with 5% CO_2 by inserting a 19 G needle, which is connected to the gas cylinder through a silicon tube, in one corner of the bag close to the point of the heat seal. The holes are resealed and the two bags are placed in the submarine incubator set at 37 °C.

On the day of oocyte collection, the retrieved oocytes are rinsed in well 1 of dish A and immediately transferred into well 2 and well 3 of the same dish. Dish A is placed again into the foil bag, heat-sealed and gassed as previously described, and returned to the submarine incubator until the time of insemination. Approximately 4 hours later dish A is removed from the bag and the oocytes are inseminated with the prepared spermatozoa. Thereafter, dish A is returned to the foil bag, which is heat-sealed and gassed again. One hour later, the two dishes are removed from the submarine incubator and the partially digested cumulus–oocyte complexes are rinsed in well 4 of dish A and transferred to well 1 of dish B [27]. Dish A can now be discarded, while a 50 μl drop of cleavage medium is dispensed into well 2 of dish B and overlaid with oil. Fertilized oocytes are transferred to this drop at the time of fertilization check, when fresh cleavage medium is placed into well 3 and well 4 of dish B in preparation for embryo transfer. The dish is placed into the submarine incubator until the time of transfer. The catheter is loaded directly from the drop in well 4 of dish B.

The main advantages of this system are stability of culture parameters (temperature, humidity, and CO_2 level) and quick recovery of these parameters after resealing of the bag. If the foil bag used for wrapping the dish is transparent, embryo observation can be performed without removing the dish from the bag. The system is safe, non-expensive, at low risk of contamination, and easy for cleaning and transport.

- **Vaginal incubation**. The method of intravaginal culture (IVC) avoids the use of CO_2 incubators by placing both gametes in a sterile vial with culture medium. The vial is sealed and placed into the vaginal cavity where it is held in place by a vaginal diaphragm [28]. The embryos are removed at the time of transfer, usually on day 2, loaded into a catheter, and immediately transferred into the patient's uterus. In this way, handling of oocytes and embryos is kept at a minimum with a concomitant reduction of expenses. More recently, new devices for IVC have been proposed [29] that make the procedure more efficient and simple with a good level of acceptance by patients and reported pregnancy rates of 20% [30].

- **Encapsulated gametes**. This is an evolution of IVC based on the use of a culturing capsule made of a biodegradable semipermeable matrix. The capsule containing oocytes and spermatozoa is transferred into the uterine cavity where it dissolves after fertilization has occurred; in this way, embryos are released directly into the uterine cavity. This approach bypasses not only the need for an incubator, but also the step of embryo transfer [31].

Minimizing risks of ART treatment

The two major complications of ART are OHSS and multiple pregnancies that, as already mentioned, can almost completely be avoided by using mild stimulation protocols and by transferring only one embryo. However, doctors running an IVF program should also be prepared to confront, and prevent whenever possible, any type of complication arising from the procedure.

- **OHSS** and its thromboembolic complications is by far the most important risk of ovarian stimulation, being responsible for a 1% hospitalization rate in Western countries [32]. The well-known list of risk factors includes both patient characteristics (young age, low body weight, polycystic ovary syndrome (PCOS) or PCO-like patients, history of OHSS, allergies) and stimulation protocol (use of GnRH agonists, use of human chorionic gonadotropin (hCG) for luteal support, size and number of mature follicles, high estradiol levels).

    The number of follicles developed during the stimulation is the major predictor of OHSS and for this reason the agonist protocol shows the highest incidence of severe OHSS [33], implying that the use of mild protocols or CC is a good strategy to prevent OHSS and to drastically reduce the cost of stimulation [16].

- **Complications following oocyte retrieval**. These complications mainly follow from bleeding or from pelvic infection and occur at a frequency lower than 1% of oocyte retrievals [34]. Common aseptic precautions and avoidance of repeated vaginal punctures to reach follicles should minimize the occurrence of this type of complications. In addition, a thin needle (18 G) would certainly be less traumatic and painful, and would facilitate having scarce blood in the follicular fluid. Due to its thinness, a steel mandrel is recommended to support the needle itself. The presence of an intense echotip enhances visualization of the needle tip even when it is used with non-sophisticated ultrasound equipment as possibly happens in low-resource settings.

- **Pregnancy complications**. It has been reported that the incidence of ectopic pregnancies after ART is around 4%, with risk factors being previous myomectomy and tubal diseases [35]. Heterotopic pregnancies have similar incidence (between 1% and 3%) and risk factors with an additional risk that varies proportionally to the number of transferred embryos [36]. These figures are expected to be higher in developing countries where tubal pathologies are especially frequent.
- **Multiple pregnancies**. The transfer of more than one embryo is associated with the occurrence of multiple pregnancies that represent the major complication in ART. According to national registries, 20–30% of ART pregnancies are multiple and this causes a series of physical, social, and economic implications for which a high price has to be paid. In addition to a 2.4- to 5.3-fold increase in perinatal mortality in twins and triplets over singletons, there is a sharp rise in neonatal expenses. There is no doubt that the solution is to transfer only one embryo, especially in young women in their first cycle, or in women with previous pregnancies. Clearly, this would cause loss of some pregnancies, but an effort should be made to change the concept of successful outcome in IVF from the measure of pregnancy rate per cycle to that of a healthy singleton baby [37]. This approach would be especially important in countries with low economical resources where facilities for neonatal intensive care are lacking.

Training

The design of the above-mentioned strategies in a reality where limitation of expenses is the priority also implies a predisposition of adequate training for the clinicians and scientists that will be involved in the corresponding activities. In addition, periodical monitoring must be planned to verify that procedures are correct and appropriate, and the results obtained are within the expectations.

Clinicians must be prepared to deal with possible complications related to ART, but also with a different approach to procedures that are planned in a peculiar way.

In turn, scientists should be prepared to adopt strategies and protocols that are based on simple conditions from which the greatest advantage must be taken irrespective of being far from the latest advances.

One of the most relevant skills requested of all involved IVF professionals, both clinicians and scientists, is the capacity to confront emergency situations for which prompt solutions must be put in place. In other words, this sort of troubleshooting ability should be a prerequisite for which specific training should be much more sophisticated and demanding compared to what is done for laboratories in Western countries.

Our experience in low cost IVF in Arusha

A group of professionals from our center had the opportunity to set up the IVF and andrology laboratories in Arusha, Tanzania, at Saint Thomas Hospital. During this phase, our doctors also had the possibility to perform 18 diagnostic hysteroscopies in women aged between 23 and 39 years. The indication was infertility mostly due to tubal occlusion or bilateral salpingectomy caused by ectopic gestations. One patient was excluded from IVF treatment due to severe scarring of the cavity, while all remaining women presented with a stenotic cervix that could possibly be consequent to traumas or vaginal infections.

Table 18.2. Outcome of 20 oocyte retrievals performed in Arusha

No. patients	20
Maternal age (M±SD), years	33.8 ± 3.8
No. collected oocytes (M ± SD)	31 (1.5 ± 0.9)
No. inseminated oocytes	31
No. fertilized oocytes (%)	17 (55)
No. transferred cycles (%)	13 (65)
No. transferred embryos (M ± SD)	17 (1.3 ± 0.5)

Table 18.3. Preliminary results with the long shelf life medium especially designed by Patrick Quinn to be used in low cost IVF programs

No. patients	23
Maternal age (M±SD), years	38.4 ± 5.0
No. collected oocytes (M±SD)	86 (3.7 ± 2.5)
No. inseminated oocytes	77
No. fertilized oocytes (%)	65 (84.4)
No. embryos (%)	60 (92.3)
N. transferred cycles (%)	18 (78.3)
No. transferred embryos (M±SD)	44 (1.9 ± 1.2)
No. clinical pregnancies (%)	4 (22.2)
No. deliveries	3

These data confirmed the importance of performing a preliminary exploration of the uterine cavity in order to avoid hopeless IVF or IUI treatments.

Two preliminary series of patients scheduled for conventional IVF were performed in Arusha including 32 infertile patients that were selected by the local doctor (Table 18.2).

Treatment was cancelled in 12 of them because of poor response, while 20 underwent oocyte collection, having a mean of 1.5 retrieved oocytes. Embryo transfer was performed on day 2 in 13 patients. Unfortunately, no pregnancies resulted despite the good morphology of the majority of the transferred embryos (59% were top quality).

Several reasons were responsible for the poor performance of the results. First of all, stimulation was problematic due to the lack of precision that women had in following the therapy. As a result, 36% of the inseminated oocytes were immature on the day of fertilization check and in one case no oocytes were retrieved. Secondly, no accurate prescreening of the couples was done and many women were admitted despite the presence of uterine pathologies, while several men refused to do a preliminary semen analysis. In the laboratory, the major problems were a high room temperature and a discontinuous energy supply that resulted in several black outs.

This experience reinforced the importance of performing a correct patient selection, of giving an accurate training to the local doctors regarding the importance of infertility diagnosis, and to correctly instruct patients about the procedures required during treatment.

We are now ready for another series of patients whose treatment has been momentarily withheld due to a local temporary restriction in energy supply that does not give enough security for the program to be run. In the meanwhile, important improvements have been evaluated, including the design by Patrick Quinn of a culture medium that could be used both for insemination and embryo culture, which is characterized by a long shelf life and storage at room temperature. This medium has already been used in a trial in one of our centers and could support clinical pregnancies and deliveries (Table 18.3). Three of the derived pregnancies were obtained after day-4 and day-5 transfer but in the next trial transfers will be performed on day 2 in the hope of increasing the rate of pregnancies.

Conclusions

There is an increasing awareness of the necessity for affordable ART programs in developing countries. It is clear now that the design and provision of low cost IVF can be achieved through modifications of traditional protocols and monitoring systems.

It will take time to convince policy makers to recognize infertility as a public health issue needing government funding. However, the feasibility of implementing low cost IVF programs in realities where childlessness has dramatic social and cultural consequences should be a strong argument in favor of supporting ART. We think that it is time now to provide this service that is socially needed and economically sustainable.

References

1. Boivin J, Bunting L, Collins JA, Nygren KG. International estimates of infertility prevalence and treatment-seeking: potential need and demand for infertility medical care. *Hum Reprod* 2007;**22**:1506–12.

2. Van Balen F, Gerrits T. Quality of infertility care in poor-resource areas and the introduction of new reproductive technologies. *Hum Reprod* 2001;**16**:215–19.

3. Dyer SJ, Abrahams N, Mokoena NE, Lombard CJ, van der Spuy ZM. Psychological distress among women suffering from couple infertility in South Africa: a quantitative assessment. *Hum Reprod* 2005;**20**:1938–43.

4. Dyer SJ, Pennings G. Considerations regarding government funding of assisted reproductive techniques in low-resource settings. *Hum Reprod* 2008; ESHRE Monographs **1**:77–84.

5. Johnson NP, Mak W, Sowter MC. Laparoscopic salpingectomy for women with hydrosalpinges enhances the success of IVF: a Cochrane review. *Hum Reprod* 2002;**17**:543–8.

6. Strandell A, Lindhart A, Eckerlund I. Cost-effectiveness analysis of salpingectomy prior to IVF, based on a randomized controlled trial. *Hum Reprod* 2005;**20**:3284–92.

7. Oliveira FG, Abdelmassih VG, Diamond MP, *et al.* Uterine cavity findings and hysteroscopic interventions in patients undergoing in vitro fertilization-embryo transfer who repeatedly cannot conceive. *Fertil Steril* 2003;**80**:1371–5.

8. Gianaroli L, Gordts S, D'Angelo A, *et al.* Effect of the inner myometrium fibroid on the reproductive outcome after IVF. *Reprod Biomed Online* 2005;**10**:473–7.

9. Molinas CR, Campo R. Office hysteroscopy and adenomyosis. *Best Pract Res Clin Obstet Gynaecol* 2006;**20**:557–67.

10. Ombelet W. IUI and evidence-based medicine: an urgent need for translation into our clinical practice. *Gynecol Obstet Invest* 2005;**59**:1–2.

11. Semprini AE, Levi-Setti P, Bozzo M, *et al.* Insemination of HIV-negative women with processed semen of HIV-positive partners. *Lancet* 1992;**304**:1317–19.

12. Bujan L, Hollander L, Coudert M, *et al.* Safety and efficacy of sperm in washing HIV-1-serodiscordant couples where the male is infected: results from the European CREAThE network. *AIDS* 2007;**21**:1909–14.

13. Loskutoff NM, Huyser C, Singh R, *et al.* Use of a novel washing method combining multiple density gradients and trypsin for removing human immunodeficiency virus-1 and hepatitis C virus from semen. *Fertil Steril* 2005;**84**:1001–10.

14. Huyser C. Affordable ART services in Africa: synthesis and adaptation of laboratory services. *Hum Reprod* 2008; ESHRE Monographs **1**:77–84.

15. Benagiano G, Gianaroli L. The constitutional court modifies Italian legislation on assisted reproduction technology. *Reprod Biomed Online* 2010;**20**:261–6.

16. Noorashikin M, Ong FB, Omar MH, *et al.* Affordable ART for developing countries: a cost-benefit comparison of low dose stimulation versus high dose GnRH antagonist protocol. *J Assist Reprod Genet* 2008;**25**:297–303.

17. Aleyamma TK, Shashikant Kamath M, Muthukumar K, Mangalaraj AM, George K. Affordable ART: a different perspective. *Hum Reprod* 2011;**26**:3312–18.

18. Inhorn MC. Global infertility and the globalization of new reproductive technologies: illustrations from Egypt. *Soc Sci Med* 2003;**56**:1837–51.

19. Trounson AO, Leeton JF, Wood C, Webb J, Kovacs G. The investigation of idiopathic infertility by in vitro fertilization. *Fertil Steril* 1980;**34**:431–8.

20. Quinn P, Kerin JF, Warnes GM. Improved pregnancy rate in human in vitro fertilization with the use of a medium based on the composition of human tubal fluid. *Fertil Steril* 1985;**44**:493–8.

21. Edwards RG. Test-tube babies. *Nature* 1981;**293**:253–6.

22. Trounson A, Wood C. In vitro fertilization results 1979–1982, at Monash University, Queen Victoria, and Epworth Medical Centres. *J In Vitro Fert Embryo Transf* 1984;**1**:42–7.

23. Jones GM, Figuereido F, Osianlis T, *et al.* Embryo culture, assessment, selection and transfer. In: Vayena E, Rowe PJ, Griffin PD, eds. *Current Practices and Controversies in Assisted Reproduction*. Geneva, World Health Organization. 2002;177–209.

24. Biggers JD, Racowsky C. The development of fertilized human ova to the blastocyst stage in KSOM(AA) medium: is a two-step protocol necessary? *Reprod Biomed Online* 2002;**5**:133–40.

25. Vajta G, Holm P, Greve T, *et al.* The submarine incubation system, a new tool for in vitro embryo culture. *Theriogenology* 1997;**48**:1379–85.

26. Thouas GA, Korfiatis NA, French AJ, Jones GM, Trounson AO. Simplified technique for differential staining of inner cell mass and trophectoderm cells of mouse and bovine blastocysts. *Reprod Biomed Online* 2001;**3**:25–9.

27. Gianaroli L, Fiorentino A, Magli MC, Ferraretti AP, Montanaro N. Prolonged sperm-oocyte exposure and high sperm concentration affect human embryo viability and pregnancy rate. *Hum Reprod* 1996;**11**:2507–11.

28. Ranoux C, Aubriot FX, Dubuisson JB, *et al.* A new in vitro fertilization technique: intravaginal culture. *Fertil Steril* 1988;**49**:654–7.

29. Bonaventura L, Ahlering P, Morris R, *et al.* The INVOcell, a new medical device for intravaginal fertilization and culture. *Fertil Steril* 2006;**86**:S164.

30. Frydman R, Ranoux C. INVO: a simple, low cost effective assisted reproductive technology. *Hum Reprod* 2008; ESHRE Monographs **1**:85–9.

31. Torre ML, Faustini M, Attilio KM, Vigo D. Cell encapsulation in mammal reproduction. *Recent Pat Drug Deliv Formul* 2007;**1**:81–5.

32. Chan WS, Dixon ME. The "ART" of thromboembolism: a review of assisted

reproductive technology and thromboembolic complications. *Thromb Res* 2008;**121**:713–26.

33. Al-Inany HG, Abou-Setta AM, Aboulghar M. Gonadotrophin-releasing hormone antagonists for assisted conception: a Cochrane review. *Reprod Biomed Online* 2007;**14**:640–9.

34. De Sutter P, Gerris J, Dhont M. Assisted reproductive technologies: how to minimize the risks and complications in developing countries. *Hum Reprod* 2008; ESHRE Monographs **1**:73–6.

35. Strandell A, Thorburn J, Hambreger L. Risk factors for ectopic pregnancy in assisted reproduction. *Fertil Steril* 1999;**71**:282–6.

36. Rojansky N, Schenker JG. Heterotopic pregnancy and assisted reproduction: an update. *J Assist Reprod Genet* 1996;**13**:594–601.

37. Kalstrom PO, Bergh C. Reducing the number of embryos transferred in Sweden: impact on delivery and multiple birth rates. *Hum Reprod* 2007;**22**:2202–7.

Chapter

19

Incubators old and new

Eduardo Kelly and Takeo Cho

Introduction

The incubator is more than a piece of equipment that keeps cells in culture warm and gassed, it is an essential element of the culture system for IVF. In this chapter we will attempt to cover the history of incubators, the variables manipulated to optimize their use, different types of incubators, and technology challenges we face.

History

In 1959 the first evidence of the possibility of in vitro fertilization (IVF) was obtained by Chang [1], when he demonstrated in rabbits that it was possible to fertilize newly ovulated eggs, incubate them, and transfer them back into adult females to result in the live birth of viable newborns. Building upon this work, and the work of others, Robert G. Edwards worked for several years to develop techniques that would provide viable oocytes for human IVF. He discovered two important findings. The first was that human oocytes require 24 hours of in vitro incubation prior to initiating maturation [2, 3]. The second was that using a buffer to stabilize pH could activate human sperm to fertilize human oocytes [4]. However, the true breakthrough came when he discovered, in conjunction with Patrick Steptoe, that controlled use of gonadotropins to produce metaphase II oocytes allowed for the laparoscopic retrieval of these oocytes from infertile women [5], and further that fertilized oocytes, under appropriate conditions, could develop into 8-cell [6], and later 16-cell [7] stage human embryos. This work culminated in the birth of the first IVF baby in 1978 [8], and led to the success rates seen in IVF today. This lifetime of work eventually led to the awarding of the 2010 Nobel Prize in Medicine to Edwards.

One of the first devices used inside conventional incubators used to culture embryos is presented in Figure 19.1.

The following is a description of the procedures used between 1976 and 1978, as described by Kay Elder (personal communication, 2011):

> The actual "incubator" was just a standard 37 degree "oven", the kind that were used in any kind of clinical lab before gas-perfused incubators were available. Each patient had their own little desiccator/culture chamber, and they were all kept inside the 37 degree oven – pretty simple, really. If I remember correctly, the gas mixture went through a water bottle and then a Millipore filter first. A standard laboratory desiccator is normally used to keep specimens in a vacuum by removing all of the air via suction through the stopcock valve at the top. Professor Robert Edwards

Culture Media, Solutions, and Systems in Human ART, ed. Patrick Quinn. Published by Cambridge University Press. © Cambridge University Press 2014.

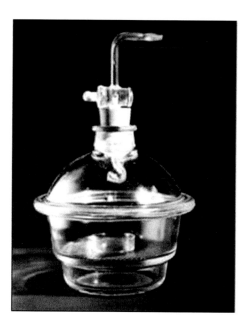

Figure 19.1 The first IVF incubator.

and his nurse Jean Purdy converted this desiccator into an embryo culture chamber by reversing the process, using the stopcock valve to perfuse the chamber with a special gas mixture suitable for in vitro tissue culture. Oocytes recovered by laparoscopy were mixed with a prepared sperm sample and transferred as droplets into a Petri dish. The Petri dish was then placed into this desiccator chamber and the lid placed so that a small gap between chamber and lid remained. The open valve was connected to the special gas mixture supply, with the gap between chamber and lid open, so that the perfused gas then displaced the air contained within the chamber, allowing it to escape. The gas supply was then stopped while sealing the chamber shut, the stopcock closed, and the chamber placed inside a 37 degree incubator to maintain the correct temperature for early embryo development during the next two days. Between 48–72 hours after mixing eggs and sperm, the early embryos were then loaded into a special catheter for transfer into the patient's womb, by a procedure similar to the insertion of an intrauterine contraceptive device (IUD).

Evolution

Significant progress has been made in the technology of incubators since the original technology described above by Kay Elder. Firstly, large incubators became available with flow meters where gas and air were injected directly into the chamber at a selected proportion. Later, incubators with carbon dioxide (CO_2) control were launched with a sensor installed capable of measuring the gas concentration inside the incubator. Gas was injected until the incubator chamber reached the desired gas concentration. During the early years of assisted reproductive technologies (ART), there were no materials or equipment that were specifically built or designed for use in humans. Most of the equipment that was used by early embryologists was derived from products used for cell culture systems, or products that were developed for veterinary medicine. In fact, it was not until 1993 that the European Medicines Agency and 1998 that the US Food and Drug Administration (FDA) began regulating IVF equipment as medical devices, requiring agency approval prior to marketing.

Today there are a variety of incubator models available, with the largest having a capacity of 220 liters and the smallest a capacity of 600 milliliters. The larger, standard incubators have the benefit of being able to handle a large number of cases (dishes) at once, have the advantage of allowing independent probes to be used, and may be fitted with high-efficiency particulate air filters–volatile organic compounds filters (HEPA-VOC) [9]. Smaller tabletop models have the advantage of being portable, use premixed gas canisters, and are able to maintain temperature and pH more easily [9]. Types of incubators also differ in the types of gases that can be adjusted. Some allow only for adjustment of CO_2, whereas others, the so called tri-gas incubators allow adjustments for both CO_2 and oxygen (O_2). The reduction of O_2 concentration is done through the injection of nitrogen (N_2) into the chamber diminishing the O_2 concentration existing in the air (from 20.95% to 5%). Incubators also differ in the way they are warmed (water-jacket vs. direct heat), whether they are humidified or not, and whether they mix gases or not. State-of-the-art models may also include an embryo observation system which allows for embryo development monitoring without exposing the embryo to changes in culture conditions. More detailed information on the varying types of incubators is provided below.

The culture system

As noted above, it is important to realize that the incubator is not just a piece of equipment responsible for warming gametes and embryos; it is an integral part of the culture system. The incubator with CO_2 or CO_2/O_2 control interacts with the culture media used, to determine the pH within the system, and is also responsible for maintaining the humidity and temperature inside the chamber. These variables are important to consider in optimizing results when using incubators, and each of these is discussed in turn, below.

Temperature

It is critical that a constant temperature is maintained in order to ensure the healthy growth of cultured cells. Since 1969, 37 °C has been accepted as the best temperature for culturing human embryos [10]. However, it has been suggested that because follicular fluid is colder than the ovarian stroma, and the temperature of the follicular fluid increases as one nears ovulation [11] that a two-temperature approach may be needed. This observation is supported by a study by Shi et al., which found that more oocytes cleaved (79.2%; P = 0.0653) and developed to morulae (43.6%; P = 0.0019) and blastocysts (27.4%; P = 0.1568) when they were matured in vitro at 38.5 °C between 0 and 10 hours, and then at 37 °C from 10 to 24 hours [12]. The authors suggest that this short period of reduced temperature may be necessary for meiosis to resume. After this, the optimal temperature of 37 °C should be maintained, as it has been demonstrated that human meiotic spindles are temperature sensitive, and changes in temperature for as little as 10 minutes can affect spindle integrity, and lead to suboptimal embryo development [13]. It has also been demonstrated that healthy oocytes can re-polymerize the spindle after being exposed to temperature changes.

There are three main heating options available for culturing dishes inside incubators, direct heat (radiant walled), water-jacketed (air convection incubator), and contact heat (no air interface). Direct heat incubators heat the interior chamber with heaters mounted on the chamber that radiate heat into the interior chamber. A water-jacketed incubator maintains temperature by means of heated elements surrounded by water that heats the interior of the chamber's walls. One of the benefits of a water-jacketed incubator is that water is an effective insulator and is able to maintain the interior temperature 4–5 times longer than a direct heat incubator in the case of a power blackout. The main benefit of a direct heat incubator is that this type of system allows for a more rapid temperature recovery when the door is opened or a power outage occurs. The third system, contact heat, allows the temperature to be transmitted directly to the culture dish, allowing fast recovery and homogeneous transmission of the temperature without air interphase. A study evaluating temperature maintenance in vitro, reported that a direct heat incubator (MINC) was superior to a large volume air convection incubator (FORMA) in temperature recovery; the MINC was able to regain temperature from 35 °C to 37 °C in 5.5 minutes, whereas the FORMA regained the same temperature in > 20 minutes [14].

Humidity

The choice of a humidified or non-humidified incubator depends on the type of tissue culture system used. If one is using "open" culture then a humidified incubator is definitely required. Culture media evaporation leads to osmolarity changes. This phenomenon could damage oocytes and embryos if it is not handled carefully and the evaporation minimized and prevented. If clinical grade mineral oil is being used as an overlay, humidity is not required and therefore a non-humidified incubator could be used [9]. Oil overlay culture system is widely used and most IVF laboratories still use humidified culture systems as a matter of precautionary measure against dramatic changes in osmolarity, pH, and temperature loss when the dishes are outside of the incubator.

For humidified incubators it is important to maintain adequate moisture inside the chamber to avoid osmolarity changes. Ideally the humidity should be maintained at 95–98%. The majority of the incubators used in IVF use evaporation to produce humidity by means of either warming humidity pans or a humidity reservoir at the bottom of the incubator.

Gas composition and pH

Carefully calibrated and controlled incubators are critical to successful IVF [9]. Unlike temperature and humidity, which are directly controlled or monitored, pH is managed indirectly by monitoring and adjusting the amount of CO_2 present in the incubator. CO_2 levels within the incubator are set for a specific percentage relative to O_2 and N_2 or air. CO_2 and pH have an inverse relationship; as CO_2 concentration decreases, pH increases. The ideal pH in a culture environment is 7.2 to 7.3 and in order to maintain that strict range in the incubator, it is therefore also necessary to maintain a strict range of CO_2 as well. These parameters should be compared with the culture media manufacturer recommendations, taking into consideration the amount of sodium bicarbonate in culture media before any changes are applied to current culture conditions.

The principle gas mixtures used are (1) 5% CO_2 in air (20% O_2) and also known as atmospheric and (2) 5% CO_2, 5% O_2 and 90% N_2, also known as 5/5/90 or physiological [15]. Although embryos can develop well in an atmospheric system, it has been suggested that since the embryos develop in vivo under low O_2 concentrations, an O_2 setting lower than ambient air may be optimal. For example, in the hamster uterus, the percentage of O_2 is 8.7% and this drops to 5.3% at the time of blastocyst formation and implantation [16]. It has been suggested that reducing the O_2 concentrations to physiological levels might result in higher quality embryos by mitigating free radical damage to the embryo [17].

Increasing evidence has been accumulating to support this hypothesis. In a study comparing atmospheric to physiological conditions, Kea reported that although there were no differences in fertilization rate, blastocyst formation, or pregnancy rates between the two gas phases, the mean embryo score on day 2 was significantly higher in the group of embryos that were treated with 5% O_2 when compared with the embryos that were treated with 20% O_2 [15]. In a controlled randomized study of 230 first cycle women undergoing routine IVF or intracytoplasmic sperm injection (ICSI) that compared embryos cultured in a 5% O_2 environment with those cultured in an atmospheric environment, the authors reported significant differences between the outcomes of the embryos in the different culture conditions. Specifically, in the 5% O_2 group there was a higher rate of implantation and live births when compared with the atmospheric group [18]. In contrast, in a study of 382 patients undergoing IVF, there were no differences reported in embryo score on day 3 or 5, blastulation rate, transfer score, implantation rate, or clinical pregnancy rate between embryos exposed to a 5% O_2 concentration and embryos exposed to a 20% O_2 concentration [19].

Air quality

The role of ambient air quality and air quality within incubators has not been extensively evaluated. It is important to remember that incubators with CO_2 control only will have 94–95% of the air inside the chamber from the air inside of the laboratory. In general, the most common air pollutants are (1) VOCs, (2) small inorganic molecules such as N_2O, sulfate and CO, (3) substances derived from building materials (aldehydes, substituted benzenes), and (4) other polluting compounds released by pesticides or aerosols [20]. In a thorough analysis of chemical air contamination (CAC) of their IVF laboratory, Cohen and coworkers found an accumulation of VOCs derived from adjacent spaces or specific laboratory products such as compressed CO_2, sterile Petri dishes, and other materials or devices known to release gaseous emissions, and that outside air may be cleaner than HEPA-filtered laboratory air [21]. They also noted several instances in which the installation of various filtration systems improved pregnancy rates. Additionally, it has been reported that clinical pregnancy and fertilization rates dropped in one center while construction was being performed, during this time it was noted that strong construction odors were detected [22].

In terms of air quality within the incubator, Cohen et al. noted that when they tested air extracted from a new incubator they found VOC concentrations >100 times higher than from used incubators from the same manufacturers. They also found that products such as anesthetic gases, refrigerants, cleaning agents, hydrocarbons, and aromatic compounds such as benzene and toluene accumulated specifically in incubators. As with the finding for ambient air, they recommend that incubators be vented with unfiltered outside air, and that allowing the emission of gases from new laboratory products prior to use should be considered [21]. Filtering may reduce contaminants as well; in a study evaluating the effects of two different types of filters for incubators it was reported that there was a 6% increase in blastocyst rate and blastocyst development when a VOC filter was used when compared with a HEPA filter [23]. In a similar vein, Wang and associates reported decreased fertilization and cleavage rates following a faulty back-flow of gas from a gas analyzer (Fyrite) [24]. In contrast, it has also been noted that there were no differences in ICSI outcome when comparing an incubation environment ISO class 8 (3 530 000 particles of $\geq 0.5\,\mu m/m^3$) to an incubation environment of ISO class 5 (3530 particles of $\geq 0.5\,\mu m/m^3$) [25].

Incubator models
Front-loading chamber incubators
Astec Penguin DH

The Penguin DH (Astec, Fukuoka, Japan) is a direct heat incubator that has both CO_2 and CO_2/O_2 models. It has a 30 liter (standard 2 shelves, maximum 4) capacity, and a temperature range of ambient temperature +5 °C to 50.0 °C (±0.1 °C). It has a CO_2 control range of 0% to 20.0% (±0.1%) and an O_2 control range of 1.0% to 89.0% (±0.5%). The humidity is set at 95% (±4 RH [relative humidity]). Depending upon the model, the CO_2 sensor is either thermal conductivity (TC) or infrared (IR), and the O_2 sensor is galvanic.

Astec Penguin AQ

The Penguin AQ (Astec, Fukuoka, Japan) is a water-jacket incubator that has both CO_2 and CO_2/O_2 models. It comes with both a 32 (standard 3 shelves, maximum 7) and 57 (standard 3 shelves, maximum 10) liter capacity, and a temperature range of ambient temperature +5 °C to 50.0 °C (±0.1 °C). It has a CO_2 control range of 0% to 19.9% (±0.1%) and an O_2 control range of 1% to 20% at 95% (CO_2 5%) (±0.5%). It is available with TC sensor or an IR CO_2 sensor and a galvanic O_2 sensor.

Thermo Forma Series II Model 3110

The Forma Model 3110 (Thermo Scientific, Ashville, North Carolina) is a water-jacketed CO_2/O_2 incubator. It has a capacity of 184 liters and a temperature range from ambient +5 °C to 55 °C (±0.2 °C at 37 °C). It has a CO_2 control range of 0% to 20% and an O_2 control range of 1% to 20%. This model comes with a choice of either a TC or an IR CO_2 sensor.

Thermo Forma Series II Model 3100

The Forma Model 3100 (Thermo Scientific, Ashville, North Carolina) is a direct heat CO_2 incubator. It has a capacity of 184 liters (standard 4 shelves, maximum 17) and a temperature range from +5 °C above ambient to 55 °C (±0.2 °C at 37 °C). It has a CO_2 control range of 0% to 20%. This model comes with a choice of either a TC or an IR CO_2 sensor.

Heracell i Series

The Heracell i series (Thermo Scientific, Ashville, North Carolina) of incubators are air jacketed incubators that range in capacity from 150 to 240 liters. They have a temperature range from +10 °C (±0.1 °C/±0.5 °C). They have a CO_2 control range of 0% to 20% (±0.1 at 0.5%), and come with a choice of either a TC or an IR CO_2 sensor with an optional zirconium O_2 sensor.

Galaxy Series

The Galaxy (New Brunswick Scientific, Edison, New Jersey) series of incubators are direct heat CO_2 incubators with capacities ranging from 14 to 170 liters with a temperature range from 4 or 5 °C above ambient to 50 °C. These incubators do not have internal fans and use convection to mix the air in the chamber. All models have a humidity range of up to 95% and a CO_2 range of 0.2% to 20% (±0.1%), and have an IR CO_2 sensor. There are options for O_2 sensor.

Sanyo MCO-175M

The MCO-175M (Sanyo, San Diego, California) is a water-jacketed CO_2 incubator. It has a capacity of 170 liters and a temperature range from +5 °C above ambient to 55 °C (± 2 °C). It has a CO_2 control range of 0% to 20% (± 0.15%), and has a TC CO_2 sensor.

Sanyo MCO-17AC

MCO-17AC (Sanyo, San Diego, California) is a water-jacketed/direct heat CO_2 incubator. It has a capacity of 164 liters and a temperature range from +5 °C above ambient to 55 °C (± 2 °C). It has a CO_2 control range of 0% to 20% (± 0.15%), and has a TC CO_2 sensor.

Incubators options

Several incubator manufacturers offer optional features to be added before purchasing the units. The list includes decontamination by heat (only available for direct heat incubators), narrow bandwidth UV light sterilization, remote monitoring, alarm systems, shelf doors, and automatic gas switch-over connection. All these options should be carefully considered before purchasing and a thorough evaluation should be made for selecting the most cost-effective configuration of the incubator.

Top-loading benchtop incubators

MINC

The MINC incubator (Cook Medical Incorporated, Bloomington, Indiana) uses a premixed canister blend of 6% CO_2, 5% O_2, and 89% N_2 or high purity 6% CO_2 in air. It has a temperature capacity of 35.0 °C to 40.0 °C in 0.1 °C increments in an ambient temperature range of +20 °C to +28 °C. It has a capacity for four culture dishes in each of two separate chambers.

G-195

The G-195 tri-gas incubator (K-System, Birkerod, Denmark) connects to pure CO_2 and or N_2 (does not require premixed canisters). It has a CO_2 range of 2% to 10% and an O_2 range of 2% to 20% and a temperature range from ambient to 49.9 °C. It has a total capacity of 40 individual culture dishes (10 chambers that can hold up to 4 dishes).

BT-37

The BT-37 incubator (Planer PLC, Middlesex, United Kingdom) has a temperature range from ambient +5 °C to 40 °C (± 0.1 °C). It uses a premixed gas canister (6% CO_2, 5% O_2 with the balance N_2), and has a capacity of 4–10 (dependent upon size) culture dishes in each of two separate chambers.

EZ Culture

The EZ Culture incubator (Astec, Fukuoka, Japan) is a dry CO_2/O_2 culture system. It has a CO_2 control range of 0% to 20% (IR sensor) and an O_2 control range of 4% to 25% (zirconia sensor). It has a temperature control range from ambient +5 °C to 40 °C (± 0.1 °C) and a capacity of either 6 or 12 standard plates depending upon the model. The system can also be configured for humidity with a range of up to 95%. The EZ Culture includes a data-logging software to be installed in a computer.

Hybrid models: contact heat/small chamber

IVF Cube

The IVF Cube (Astec, Fukuoka, Japan) is a drawer type, CO_2/O_2 incubator. It has a CO_2 control range of 0% to 10% (IR sensor) and an O_2 control range of 4% to 10% (galvanic sensor). It has a temperature control range from ambient +5 °C to 40 °C (±0.1 °C) and a humidity range of up to 95% and a capacity equivalent to two to four 4-well multidishes, three to six 60×15 mm dishes, or five to twelve 30×15 mm dishes per drawer (total four drawers). Each individual drawer has an independent temperature, CO_2, and O_2 control. The incubator has a gas mixer included needing gas feedings for CO_2 and N_2 only. No premix gas is needed. The IVF Cube combines direct contact temperature transmission to the culture dishes with a very small culture chamber in each of the four independent drawers.

Embryo observation systems

Embryo observation systems use microscopes and cameras within the incubator which allow the monitoring of embryogenesis without having to take the embryos out of the incubator, thereby reducing the stress of environmental changes from frequent door opening and closures. Because the number of door openings and closings is reduced there is also a reduction in gas consumption and a reduction in the risk of contamination. These systems also offer a novel approach for developmental and reproductive research in that they enable both retrospective and prospective analyses of embryo development [26].

One concern about the use of time-lapse embryo observation systems is the light that the embryos are exposed to when the digital images are obtained. Takenaka *et al.* reported that cool white fluorescent light produced more reactive oxygen species in mouse and hamster zygotes than did warm white fluorescent light [27]. However, a study that compared embryos cultured in a standard incubator with embryos cultured with time-lapse observations every 15 minutes revealed no significant differences in the fertilization rate or in the rate of excellent cleaved embryos between the two groups [28]. The use of these time-lapse systems has also been reported to not impair embryo quality, blastocyst development or viability [29].

Some examples and specifications of marketed embryo monitoring systems for clinical and research use are presented below.

The EmbryoScope™ Embryo Monitoring System

The EmbryoScope Monitoring System (Unisense FertiliTech A/S, Aarhus, Denmark) is a tri-gas incubator that has a capacity for 6 disposable trays that can hold 12 embryos each. It has a temperature range from 30 °C to 45 °C (±0.2 °C), an O_2 range from 5% to 20% ± 2%, and a CO_2 range from 2% to 10% ± 0.2%. The gas volume is regenerated/purified every 10 minutes. VOCs are removed by an active carbon filter and particles are removed by a HEPA filter.

The system has a built-in Hoffman Modulation microscope with a contrast phase objective specialized for 635 nm illumination, and a Leica camera designed to operate at 635 nm, with a resolution of 1280×1024 pixels. It is a time-lapse system that has a 20-minute cycle time for six slides with a 5-minute cycle time possible with a single slide. The camera works with an IR light specially designed to minimize embryo exposure.

CCM-IVF

The CCM-IVF Embryo Observation System (Astec, Fukuoka, Japan) is a 30 L direct heat, natural evaporation incubator with a temperature control range from ambient temperature (+5 °C), up to 50 °C (±0.1 °C), a CO_2 control range of 0% to 20% (±0.1%), and an O_2 control range of 1.0% to 89.0% (±0.5%). The system has an IR CO_2 sensor and a galvanic battery O_2 sensor.

The camera unit has a resolution of 1.3 mega pixels (1280 × 1024) with a CMOS (complementary metal oxide semiconductor) image sensor and has a field of view of 660 µm × 530 µm and a time-lapse interval of 1 minute to 24 hours. The camera works with an IR light specially designed to minimize embryo exposure.

Natural incubators

It has been proposed that gamete and embryo incubation can be successfully done using the woman's vagina as an incubator chamber [30]. Intravaginal culture (IVC) is a method by which retrieved oocytes are placed with sperm in a tube containing commercial culture medium and then cultured in the vagina. In one technique, the oocytes are placed, regardless of level of maturity in one or more 3 mL tubes completely filled with culture media and fertilized. The tube(s) are then placed into the posterior vaginal cul-de-sac, kept in place with a diaphragm, and cultured for 44 to 48 hours. The resultant embryos are then transferred [30]. In a similar method, the oocytes are fertilized in an air-free plastic capsule which is placed into the vagina. In this study, 22 patients were treated with IVC and 23 were treated with standard IVF, the pregnancy rate was 22.7% in the IVC group and 17.4% in the IVF group [31]. One such product, INVOcell™ which is a capsule, is commercially available in parts of South America, Africa, Europe, Canada, and the Middle East. Preliminary findings report lead embryos of between 6 and 14 cells, fertilization rates of 48%, and a 31% pregnancy rate [32].

Technology challenges

Oxygen sensors

There are two types of O_2 sensors used in incubators, galvanic (paramagnetic method) or zirconia. Zirconia sensors are solid-state sensors, which are very precise, do not need to be continuously calibrated, and are relatively maintenance free. However, they sometimes experience condensation in the sensor when the incubator is powered off with humidity still inside the chamber. Galvanic sensors are also practically maintenance free but have a battery in the sensor, so the sensor has to be calibrated periodically as the battery deteriorates.

Carbon dioxide sensors

When the door of the incubator is opened, air with 0.05% CO_2 and 20.95% O_2 enters the chamber. CO_2 escapes from the chamber. When the CO_2 sensor detects a drop in the level of CO_2, CO_2 is automatically injected to raise the level. There are two types of sensors available to detect changes in CO_2 levels, TC and IR.

TC sensors measure the resistance between two thermistors, one of which is inside of the incubator and the other of which is enclosed. When there is CO_2 present in the incubator the resistance between the two thermistors is changed and the TC sensor

Table 19.1. Comparison of thermal conductivity and infrared sensors

	Thermal conductivity	Infrared
Measures	CO_2 and humidity	CO_2
Temperature	Can be affected by temperature changes	Not affected by temperature changes
Humidity	Can be affected by changes in humidity	Not affected by changes in humidity
Recovery time after door opening	Longer	Shorter
Price	Inexpensive	Somewhat expensive
Lifespan	Longer	Shorter

measures the change in resistance. TC sensors are often considered more stable than IR sensors because of their simple structure, but they need to coexist with relatively high humidity (>90%) in order to function very precisely. IR sensors use an optical sensor to detect CO_2. In this type of sensor, an air sample from the chamber is passed between the light source (emitter) and the sensor. The amount of IR absorbed is relative to the level of CO_2 in the air sample. Table 19.1 lists the benefits and disadvantages of each of these sensors.

Altitude

Height above sea level influences CO_2 levels in the incubator; therefore, adjustments in CO_2 concentration need to be made. This is particularly important to keep in mind if one is considering purchasing an incubator with an automatic O_2 sensor reference to air in a high altitude location. The relative concentration of O_2 in the air at high elevations is essentially the same as it is at sea level, approximately 21%. However, because air pressure is lower at high altitudes, this also lowers the partial pressure of all gases, including O_2, CO_2, and N_2. At high altitudes, where there is low air pressure, a higher CO_2 concentration is required to achieve the correct partial pressure (ppCO_2) to maintain the bicarbonate ions in solution and the pH at 7.2–7.3 [33].

Gas analyzers

The use of gas analyzers is a great help for the IVF laboratory. The problem is that analyzers should be calibrated against a fixed reference (certified gas mix) to be most accurate. The use of Fyrite analyzers in IVF should be avoided due to the lack of consistent precision and due to potential toxicity for the embryos and operators.

There are tabletop and handheld gas analyzers specifically designed for incubators that are a great addition to the laboratory QC instruments if they are calibrated and well maintained.

Conclusion

Incubator technology has grown exponentially since the late 1960s. Beginning as an improvised glass chamber, now the incubator is a pivotal component of the entire IVF culture system. The sophisticated systems of today offer multiple options to suit any requirements, ranging from large models capable of storing multiple culture dishes to desktop versions offering separate drawers for individual patients, each with the capacity to be calibrated individually. While larger units have the ability to incubate a large number of cases at one time, they may have larger temperature and CO_2 excursions following door openings than do smaller units. An additional benefit of the smaller benchtop units is that some models provide space for individual patients, and as such, potentially reduce the risk of contamination.

State-of-the-art technology including microscopes and cameras inside incubators also now makes it possible to observe and document embryo growth without removing the culture dishes from the incubator and offers the ability to monitor embryo growth remotely. These technologies also have the added benefit of reducing embryo stress by reducing the number of door openings, thereby decreasing the resultant fluctuations of temperature, CO_2, O_2, and pH. These new technologies are providing the embryologist different options to mimic in vitro culture conditions closer to those in vivo in favor of better outcomes in assisted reproduction.

Acknowledgements

The authors would like to thank Ms. Kate Banks for assisting in the writing of this chapter and Kay Elder for her contribution.

References

1. Chang MC. Fertilization of rabbit ova in vitro. *Nature* 1959;**184**(Suppl 7):466–7.

2. Edwards RG. Maturation in vitro of mouse, sheep, cow, pig, rhesus monkey and human ovarian oocytes. *Nature* 1965;**208**:349–51.

3. Edwards RG. Maturation in vitro of human ovarian oocytes. *Lancet* 1965;**2**:926–9.

4. Edwards RG, Bavister BD, Steptoe PC. Early stages of fertilization in vitro of human oocytes matured in vitro. *Nature* 1969;**221**:632–5.

5. Steptoe PC, Edwards RG. Laparascopic recovery of preovulatory human oocytes after priming with gonadotropins. *Lancet* 1970;**1**:683–99.

6. Edwards RG, Steptoe PC, Purdy JM. Fertilization and cleavage in vitro of preovulatory human oocytes. *Nature* 1970;**227**:1307–9.

7. Steptoe PC, Edwards RG, Purdy JM. Human blastocysts grown in culture. *Nature* 1971;**229**:132–3.

8. Steptoe PC, Edwards RG. Birth after the reimplantation of a human embryo. *Lancet* 1978;**2**:366.

9. Elder K, Dale B, Harper J, Huntriss J. *In-Vitro Fertilization*. Cambridge, Cambridge University Press, 2011.

10. Brinster RL. In vitro cultivation of mammalian ova. *Adv Biosci* 1969;**4**:199–233.

11. Grinsted J, Kjer JJ, Blenstrup K, Pedersen JF. Is low temperature of the follicular fluid prior to ovulation necessary for normal oocyte development? *Fertil Steril* 1985; **43**(1):34–9.

12. Shi DS, Avery B, Greve T. Effects of temperature gradients on in vitro maturation of bovine oocytes. *Theriogenology* 1998;**50**(4):667–74.

13. Wang WH, Meng L, Hackett RJ, Odenbourg R, Keefe DL. Limited recovery of meiotic spindles in living human oocytes after cooling-rewarming observed using polarized light microscopy. *Hum Reprod* 2001;**16**(11):2374–8.

14. Cooke S, Tyler JPP, Driscoll G. Objective assessment of temperature maintenance using in vitro culture techniques. *J Assist Reprod Genet* 2002;**19**(8):368–75.

15. Kea B, Gebhardt J, Watt J, *et al.* Effect of reduced oxygen concentrations on the

outcome of in vitro fertilization. *Fertil Steril* 2007;**87**(1):213–16.

16. Fischer B, Bavister BD. Oxygen tension in the oviduct and uterus of rhesus monkeys, hamsters and rabbits. *J Reprod Fertil* 1993;**99**(2):673–9.

17. Burton GJ, Hempstock J, Jauniaux E. Oxygen, early embryo development and free radical-mediated embryopathies. *Reprod Biomed Online* 2003;**6**(1):84–96.

18. Meintjes M, Chantilis SJ, Douglas JD, *et al.* A controlled randomized trial evaluating the effect of lowered incubator oxygen tension on live births in a predominantly blastocyst transfer program. *Hum Reprod* 2009;**24**(2):300–7.

19. Nanassy L, Peterson CA, Wolcox AL, *et al.* Comparison of 5% and ambient oxygen during days 3–5 of in vitro culture of human oocytes. *Fertil Steril* 2010; **93**(2):579–85.

20. Locke DC, *et al.* Detemination of C1 through C5 atmospheric hydrocarbons. In: Lodge JP Jr., ed. *Methods of Air Sampling and Analysis.* New York, Academic Press, 1990.

21. Cohen J, Gilligan A, Esposito W, Schimmel T, Dale B. Ambient air and its potential effects on conception in vitro. *Hum Reprod* 1997;**12**(8):1742–9.

22. Boone WR, Johnson JE, Locke AJ, Crane MM 4th, Price TM. Control of air quality in an assisted reproductive technology laboratory. *Fertil Steril* 1999;**71**(1):150–4.

23. Higdon HL, Blackhurst DW, Boone WR. Incubator management in an assisted reproductive technology laboratory. *Fertil Steril* 2008;**89**(3):703–10.

24. Wang H, Wang R, Liu J. Decreased in vitro fertilization and cleavage rates after equipment error during CO_2 calibration. *Fertil Steril* 2000;**73**(6):1247–9.

25. Souza Mdo C, Mancebo AC, da Rocha Cde A, *et al.* Evaluation of two incubation environments – ISO class 8 versus ISO class 5 – on intracytoplasmic sperm injection cycle outcome. *Fertil Steril* 2009; **91**:1780–4.

26. Yamagata K, Suetsugu R, Wakayama T. Long-term, six-dimensional live-cell imaging for mouse preimplantation embryo that does not affect full-term development. *J Reprod Dev* 2009; **55**:343–50.

27. Takenaka M, Horiuchi T, Yanagimachi R. Effects of light on development of mammalian zygotes. *Proc Natl Acad Sci U S A* 2007;**104**(36):14289–93.

28. Nakahara T, Iwase A, Goto M, *et al.* Evaluation of the safety of time-lapse observations for human embryos. *J Assist Reprod Genet* 2010;**27**:93–6.

29. Cruz M, Gadea B, Garrido N, *et al.* Embryo quality, blastocyst and ongoing pregnancy rates in oocyte donation patients whose embryos were monitored by time-lapse imaging. *J Assist Reprod Genet* 2011; **28**(7):569–73.

30. Ranoux C, Dubuisson JB, Foulot H, Aubriot FX. Intravaginal culture and embryo transfer. A new method for the fertilization of human oocytes. *Rev Fr Gynecol Obstet* 1987; **82**(12):741–4.

31. Sterzik K, Rosenbusch B, Sasse V, *et al.* A new variation of in-vitro fertilization: intravaginal culture of human oocytes and cleavage stages. *Hum Reprod* 1989; **4**(8 Suppl):83–6.

32. Bonaventura L, Ahlering P, Morris R, *et al.* The Invocell, a new medical device for intravaginal fertilization and culture. *Proceedings of The American Society of Reproductive Medicine Annual Meeting* 2006;**86**(Suppl 2):S164.

33. Mortimer D, Quinn P. Bicarbonate-buffered media and CO_2. *Alpha Newsletter* 1996;**4**.

Incubator management

William R. Boone and H. Lee Higdon III

Introduction

When it comes to controlling the environment of gametes/embryos and thus success of Assisted Reproductive Technology (ART), the main variable is the incubator. It is not sufficient simply to turn on this artificial uterus and expect it to produce a viable product. Instead, to maximize success, the incubator needs to be monitored continuously.

Here we review the general topic of incubator management as it pertains to ART. In this article, we discuss experiments with human and cattle gametes and embryos as well as gametes and embryos of other eutherian mammals. We consider such parameters as temperature, humidity, air quality, gas concentration, electromagnetic waves, and incubator design.

While we realize that many managers of incubators have their own sacrosanct cleaning protocols, we have included, in this chapter, our methodologies for the reader to consider. Once an acceptable incubator environment has been established, it is best to perform minimal cleaning to limit the potential introduction of new variables. In addition, we discuss a test to determine when to implement changes within the incubator. At the end of the chapter, we list specific "Dos and Don'ts" that we found helpful in our ART practice.

Control of air quality within the incubator

Most ART incubators in use today obtain their air from the surrounding environment. Therefore, particles and volatile organic compounds (VOCs) that make up part of the environmental air should be considered when managing the incubator.

Particle counts

Because bacteria and other contaminants can attach themselves to particles, a reduction in particles equates to an increase in air quality. While particle counts may not be related directly to fertilization rate or pregnancy outcome, there are some indirect data to indicate that as laboratory air becomes cleaner (reduced particle counts), ART outcome improves [1]. With the addition of high-efficiency particulate air (HEPA) filtration and ultra-low penetration air (ULPA) filtration in heating, ventilating, and air conditioning (HVAC) systems, particle counts can be reduced.

Anecdotal stories abound concerning reduced embryo quality and pregnancy rates when the laboratory is near a construction site or when chemicals are stored in the

Culture Media, Solutions, and Systems in Human ART, ed. Patrick Quinn. Published by Cambridge University Press. © Cambridge University Press 2014.

laboratory. The stories often describe an increase in embryo quality and pregnancy rates when construction is completed or when chemicals are removed from the environment that surrounds the incubator. However, it only has been in the last 15 or so years that scientists have reported a correlation among air quality, fertilization, and embryo development.

Our air-quality story is similar to that of other ART laboratories. In the early 1990s, our clinical pregnancy rates were similar to or better than the national average in the United States, but we saw these values take a drastic drop in 1994. Because our patient population had not changed, our personnel were the same, and the culture media and the way we handled gametes were still the same, we went in search of a culprit. The new variable was construction juxtaposed to our embryology laboratory. We were able to detect odors from paints, sealants, and floor glues. Dust and other particulates surrounded the laboratory. To add insult to our already injured air quality, the emergency room had been relocated and diesel fumes from arriving ambulances could be detected in the laboratory.

We provided evidence to the hospital administration that these odors, also known as volatile organic compounds (VOCs), inhibited mouse embryo development [2]. With this proof, the hospital administration provided funds to construct a cleanroom that had an air-handling unit separate from the rest of the hospital and contained ULPA filters [1, 3]. Within a year, the downward trend had been reversed and within 3 years, we significantly improved fertilization rates from 60.2% to 69.2% and noted a significant rise in clinical pregnancy rate from 16.2% to 58.7%. The 0.3 µm particle counts in the cleanroom were reduced greatly when compared to particle counts in the juxtaposed operating room (12.7 counts/ft^3 versus 455 000 counts/ft^3).

Volatile organic compounds

While we could not directly correlate volatile organic compounds (VOCs) and pregnancy rates, as the "newness" of the laboratory wore off with each cleaning, embryo quality and pregnancy rate improved. By the third year, we had surpassed our preconstruction pregnancy rate. The belief that there is a "curing time" for facilities has some credence because Von Wyl and Bersinger reported a decline in VOCs after 6 months of utilization of a new facility [4]. In addition, Cohen and colleagues reported that new incubators produced >100 times more VOCs than did older incubators [5].

To investigate VOC toxicity, we performed a prospective, randomized trial between four new incubators [6]. We compared the development of mammalian embryos in VOC-filtered incubators to embryos developed in traditional HEPA-filtered incubators. Approximately 200 bovine oocytes were equally distributed among four incubators, which were set at 7% carbon dioxide (CO_2), 5% oxygen, and 88% nitrogen. We repeated this experiment 11 times. Incubators that were initially fitted with VOC filters were fitted with HEPA filters during the second part of the study, and incubators that initially contained HEPA filters were fitted with VOC filters.

We evaluated the fertilization rates and embryo development rates from the above-mentioned study. When we combined the data between replications and incubators, the fertilization rate did not differ for VOC-filtered, incubated oocytes compared to the fertilization rate for HEPA-filtered, incubated oocytes (69.3% versus 67.7%, respectively). However, we examined the blastocyst rate between those embryos incubated in the VOC-filtered environment and those incubated in the HEPA-filtered environment and discovered a 6% increase in blastocyst rate for incubators fitted with VOC filters. This difference was significant. In addition, odds ratio analysis indicated that embryos cultured in an incubator with VOC filtration were 2.6 times more likely to develop to blastocysts than were embryos housed in incubators with HEPA filtration. These data would imply that VOC filters should be installed inside incubators used to culture embryonic cells.

In contrast to this study, when Merton and coworkers added intra-incubator, carbon-activated air filtration systems to incubators, they did not see an improvement in embryo stage or grade, or percent blastocyst development among cattle embryos [7]. However, when transferred to recipients, the cattle embryos did produce a significant increase in pregnancy rates. These data imply that filtering the air that enters an incubator can improve outcome.

Unfortunately, even the use of filtration devices may not completely eliminate embryo toxicity. There is some research to indicate that incubators which contained filters still harbor VOCs [8] and cleanrooms with filters can still contain VOCs, which can reduce pregnancy rates [9].

In summary, while not all laboratories are plagued with poor quality air [10], all laboratory personnel need to be cognizant of air quality that surrounds in vitro cultured gametes and embryos. Ways to determine air quality can include evaluation of particle counts and VOCs that may be present in the air. One has to remember that ART success may depend upon variables such as air quality, which is not easily detected by our five senses. Therefore, one must rely on sensitive instruments to evaluate the surrounding environment.

Control of relative humidity within the incubator

In the early years of embryo culture, laboratory personnel exposed culture media directly to air within the incubator. To prevent rapid evaporation of water from media, embryologists had to ensure that the environment contained a high moisture level. Water loss via evaporation would increase osmolality of the media, which could be detrimental to cells [11]. Embryologists had to monitor relative humidity (RH) closely to prevent such an increase in osmolality.

When laboratory personnel learned to overlay culture media with oil, the need for high RH within the incubator became a non-issue. Oil acted as a barrier to prevent water loss from culture media. However, addition of moisture to the incubator environment remains dogma.

When embryologists place a pan of water in the bottom of the incubator and allow air to flow over the water, a high RH within the incubator can be obtained. For years, people in the poultry industry have obtained high moisture in the incubators used to hatch eggs when they place a wick in the water pan. With passage of air over the wick, elevated moisture in the incubator is reached more quickly. However, air within the incubator will be saturated with moisture eventually, with or without a wick in the water pan. The downside to a wick is that it is usually made of cloth, which attracts bacteria and other unwanted organisms.

If bacterial and fungal growth is to be prevented, maintenance of water pans is crucial. Laboratory personnel have learned to place copper in the water pan to reduce the potential for water-borne bacteria and fungal growth. Because of potential contaminants, we discard old water, wipe the pan clean, and add fresh, warmed, distilled water to the pan on a weekly basis.

In summary, while relative humidity is not a critical issue if laboratory personnel overlay culture media with oil, they continue to place water pans in incubators. This ritual has the potential for introducing bacterial and fungal contamination if water is not changed on a frequent basis.

Control of gas concentration within the incubator

While control of pH through CO_2 levels has been discussed in a previous chapter, methods used to determine CO_2 levels need evaluation. Often times, laboratory personnel monitor incubator CO_2 levels with Fyrite analyzers (Bacharach, Inc., Pittsburgh, PA). While this instrument provides laboratory personnel with data, we found that CO_2 values fell outside the acceptable range 11.7% and 6.7% of the time when we used the Fyrite analyzer to evaluate two incubators [12].

The Fyrite analyzer differed significantly from the more accurate infrared CO_2 monitor that we used. The following factors attributed to variation between these instruments: 18.5% was caused by investigator, 40.25% was caused by incubators, and the remaining 41.3% was attributed to random error [13]. This instability led us to change from the Fyrite with an accuracy of ±0.5% to the infrared instrument (Ohmeda, Louisville, CO, Model 5200) with an accuracy of ±0.1%.

In summary, CO_2 concentration in the incubator environment controls the pH of the culture media and thus this gas needs to be monitored accurately. An infrared instrument provides more accuracy to measure such gas than a Fyrite.

Electromagnetic waves

Because incubators operate on alternating current, they generate electromagnetic fields (EMFs). These magnetic fields can penetrate most materials, including plastic, and are blamed for such diseases as leukemia, lung cancer, and fetal loss. In addition, EMFs can alter slime molds, bone cells, salivary gland cells, and lymphocytic cells [14]. Furthermore, depending upon the electrical intensity and magnetic intensity, EMFs altered embryo development in sea urchins and chicks [14].

Reproductive cells are not immune to EMFs. Wamil and associates exposed sperm penetration assay dishes to four magnets of alternating polarity and observed a reduced sperm penetration potential [15]. Zusman and associates exposed late morula and early blastocyst mouse embryos to various hertz (Hz; units of electrical intensity) and time [16]. They discovered that some levels of electrical current are more teratogenic than others, with 70 Hz being more harmful than 20 Hz. In addition, they found 20 Hz to be more teratogenic than 50 Hz in mouse embryos. These same scientists reported decreased rat embryo crown–rump length and fewer somites when they exposed 10.5 day embryos to EMFs. Furthermore, rat embryos had loss of forelimb buds and an increase in concaveness if exposure lasted for 70 hours. These variations may be caused by species differences, embryo cell stage or frequency, or intensity of the electrical current [16].

In contrast to the aforementioned negative effects, other scientists reported no detrimental effects from exposure to EMFs. With the use of chick embryos as the model, Zervins exposed embryos to 26 kHz, while Maffeo and associates used 10 Hz, 100 Hz and 1000 Hz with no known detrimental effects [17–19]. Martin found similar results if chick embryos were exposed within the second 24 hours of development. However, if chick embryos were exposed to an EMF within their first 24 hours of development, teratogenic effects were noted [20].

In a recent article, Mild and associates reported the values for EMFs in incubators were much different from those found in the normal environment. They reported 0.05–0.1 μT (microtesla; 0.1 μT = 1 milligaus) in the normal environment, while inside cell culture incubators the values registered tens of μT [21].

Because of potential harm from EMFs, it would be prudent to determine to what extent laboratory incubators emit such fields and if the intensity of EMFs varies from place to place within an incubator. If results of such a survey indicate there is potential harm, gametes might simply be moved as far from the electrical current as possible. Furthermore, Turczynski and coworkers suggested that Mu metal (nickel, iron, copper, and molybdenum alloy) can be mounted inside incubators to shield cells from magnetic fields [14].

In summary, it would appear as though there is potential harm to early embryonic development if EMFs of specific intensity and longevity are allowed to come in contact with such cells. It would appear that more research in this area is warranted.

Incubator design

During our study of HEPA versus VOC filters, we discovered that regardless of filter type, one of four new incubators outperformed the other three incubators for fertilization rate (77% versus 63%, 65%, and 68%, $P < 0.0001$) [6]. While the reason for this variation remains to be elucidated, data do indicate that even though incubators may appear similar, they may perform quite differently. This would lend credence for laboratory personnel to test every incubator with control materials (i.e., mouse embryos) before they start experiments or routine culture.

During the above-mentioned study, we discovered not only did clinical pregnancy rate among incubators vary, but also the shelves within an incubator provided differing clinical pregnancy rates [6]. These variations were significant enough that we now arrange oocytes and embryos on specific shelves within incubators.

Currently there are two major types of incubators – front-loading incubators and top-loading incubators. While the standard, front-loading incubator has more space available for embryo culture, it has a major disadvantage. Upon opening the door, the internal environment is altered quickly with loss of heat, relative humidity, and gas concentration. This environment is not easily reconstituted, often requiring 20 minutes [22] or more [23, 24] to re-equilibrate. With multiple door openings comes an even more dramatic alteration in internal environment [24–26].

Boone and Shapiro discovered that if they added a plastic partition to the lower portion of the door opening, "roll out" of gas decreased and time required to re-equilibrate CO_2 to 5% was reduced from 75 minutes to 40 minutes [23]. On some models of incubators, "Dutch" doors have been added to reduce change in internal environment of the incubator when the door is opened.

While manufacturers initially built front-loading incubators for tissue culture work, they built top-loading incubators for in vitro culture of mammalian embryos. Top-loading incubators reduce loss of gas, humidity, and heat when laboratory personnel open the doors. Mortimer and coworkers, along with Fujiwara and associates, demonstrated significant improvement in embryo quality and clinical pregnancy rate with the top-loading incubators versus the front-loading incubators [22, 27]. However, more studies are needed to validate these findings.

In summary, the design of incubators can alter in vitro development of cells. While culture environment within the incubator can be altered drastically by simply opening the incubator door, internal design of the incubator can also alter successful development of cells regardless of the number of door openings. With the advent of incubators being designed specifically for mammalian embryo culture, one can hope higher quality embryos will be developed and available for transfer or cryopreservation.

Dos and don'ts of incubator management

1. Always read warrantees and manuals that come with the incubator before you use the equipment.
2. Do not assume digital displays are correct. Obtain back up instruments for temperature, relative humidity, and gas measurements.
3. If water is added to the incubator to increase relative humidity within the incubator chamber, change the water on a regular basis and use distilled water in the pan.
4. Establish a schedule for the removal, cleaning, and replacement of shelves and side walls. Autoclave these parts, if possible, before reinstalling them.
5. Replace air filters on a routine basis.
6. Routinely run bioassays in incubator chambers to insure they operate properly. In addition, bioassays should follow any maintenance performed on the incubator.
7. If you have access to microbiologists who can supply, culture, and read agar plates, place such plates in the incubator overnight on a routine basis to detect unwanted bacterial and fungal growth within the chamber.
8. Do not place any unnecessary plasticware or other containers inside incubators as they may introduce unwanted off-gassing.
9. Do not use tape to label dishes or containers that will be placed into the incubator. Tape may attract mold.
10. Do not label dishes or containers that will be placed into the incubator with felt-tipped markers. The ink from the markers can produce VOCs.
11. Keep a log of temperatures, relative humidities, and gas levels within the incubator chamber. Obtain these values at approximately the same time every day so you can troubleshoot if necessary. Remember, the outside environment can alter chamber environment, so collect room temperatures and relative humidity as well.
12. With the commercial availability of sequential media and other newer media, it is essential that laboratory personnel understand the conditions under which the chosen type(s) of culture media are used.
13. Incubators are sensitive. Try to maintain the incubator within close tolerances for the best performance. It may require technical support from the manufacturer to accomplish this.

References

1. Boone WR, Higdon HL III, Skelton WD. How to design and implement an assisted reproductive technology (ART) cleanroom. *Clin Embryologist* 2007;**10**:5–17, vi.

2. Johnson JE, Boone WR, Bernard RS. The effects of volatile compounds (VC) on the outcome of in vitro mouse embryo culture. *Fertil Steril* 1993;**60**(Suppl 1):S98–9.

3. Boone WR, Johnson JE, Locke A-J, Crane MM IV, Price TM. Control of air quality in an assisted reproductive technology laboratory. *Fertil Steril* 1999;**71**:150–4.

4. von Wyl S, Bersinger NA. Air quality in the IVF laboratory: results and survey. *J Assist Reprod Genet* 2004;**21**:347–8.

5. Cohen J, Gilligan A, Willadsen S. Culture and quality control of embryos. *Hum Reprod* 1998;**13**(Suppl 3):137–47.

6. Higdon HL III, Blackhurst DW, Boone WR. Incubator management in an assisted reproductive technology laboratory. *Fertil Steril* 2008;**89**:703–10.

7. Merton JS, Vermeulen ZL, Otter T, *et al.* Carbon-activated gas filtration during in vitro culture increased pregnancy rate

following transfer of in vitro-produced bovine embryos. *Theriogenology* 2007;**67**:1233–8.

8. Geisthövel F, Ochsner A, Gilligan AV. Environmental evaluation of assisted reproduction techniques laboratories in Germany and the United States of America. In: Kumar A, Mukhopadhyay AK, eds. *Follicular Growth, Ovulation and Fertilization: Molecular and Clinical Basis.* New Delhi, India, Narosa Publishing House. 2001;184–98.

9. Worrilow KC, Huynh HT, Gwozdziewicz JB, Schillings WA, Peters AJ. A retrospective analysis: the examination of a potential relationship between particulate (P) and volatile organic compound (VOC) levels in a class 100 IVF laboratory cleanroom (CR) and specific parameters of embryogenesis and rates of implantation (IR). *Fertil Steril* 2001;**76**(Suppl 1):S15–16.

10. Battaglia DE, Khabani A, Rainer C, Moore DE. Prospective randomized trial of incubator CODA filtration units revealed no effect on outcome parameters for IVF. *Fertil Steril* 2001;**75**(Suppl 1):6S.

11. Ozawa M, Nagai T, Kaneko H, *et al.* Successful pig embryonic development in vitro outside a CO_2 gas-regulated incubator: effects of pH and osmolality. *Theriogenology* 2006;**65**:860–9.

12. Johnson JE, Boone WR, Lee ST, Blackhurst DW. Using Fyrite to monitor incubator carbon dioxide levels. *J Assist Reprod Genet* 1995;**12**:113–17.

13. Boone WR, Johnson JE, Lee ST, Detry MA, Blackhurst DW. Sources of variation in measurements of carbon dioxide levels inside incubators. *J Assist Reprod Genet* 1996;**13**:606–8.

14. Turczynski C, Frilot C, Sartor S, Webster B, Marino A. Electro-magnetic fields: a quality control issue for the IVF laboratory. *Embryol Newsletter* 1997;2–11, vi.

15. Wamil BD, Holcomb RR, Wamil AW, Rogers BJ, McLean MJ. Effect of static magnetic fields on human sperm penetration. *Fertil Steril* 1992;**58**:S166.

16. Zusman I, Yaffe P, Pinus H, Ornoy A. Effects of pulsing electromagnetic fields on the prenatal and postnatal development in mice and rats: in vivo and in vitro studies. *Teratology* 1990;**42**:157–70.

17. Zervins A. Chick embryo development in a 26-KHz electromagnetic field. *Am Ind Hyg Assoc J* 1973;**34**:120–7.

18. Maffeo S, Brayman AA, Miller MW, *et al.* Weak low frequency electromagnetic fields and chick embryogenesis: failure to reproduce positive findings. *J Anat* 1988;**157**:101–4.

19. Maffeo S, Miller MW, Carstensen EL. Lack of effect of weak low frequency electromagnetic fields on chick embryogenesis. *J Anat* 1984;**139**:613–18.

20. Martin AH. Magnetic fields and time dependent effects on development. *Bioelectromagnetics* 1988;**9**:393–6.

21. Mild KH, Wilén J, Mattsson MO, Simko, M. Background ELF magnetic fields in incubators: a factor of importance in cell culture work. *Cell Biol Int* 2009;**33**:755–7.

22. Fujiwara M, Takahashi K, Izuno M, *et al.* Effect of micro-environment maintenance on embryo culture after in-vitro fertilization: comparison of top-load mini incubator and conventional front-load incubator. *J Assist Reprod Genet* 2007;**24**:5–9.

23. Boone WR, Shapiro SS. Quality control in the in vitro fertilization laboratory. *Theriogenology* 1990;**33**:23–50.

24. Avery B, Melsted JK, Greve T. A novel approach for in vitro production of bovine embryos: use of the Oxoid atmosphere generating system. *Theriogenology* 2000;**54**:1259–68.

25. McKiernan SH, Bavister BD. Environment variables influence in vitro development of hamster 2-cell embryos to the blastocyst stage. *Biol Reprod* 1990;**43**:404–13.

26. Gardner DK, Lane M. Alleviation of the '2-cell block' and development to the blastocyst of CF1 mouse embryos: role of amino acids, EDTA, and physical parameters. *Hum Reprod* 1996;**11**:2703–12.

27. Mortimer D, Henman MJ, Jansen RPS. *Development of an Improved Embryo Culture System for Clinical Human IVF.* Brisbane, Cook Australia, 2002;1–38.

Chapter

21

Summary and conclusions

Patrick Quinn

As more awareness grows of the possible effects of assisted reproductive technology (ART) media and how they are used may impact outcomes in human ART, there have been calls for more rigorous control of media ingredients within the ART industry. As regulatory bodies become more aware of this situation, changes may be enforced on the industry rather than allowing us to make changes ourselves.

There are many examples of unexpected consequences from technology or regulation gone awry. One example of culture medium problems of which I am very aware as I was part of it [1] was the addition of human serum to medium for the culture of ovine embryos and the consequent large offspring syndrome [2]. An example of regulation gone amiss was the stipulation in Italy in 2004 that only three of the retrieved oocytes in an ART cycle could be fertilized and all of the embryos had to be replaced in the uterus. Modification of this law in 2009 allowed more than three oocytes to be fertilized, a choice of the number of embryos transferred, and no prohibition of embryo cryopreservation and since that time there have been increases in the ART results obtained [3].

A more recent example of things that have gone wrong in the ART lab is the case of metabolomics profiling to choose the best embryos for transfer. Despite initial studies showing a strong association between a good metabolomic profile and the viability of human embryos transferred, subsequent prospective trials did not validate the added value of this technology in choosing embryos for transfer. In one trial the ongoing pregnancy rates from metabolomic profiling alone were no different from those obtained when embryo selection was based on morphological evaluation alone [4]. Similarly, in another prospective randomized trial, a similar outcome resulted, with no significant differences in birth rate between embryos selected by morphology alone or metabolomic profiling plus morphology [5]. These results indicate that the disconnect between metabolome and other omic profiles of embryos and their morphology, championed by the likes of Gardner and Wale [6], may work both ways and as embryo culture conditions continue to improve, selection of good embryos based on morphology combined with profiling technologies such as morphokinetics, oxygen consumption, and other metabolic parameters such as glucose uptake and metabolism may be a good compromise. The problem(s) of metabolomic profiling in the studies mentioned above [4, 5] seems to be a technical one and the concept of such technology still seems worthwhile to pursue. There are numerous other examples and further possibilities of problems and are as elaborated in several recent articles [7, 8]. The examples above reinforce the requirement that the use of embryo selection protocols at

Culture Media, Solutions, and Systems in Human ART, ed. Patrick Quinn. Published by Cambridge University Press. © Cambridge University Press 2014.

the expense of the patient needs evidence-based proof of clinical usefulness. I am sure that the proponents of morphological kinetic profiling of early embryo cleavage rates and of more thoroughly researched tools such as glucose uptake by day 4 human embryos [6] are well aware of the need for prospective randomized trials.

An ESHRE working group has been created to interact with ART companies. The positions of the working group are (1) companies should disclose the composition and preferably the formulation of each medium that is used clinically. This collegial approach was once the norm before the commercialization of ART media and has been commented on [8], (2) new formulations should have a scientific basis, (3) a standard minimum QC certificate should be shared by all companies that should use the same standard operating procedures, (4) a more relevant test should be designed, and (5) great caution should be taken regarding the addition of growth factors or hormones to culture medium until more is known about possible effects on the epigenome [9]. Some of these proposals have already been initiated and mentioned in this book, especially aspects of a more refined QC testing of media.

It is hoped that the chapters in this book will help readers attain a greater knowledge and awareness of what goes on in designing and using ART media and solutions. It should always be kept in mind that the ART laboratory and ART media are only part of an ART program and that everything is interconnected [9]. The laboratory and in particular the media have been an easy target to blame when things go wrong. The best way to progress with quality improvement is to document everything and to keep an open mind.

References

1. Walker SK, Seamark RF, Quinn P, *et al.* Culture of pronuclear embryos of sheep in a simple medium. In: *Proceedings of the 11th International Congress on Animal Reproduction and Artificial Insemination, Dublin, Ireland.* 1988;4:483–5.

2. Thompson JG, Gardner DK, Pugh PA, *et al.* Lamb birth weight is affected by culture system utilized during in vitro pre-elongation development of ovine embryos. *Biol Reprod* 1995;53:1385–91.

3. Levi Setti PE, Albani E, Cesana A, *et al.* Italian constitutional court modifications of a restrictive technology law significantly improve pregnancy rate. *Hum Reprod* 2011;26:376–81.

4. Hardarson T, Ahlstrom A, Rogberg L, *et al.* Non-invasive metabolomic profiling of Day 2 and 5 embryo culture medium: a prospective randomized trial. *Hum Reprod* 2012;27:89–96.

5. Vergouw CG, Kieslinger DC, Kostelijk EH, *et al.* Day 3 embryo selection by metabolomic profiling of culture medium with near-infrared spectroscopy as an adjunct to morphology: a randomized controlled trial. *Hum Reprod* 2012;27:2304–11.

6. Gardner DK, Wale PL. Analysis of metabolism to select viable human embryos for transfer. *Fertil Steril* 2013;99:1062–72.

7. Harper J, Magli MC, Lundin K, *et al.* When and how should new technology be introduced into the IVF laboratory? *Hum Reprod* 2012;27:303–13.

8. Biggers JD. Ethical issues and the commercialization of embryo culture media. *Reprod Biomed Online* 2000;1:74–6.

9. Gianaroli L, Racowsky C, Geraedts J, *et al.* Best practices of ASRM and ESHRE: a journey through reproductive medicine. *Hum Reprod* 2012;27:3365–79.

Index

Note: page numbers in *italics* refer to figures and tables

Printed in the United States
By Bookmasters

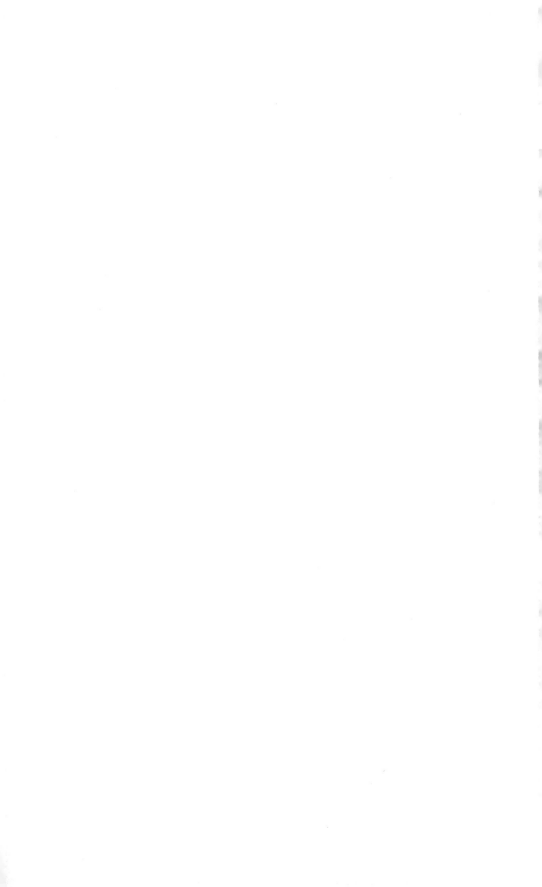